Wheelchair Users and Postural Seating

For Churchill Livingstone

Editorial director: Mary Law
Project manager: Valerie Burgess
Project development editor: Valerie Bain
Design direction: Judith Wright
Project controller: Pat Miller
Illustrator: Ethan Danielson
Copy editor: Pat Croucher
Indexer: Janine Fearon
Sales promotion executive: Hilary Brown

Wheelchair Users and Postural Seating

A Clinical Approach

Rosalind Ham MSc FCSP CertEd SRP
Superintendent Physiotherapist/Wheelchair Service Manager,
Newham Community Health Services NHS Trust,
St Andrews Hospital London, UK

Patsy Aldersea DipCot SROT
Occupational Therapist/Wheelchair Service Manager,
Merton and Sutton Community NHS Trust,
Carshalton, Surrey, UK

David Porter BSc MSc MIPEM
Clinical Engineer/Wheelchair Service Manager,
Oxfordshire Wheelchair Service at the Mary Marlborough Centre,
Nuffield Orthopaedic Centre NHS Trust, Oxford, UK

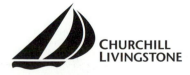
CHURCHILL
LIVINGSTONE

NEW YORK EDINBURGH LONDON MADRID MELBOURNE SAN FRANCISCO TOKYO 1998

CHURCHILL LIVINGSTONE
Medical Division of Pearson Professional Limited

Distributed in the United States of America by Churchill
Livingstone, 650 Avenue of the Americas, New York, N.Y.
10011, and by associated companies, branches and
representatives throughout the world.

First published 1998

ISBN 0 443 05472 X

British Library Cataloguing in Publication Data
A catalogue record for this book is available from the British
Library.

Library of Congress Cataloging in Publication Data
A catalog record for this book is available from the Library
of Congress.

Note
Medical knowledge is constantly changing. As new
information becomes available, changes in treatment,
procedures, equipment and the use of drugs become
necessary. The author and the publishers have, as far as it is
possible, taken care to ensure that the information given in
this text is accurate and up to date. However, readers are
strongly advised to confirm that the information, especially
with regard to drug usage, complies with latest legislation
and standards of practice.

The
publisher's
policy is to use
**paper manufactured
from sustainable forests**

Produced by Longman Singapore Publishers (Ptd) Ltd
Printed in Singapore

Contents

Preface

The provision of wheelchairs in the UK has changed considerably over the last decade. Prior to the McColl Report (1986), the issue and provision of wheelchairs was centrally organized and funded through the government Department of Health and Social Services (DHSS). This was by means of a standard prescription form that included the range of models and accessories that were available at the time. The form may have been completed by a therapist, general practitioner, hospital doctor or technical officer (TO, now known as a rehabilitation engineer [RE]) but a doctor's signature was necessary. The range of models and accessories available from the state was limited and described and illustrated in an accompanying booklet (MHM 408).

The process of supply was coordinated at a regional artifical limb and appliance centre (ALAC) by clerks. Individuals who required alterations to the standard models were seen by a TO who drew up and organized such modifications. These modifications were made by a local approved repairer who also carried out all repairs, some deliveries and collections of the wheelchairs. Deliveries were also arranged by the General Post Office and other couriers, so often the wheelchair was delivered without checking basic instruction or the correct positioning of the user.

The number of people who had wheelchairs on issue from the state in 1986 was 420 000. However, over the last decade, the number of people with mobility problems and those requesting wheelchairs has increased, for example, in 1994 alone, the number of wheelchairs issued was 193 719. This increase in demand is due to a number of factors, in particular:

- advances in medicine

- improvements in health care
- improved survival rates following trauma
- an increase in the elderly population
- a greater number of infants with disabilities surviving
- the practice of community rather than institutional care
- the closing of learning disability (mental handicap) institutions
- social policies that have improved access in the environment for people with mobility problems.

Such changes have led to an increase in demand of approximately 15% per annum in recent years.

Special seating was hardly mentioned in rehabilitation circles until the mid 1980s because the demand was not there. But as more severely disabled people survive, the demand and need has increased. However, little evaluation into the use and benefits of special seating has taken place so far.

Following the McColl Report, changes were seen in the service as it moved through the Disablement Services Authority (DSA), who managed the transition of the service in the late 1980s, into the National Health Service (NHS) in April 1991. Since then, wheelchair services in England and Wales have been organized differently. In some regions, the service is organized by rehabilitation engineers who may or may not hold the budgets centrally in their regions. In other regions, the services are managed and run on a very local level by therapists (both occupational and physiotherapists). Some regions top slice the seating budget to one centre, while in other regions the budget is devolved totally to the local service for wheelchairs and special seating. Such services may or may not purchase regional speciality services (for example, special seating and rehabilitation engineering staff) but may prefer to work with local staff and local commercial companies.

Today, NHS wheelchair services are busier than ever. The public's expectations are high and the demands on the staff for knowledge, expertise, time available, speed of service and supply are increasing at an alarming rate. Purchasers are demanding evidence-based practice, yet many wheelchair services are unable to recruit and retain staff, are staffed by part-timers, and in general, have little time for evaluation, audit or retrospective review of equipment supplied. Study time to increase knowledge on the many various conditions that are seen is also rare, and study leave for health care professionals is also difficult, to both take and organize, and to gain funding for.

Identifying the need for a concise text to assist health care professionals working in this area of practice, this book has been written by professionals from three different disciplines who are working in the wheelchair service. It is therefore intended to be a working handbook for both professionals and students working with wheelchair and special seating devices; to provide a reference book in one volume; to cover the many medical conditions seen in the service; to increase their knowledge in day-to-day problems; to provide a source for advice and information to give to users; and to provide a bibliography. The text covers a wide range of topics from: background information to the service, biomechanical principles of seating, medical conditions commonly seen, through to practical wheelchair and seating suggestions. We hope that fellow professionals find it a useful text in their departments.

R. H., P. A., D. P.

Acknowledgements

We would like to thank the staff of Churchill Livingstone for their kindness, patience and help during the production of this book.

We would also like to thank the many users, commercial companies and publishers who have allowed us to use their photographs and material as illustrations.

Finally, we would all like to thank our partners and families who have been so tolerant of our lack of company, late nights and working at week-ends. We promise we will make up the lost time!

Background science

SECTION CONTENTS

1

Wheelchair development and service provision

WHEELCHAIR DEVELOPMENT

Developing designs to meet the need

Wheelchairs in one form or another have been in use for many centuries, with one of the earliest models recorded by an engraving on a Chinese sarcophagus dated 6 AD (Kamenetz 1969). Self-propelling chairs were a later invention, but by the time of the American Civil War records show that the war wounded used wooden chairs with large front wheels and small rear castors (Bennett-Wilson 1995). Photographs taken at the turn of the century show more elegant wooden and cane seated wheelchairs being used at the Paris Exhibition (Fig. 1.1), though the users were more likely to be gout sufferers or the wealthy elderly and frail as few severely disabled people survived for long and were rarely taken out in public. Over the years, changes in design and structure reflected the introduction of new materials, advances in medical science, improvements in access and the environment, and changes in social attitudes. The arrival of the automobile resulted in demand for a portable model. In 1932, following a mining accident, Herbert A. Everest, an American mining engineer, collaborated with Harry C. Jennings, a mechanical engineer, to design and manufacture a relatively 'lightweight' folding wheelchair (Bennett-Wilson 1986). Although some improvements have been made to this earlier design, reflecting advances in technology and a concern to meet the increased specific demands of recent wars, nevertheless the folding design of Everest and Jennings, which

3

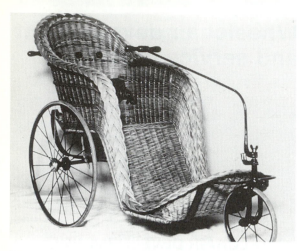

Figure 1.1   Attendant-pushed cane wheelchair used at the turn of the century in Europe. (Reproduced from Department of Health 1991, with permission.)

consists of a cross bar connecting two side frames and fitted with flexible seat and back supports (Fig. 1.2), continues to be used as a basis for the standard non-powered wheelchairs of today (Bennett-Wilson 1995).

Electrically powered wheelchairs

Electrically powered wheelchairs first appeared during the First World War when an engine was

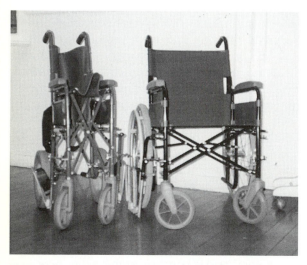

Figure 1.2   Basic wheelchair design with cross bar frame, flexible seat and back support and central folding mechanism.

added to an ordinary lever-propelled wheelchair (McColl 1986), though there was no real demand for powered wheelchairs until some 30 years later. Most improvements have been made in response to need as advances in medical knowledge resulted in a greater survival rate and better quality of life, particularly for people with poliomyelitis and spinal cord injuries (Bennett-Wilson 1995). Further design improvements were made in the USA during the 1970s as large numbers of injured war veterans returned from Vietnam. In 1956 the first electric indoor wheelchair appeared in England though these were not issued by the wheelchair service until 1964 (Walmsley 1996). Attendant-controlled powered wheelchairs for outdoor use were also available from the late 1960s. Known as the 28B, these were large, cumbersome, difficult to manoeuvre and generally unpopular. They were condemned on safety grounds and removed from most services in 1992. Various other developments have taken place in both the design of powered wheelchairs and improvements in the control boxes. These are discussed in more detail in Chapter 13.

Non-powered wheelchairs

The self-propelled basic wheelchair (Fig. 1.2) has always been the most practical general purpose design of non-powered wheelchair. Lever-propelled wheelchairs, whilst requiring the least effort for maximum power and movement, are unsuited to indoor use and difficult to transport. The earlier models (Fig. 1.3), designed for paraplegics, were modified and nowadays are of similar size and appearance to an outdoor powered wheelchair, but nonetheless are rarely used due to their bulk, weight and the large turning space they require.

In the late 1940s emphasis placed on the advantages of allowing disabled people to participate in sporting activities, initially at the Spinal Injuries Unit at Stoke Mandeville in England and later in the USA (Bennett-Wilson 1995), resulted in the production of lightweight, active user wheelchairs. Many of the features from these models proved to be beneficial to other users and have been introduced on a wide range of mass-

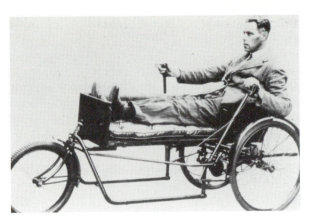

Figure 1.3 Early design of the lever propelled wheelchair used with paraplegics and amputees. (Reproduced from Department of Health 1991, with permission.)

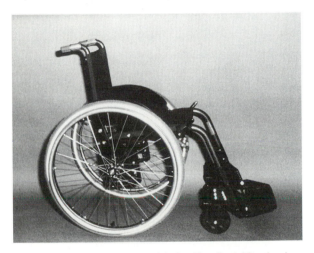

Figure 1.4 Active user wheelchair with adjustable wheel and seat position to suit individual performance. (Reproduced from Department of Health 1991, with permission.)

produced high-performance models that can be adjusted to suit individual need (Fig. 1.4) However, the high cost when lighter weight materials are used is reflected in the price, and places them beyond the means of the majority of wheelchair users. Meanwhile, sports wheelchairs have become highly specialized and are finely tuned to suit the specific need of each individual sports person.

Design development in Britain

For many years development of the wheelchair in Britain was restricted by government control over design specifications. Before 1948 many of the chairs were non-folding with a wooden frame, seat and back and often three wheels which allowed turning in a very limited space, but they were unstable and totally unsuited to outdoor use. Ministry wheelchairs were first issued in 1917 and only available for war-wounded servicemen. During the Second World War, wounded civilians were included in government provision. A brief history is provided in Box 1.1. From 1948 until the reorganization of the wheelchair service in the late 1980s, the British market was dominated by the standard DHSS (Department of Health and Social Service) models, commonly known as the Model 8 (self-propelling) and Model 9 (attendant-pushed) wheelchairs. In order to keep costs to a minimum, the scientific and technical branch of the Health Department (DHSS) provided all specifications for a standard wheelchair frame. The design, together with detailed engineering specifications, were given to the wheelchair manufacturers who contracted to mass produce a range of standard models for the service in the UK only (Walmsley 1996). Quality control was undertaken by the government testing centre at Blackpool, which later became the wheelchair division of the Medical Devices Agency, a centre of expertise in matters relating to safety, quality and performance of wheelchairs (see Glossary).

Government control of precise specifications and design resulted in:

- bulk production of low-cost wheelchairs
- simplification of reconditioning, with interchangeable parts from all manufacturers
- an opportunity for engineering firms with no design capacity to produce chairs cheaply.

On the other hand, a central design:

- restricted the range of chairs and choice available to users
- discouraged development of research and development ideas by manufacturers
- provided an opportunity for a monopoly of materials and parts
- delayed the introduction of design changes due to an inflexible and uncompetitive system.

Box 1.1   Development of wheelchair provision in England

Date	Service users and description	Service provider
1914–18	State provision to war-wounded servicemen	Earl Kitchener memorial fund
1918–39	Servicemen only. Mainly amputees and spinal injuries. Civilians purchased own wheelchairs, using a charity. Otherwise went without	Ministry of Pensions with Earl Kitchener Fund and British Red Cross until 1919
1939–48	War-wounded servicemen. Also civilians disabled in Second World War	Ministry of Pensions
1948–53	Introduction of NHS-entitled provision to all civilians as well as servicemen	Responsibilities of Ministry of Pensions extended
1953–87	All permanently disabled people with a mobility problem. Service based in ALACs	Ministry of Health. Responsibility passed to Department of Health and Social Security 1968
1964	Introduction of indoor powered wheelchair	
1967	Introduction of 28B attendant-controlled outdoor powered wheelchair	
1986	Publication of McColl Report	
1987–91	DSA established. Reorganization with closing of some ALACs and resiting of others. All users allocated to local service provider (Trust) and local contract repairer	DSA responsible for transfer of service from DHSS to NHS with further transfer from RHAs to DHAs. Special seating provided at regional or supra district level
1989–91	Pilot scheme for indoor/outdoor attendant-controlled powered wheelchairs in Northern and North West Regions. Strict criteria. Discontinued 1992 due to lack of funding	Funding provided by DSA for 3-year trial only
1991–96	Guidelines for provision as before, though some variations in local criteria. Increased range of wheelchairs available. Some inequality in service standards and range of equipment	DSA dissolved. 163 service providers in England based on Trust sites. A few on shared site with Joint loans store/Red Cross/DLC/incontinence service/DIAL
1992	Provision of in/outdoor powered wheelchairs in Scotland only. Strict criteria initially	Funding from Scottish Health Dept initially for 3 years then extended
1993–96	DoH project on NHS Wheelchair Services based at College of Occupational Therapists	DoH Section 64 Grant. Report published April 1996
Feb. 1996	Announcement of two new schemes to commence during 1996. In/outdoor user-controlled powered wheelchairs and voucher scheme in England. Criteria set locally based on DoH guidelines	£50m available from Government for period of 4 years to introduce new schemes. £27m for powered wheelchairs. £23m for voucher scheme in England only

---

Government emphasis was placed not only on low cost but also on stability and safety rather than the independence and function of the user. Though acceptable to the majority of less able users who were prepared to accept limited mobility, this was a constant source of frustration to the smaller group of users who had both the ability and the motivation to become more active, and also to the more severely disabled who required individual modifications for postural support and comfort.

During the 1980s, following criticism from users, new designs were commissioned for the wheelchair service and in 1987 a number of new chairs were introduced by the Disablement Services Authority (DSA), a special authority established to manage the wheelchair service during a period of reorganization between 1987 and 1991. In the main these 'new models' were based on the original specification with a similar level of performance, though offering a wider range of colours and additional features. Many of the new models were soon discontinued, as the extended colour range provided no improvement in performance for the user but increased the cost of the reconditioning process as the parts were no longer interchangeable on all chairs.

In the late 1980s the Remploy Roller (Fig. 1.5) was introduced to the NHS range. This had a more pleasing appearance and also the facility to alter the centre of gravity and reduce the stability of the chair by adjusting the position of the rear

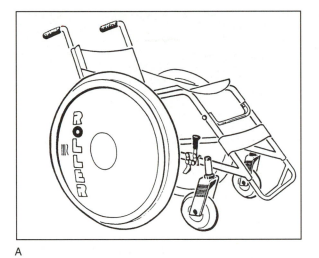

A

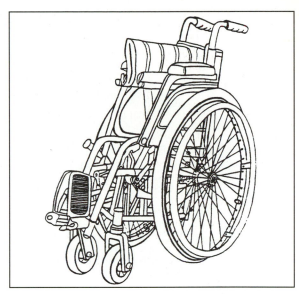

B

Figure 1.5 The Remploy Roller. (A) The original model with rigid frame and adjustable wheel position has been part of the NHS range since 1987. (B) The centre folding version became available at a later date. (Illustrations provided by Remploy Healthcare.)

wheels. This enabled active users, with sufficient trunk stability and arm strength, to tilt the chair rearwards sufficiently to clear rough ground or climb a shallow step. Though less adjustable and having lower performance specifications than the increasing range of new technology wheelchairs which appeared on the market at this time, it provided a compromise between improved appearance and manoeuvrability for the user whilst maintaining a reasonable purchase price for the NHS. To date the Roller, with a choice of 'fixed' or 'folding' frame, and the more recently produced Meteor (Fig. 1.6) with its own unique style of folding mechanism, remain the two active user style of wheelchair most commonly seen in the NHS range.

It is clear that the previously described low-cost system of central organization and single design specification which concentrated on safety rather than function had an adverse effect on the funding for the present service (Disablement Services Authority 1989–90). Since the time of the reorganization in 1991, the low level of funding (Hunter & Walker 1993) has left the service providers unable to fully meet the challenges and opportunities available through improved technology and the changing clinical and social needs of disabled people (Smith & Goddard 1994).

PROVISION WORLD WIDE

Whilst the cost of providing wheelchairs has been rising due to improved technology, there has been a concurrent world-wide escalation in demand due to:

- improvements in medical science resulting in a greater survival rate of people with congenital or acquired disability
- a world-wide ageing population
- higher expectations and increased opportunities for disabled people
- greater awareness of the benefits of new technology
- improved access and travel facilities, enabling those with mobility problems to get out and about
- change of attitudes and greater recognition of the needs and abilities of disabled people.

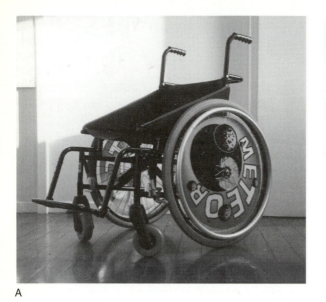
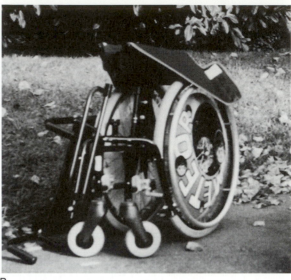

A   B

Figure 1.6 (A, B) The adult size Meteor, used by many wheelchair services, combines the features of both a rigid frame and centrally folding wheelchair.

World-wide statistics

Whilst looking at statistics and considering the question 'who are wheelchair users?', it may be helpful to bear in mind the International Classification of Impairments, Disabilities and Handicaps (ICIDH) published by the World Health Organization (WHO) (1980), which describes the phenomena of disablement as:

Impairment   the dysfunction of an organ or process of the body of a person which may lead to

Disability   the loss or reduction of normal ability to perform a particular activity, which may lead to

Handicap   which is the disadvantage experienced by the impact of the impairment of disability on the particular individual related to their desires and needs and in the context of their social life and environment.

In the USA in 1985 there were reported to be more than 750 000 wheelchair users on a daily basis (Bennett-Wilson 1986). This figure did not include those in a nursing home or hospital or with a short-term need. By 1990 this figure had risen to 1.2 million users, of whom 300 000 were disabled due to a spinal cord injury and 500 000 were in nursing homes (Phillips & Nicosia 1990), whilst recent figures (Gall et al 1997) state there are 1 411 000 wheelchair 'riders' in the USA. Figures provided by Dolfus (1988) and shown in Table 1.1 enable comparisons to be made for Europe.

It is clear from these figures that the UK has a higher number of wheelchair users per 100 000

Table 1.1 Figures given by P. Dolfus at Dundee Wheelchair and Seating Conference 1988 comparing numbers of wheelchair users in six European countries

Country	Population	Users (estimated (nos)	Powered wheelchairs (no.)
UK	55 900 000	330 000*	3225
France	53 000 000	60 000	1500
Germany	61 300 000	240 000	
Holland	14 200 000	60 000	
Belgium	9 900 000	20–25 000	
Sweden	8 300 000	30 000	1030

*This does not agree with the estimate of 420 000 (McColl 1986).

Table 1.2 Figures taken from government statistics for England: 1989–95 (Department of Health 1994–95)

	1989–90	1992–93	1993–94	1994–95
New wheelchairs issued (no.)	170 000	182 066	185 971	203 160
Per 100 000 population (no.)		376	383	417
Special seating figures (no.)		13 246	14 502	14 616

population than other European countries. This may reflect the differing policies and criteria used for providing wheelchairs in each country. In the past both France and Sweden have been willing to issue more than one wheelchair to each user, though during the 1990s the growing recession has placed restrictions on national budgets across Europe and many countries are consequently experiencing difficulty in maintaining the high level of provision. Other international differences relate to regulations imposed in some countries on the period of time permitted before replacement of a wheelchair. This is in the region of 3–5 years in France, depending on the type of wheelchair, and 7 years in Sweden, whereas in England, review and reassessment can take place at any time depending on the individual circumstances. Unlike the UK, many countries provide only to full-time users.

THE WHEELCHAIR POPULATION IN THE UK

For 1989, the Office of Population Censuses Surveys (1989) stated that out of the 6.2 million adults in the UK with some form of disability, 4.5 million had a mobility problem.

The absence of relevant statistics, as well as agreed standards and criteria for the collection of information, restricts comparison of the level of wheelchair provision and quality for users not only between services within the UK but also with other countries. In the Yorkshire region the total number of wheelchair users rose from 34 831 in 1989–90 to 45 502 at the end of 1991, an increase of 30.6% (Baughan 1992). A report from the National Audit Office (1992) stated that the NHS supplies approximately 160 000 wheelchairs per year at a cost of over £40m; this is

Table 1.3 A steady increase has been recorded in the total number of wheelchair users in England over a 27-year period

	1968	1973	1988	1995
Wheelchair users (no.)	68 000	425 000	500 000	770 000

estimated to rise rapidly in the coming years (Stewart 1992, Bar 1993).

As can be seen in Tables 1.2 and 1.3, figures published for England by the Government Statistics Department since devolution of the service indicate an increasing number of new wheelchairs issued each year.

Figures collected in England and Scotland in 1990 show the following numbers of wheelchairs per 100 000 population:

- England (Department of Health 1990) – 930
- Scotland (Hunter & Walker 1993) – 1000.

Although more accurate figures are now available from individual services in England, few reliable figures on disability in relation to wheelchair users have been published. Account must also be taken of the fact that, due to poor record keeping prior to 1991, figures available include many inactive users. In addition, government figures do not include the ever growing number of private wheelchair users. The only attempt to estimate the private market was made by the Muscular Dystrophy Group during their campaign, 'Batteries not included' (Kerridge 1993), which looked at the number of privately purchased indoor/outdoor powered wheelchairs. Based on their research they concluded that some 40 300 people in the UK would benefit from the provision of an indoor/outdoor powered wheelchair, with an annual demand of 14 000 in England and Wales.

Age and medical conditions of wheelchair users

World-wide statistics show that on average 70% of all wheelchair users are over 60 years of age (Fenwick 1977, Kettle & Rowley 1990). Figures collected from 89% (129) of wheelchair services in England in 1996 (National Prosthetic and Wheelchair Services Report 1993–1996) indicated that this figure was nearer 73%, with the majority being female. Although only some 7% of NHS registered users are classified as 'active, independent, full-time users', this group, who are mainly under the age of 60, though smaller in numbers, requires a greater amount of professional time for assessment and review as well as a higher proportion of funding to meet their complex, ever-changing and on-going needs.

Figures from Scotland (Hunter & Walker 1993) taking all age groups into consideration, indicate the following disability distribution:

● neurological disorders – 50%
● arthritis (mainly osteoarthrosis) – 30%
● amputees – 6%
● spinal cord injuries – 4%.

Figures recorded from the Welsh wheelchair service (Bar 1993) showed that there were considerable differences in disability distribution between the over and under 60 age groups. This difference is due partly to the age of onset and development of the disabilities recorded.

Over 60 years of age the five most common disorders were:

● osteoarthritis – 28%
● cardiorespiratory disorders – 24%
● strokes – 25%
● cancers – 11%
● amputees – 5%.

However, in the under 60 years of age group the two most common disabilities were:

● cerebral palsy – 20%
● multiple sclerosis – 8%.

Spinal cord injury and head injury were also more common in the younger age group.

The multiple sclerosis figures reflect other disability statistics where these numbers are consistently higher in the younger age group. In a group of patients with multiple sclerosis, Badley & Wood (1988) reported 87.3% were in the 16–64-year-old age group compared to 12.7% in the 65 years and over age group.

THE WHEELCHAIR SERVICE IN ENGLAND SINCE 1987

The structure of government provision showed little change from 1917 until the present time, when emphasis shifted from the service being 'equipment' orientated to being 'people' centred.

In response to growing criticism, the government, in 1984, set up an independent review of the ALAC (Artificial Limb and Appliance Centre) services in England. In 1986 the review body, chaired by Professor (now Lord) Ian McColl, a Consultant in Surgery at Guy's Hospital, London, published a critical report which made 48 recommendations for improvement; the main recommendation being a total reorganization of the service and transfer of responsibility from the Department of Health and Social Services (DHSS) to a special authority. In the event, the government decided to move the service into the National Health Service (NHS). The first stage in this reorganization (1987) was to establish the Disablement Services Authority (DSA) for an interim period of 3½ years. The DSA was a special health authority chaired by Lord Holderness with Lord McColl as vice-chairman. It had three main responsibilities:

● To provide a service during the interim period until integration with the NHS was achieved.
● To build upon improvements taking place in the service.
● To plan transfer of the service to the territorial health authorities (NHS regional and district health authorities) by 1 April 1991.

Since devolution has taken place, significant variations in both quality of service and pattern of provision have developed across England. These differences are due to a number of reasons, including:

- local patterns in provision of rehabilitation services
- availability of space and suitable sites
- inequality in levels of funding reflecting the priorities of local policy makers
- pressure from local user groups for a preferred pattern of service
- on-going changes and instability within the NHS with development of Trusts following implementation of the NHS & Community Care Act 1990.

The changes in 1991 had less effect in Scotland, Wales and Northern Ireland, though some re-organization has since taken place in these services.

The principle of reorganization was to remove control from a central body and allow funding decisions to respond to and reflect local needs through a contracting process. There developed what is known as a purchaser/provider split, with health authorities as purchasers contracting a range of health services from the trusts. This included the provision of wheelchairs (Lee 1996). Continuing changes in NHS policies have de-volved budgets to GPs, who are now becoming fundholders, and over a total period of time have become purchasers for a range of services and equipment including wheelchairs. Whilst the 'internal market' process has resulted in notice-able benefits for some service users, it has created a costly, fragmented and inequable service for many others who find that the level and quality of wheelchair provision is dependent on locality and available funding rather than individual need.

On the other hand, since reorganization wheelchair provision has become more closely integrated with other rehabilitation services – occupational therapists and physiotherapists now play a more active role in wheelchair assess-ment and prescription and there is a closer working relationship between health and social services, though service patterns vary consider-ably around the country.

Another noticeable improvement in some services has been the increase in the range of models of wheelchairs and special seating. This obviously has a cost implication and the choice available to users varies considerably between the different services resulting in a sense of inequality and a feeling that what you get is dependent on where you live and not on what you actually need (Smith & Goddard 1994).

Since 1964 the UK wheelchair service has provided powered wheelchairs for indoor use only. This limited policy was criticized in the McColl report (McColl 1986) and in 1989 one-off funding was identified by the Disablement Services Authority (DSA) for a 2-year pilot scheme, enabling provision of indoor/outdoor powered wheelchairs to users in the Northern and North West Health Regions (Disablement Services Authority 1990). Though generally successful, the pilot schemes were discontinued due to lack of adequate funding being made available after 1991. Pressure from the Muscular Dystrophy Group campaign 'Batteries not included', which was supported by many volun-tary and professional groups as well as members of parliament, culminated in the government allocating the wheelchair service in England a sum of £50m over a period of 4 years from 1996. The money is divided between two schemes (Table 1.4): one to provide powered indoor/outdoor wheelchairs to severely disabled people (Health Service Guidelines 1996a) (see Ch. 13) and the other to introduce a voucher scheme (Health Service Guidelines 1996b) (Box 1.2). Since 1992 Scotland has been providing a limited number of indoor/outdoor powered wheel-chairs (Scottish Office 1992), though Wales and Northern Ireland have yet to make this decision.

Service structure

The number of users within a service will range from as few as 1500 to 15 000 or more, though the larger providers are likely to hold a contract with more than one health authority (purchaser) and are usually, but not always, based at a regional centre. The majority of services are based on a trust (hospital) site, though some have moved on to a shared site with other associated services, as shown in Figure 1.7. The wheelchair service

---

Box 1.2 Information on the introduction of the Voucher Scheme in England 1996

Background

The idea of introducing a voucher scheme for wheelchair users is not new and has been raised on several occasions in the past before it appeared as a recommendation in the McColl Review (McColl 1986), which stated that a cash option should be introduced for disabled people to change or enhance provision available through ALAC (now NHS). This could be used by those who accepted the available equipment to pay for non-essential items which they required to satisfy personal preference or, alternatively, to buy their wheelchair privately.

The report recommended that the cash or voucher option should reflect the cost of the prescribed wheelchair together with 'handling' charges that would normally be incurred. McColl also advised that the user would take full responsibility for all repairs and maintenance and that no further wheelchair or voucher would be supplied for a period of 5 years even 'if the money were mis-spent'.

'Good News' announcement

Until 1995, this recommendation had not been acted upon, but a question raised in Parliament at the time of the 'Batteries not included' campaign (Muscular Dystrophy Group 1994) led to an internal review of the wheelchair service and a ministerial announcement of 'Good News' on 23 February 1996.

The announcement informed wheelchair users that money had been made available for two new schemes: provision of Electrically powered indoor/outdoor wheelchairs (EPIOCs) and introduction of a voucher scheme. Whilst the provision of EPIOCs has been fully supported by professionals and users alike, there have been mixed feelings regarding the proposed voucher scheme which is yet to be fully implemented (1997). Local criteria will be based on guidelines (HSG (96) 53), which state that there will be three options from which wheelchair users can choose:

1. To accept the wheelchair prescribed as at present with free maintenance, repairs and review.
2. **Independent option.** To contribute to the cost of a more expensive wheelchair of their choice; to own the wheelchair and be responsible for maintenance and repair. This will be VAT exempt.
3. **Partnership option.** To contribute to the cost of a more expensive wheelchair of their choice from a range selected by the local wheelchair service. The NHS will own the wheelchair and be responsible for its maintenance and repair. It will therefore be subject to VAT.

Although it is recommended that on average a voucher should last 5 years, it is expected that the local service will determine an appropriate period for each individual user, taking into account their clinical condition.

Table 1.4 Allocation of £50m over 4-year period in England for the introduction of two new wheelchair schemes

	1996–97	1997–98	1998–99	1999–2000
Indoor/outdoor scheme	£6m	£6m	£7m	£8m
Voucher scheme	£2m	£5m	£8m	£8m

manager may come from a clinical or administrative background. The majority of services employ a coordinator who is responsible for the administrative and clerical side of the service, together with a dedicated wheelchair therapist who will build up an expertise and knowledge in posture, mobility and equipment matters. Assessments may be carried out either in the user's home or in a clinic situation. The clinic is generally reserved for the more complex assessments but can act as a forum for sharing expertise and exchanging ideas which may benefit the user (Jarvis 1985).

All registered NHS wheelchair service users have access to a free repair and maintenance service. The responsibilities of the individual staff vary from service to service but are, in general, as detailed below.

Wheelchair service staff and their responsibilities (Fig. 1.8)

Wheelchair therapist

This member of staff is an occupational therapist or physiotherapist with a particular interest and expertise in posture and mobility. The responsibilities cover all clinical matters, including assessments and reviews carried out either independently or with the rehabilitation engineer or another therapist in a clinic or home situation; prescribing for standard, non-standard and specialist needs including pressure-relieving cushions, accessories and modifications; providing

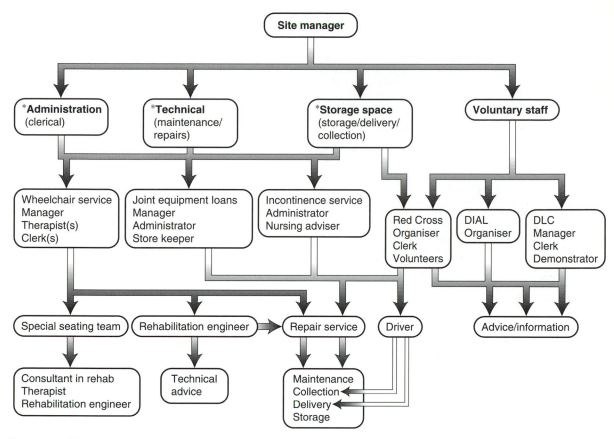

Figure 1.7   Example of 'one-stop' provision on shared site with shared funding. Shared space should include: parking/reception/disabled facilities/staff facilities. *Degree of sharing between these services will vary depending on overall structure of services.

information and advice on a wide range of wheelchair-associated matters; training users, carers, therapists and other health and community professionals. Depending on the complexity of the wheelchair user's needs, the therapist will liaise closely with other agencies, including social services, regarding access and modifications to the home. There will be close communication with relevant family members, as well as a range of statutory and voluntary services when appropriate. The duties of some wheelchair therapists will include managerial responsibility for budget control, ordering of equipment, preparing contracts for service provision, technical support and the repair service.

Wheelchair coordinator/clerical assistant

Depending on the service structure, this may be a clerical post with responsibility for appointments, database information, producing reports, maintaining stock levels, liaising with the repairer, day-to-day ordering of user equipment, answering queries and providing general information and advice. On the other hand it may be combined with the additional duties of a therapy helper with responsibility for assessing individuals requiring standard transit attendant-pushed wheelchairs and standard cushions. This includes issuing the wheelchair and instructing the user and carer in the handling, care and daily

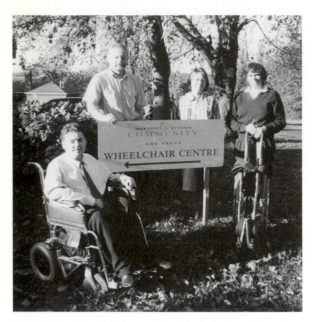

Figure 1.8 Wheelchair service staff: clerical assistant; rehabilitation engineer; coordinator; therapist.

maintenance of their wheelchair. Frequently the coordinator has sole charge of a department whilst the therapist is out on home visits, at clinics and meetings.

Rehabilitation engineer

There is often confusion regarding the titles and roles of engineers and technicians in the wheelchair service. The majority of services negotiate a contract with either a regional centre or medical physics department to provide technical support. In general the rehabilitation engineer is employed on a part-time basis and may be shared between two or more wheelchair services. The role of the rehabilitation engineer is to provide technical support and advice to both user and therapist when assessing for modifications, nonstandard equipment, powered wheelchairs or postural support; producing technical drawings for special modifications; advising on new equipment; reporting faults and checking the safety of all wheelchair equipment as well as undertaking quality control at the repairers; checking the standard of repairs, reconditioning, modifications and advising the repairer on any queries

regarding technical work for the wheelchair service and its users. Some wheelchair services independently employ a rehabilitation engineer or obtain technical advice through the contracted repair service.

Clinical engineer

A clinical engineer is a graduate or postgraduate bioengineer who has trained, and acquired a certificate of competence in medicine and biology, from the Institute of Physics and Engineering, to work as a clinical engineer. As the title suggests, the clinical engineer is able to link both clinical and engineering knowledge and expertise, and in certain circumstances, may be able to carry out assessments independently with reference to a therapist mainly regarding environmental and practical issues.

Few services in England employ a clinical engineer, though they are invaluable in the wheelchair service where the two fields are so intimately linked. Seating teams in particular can greatly benefit from the inclusion of a clinical engineer as a member of their assessment team.

Contracted repairer

Every service holds a contract for repairs, generally for a 3-year period of time. All registered wheelchair users have direct access to the repairer for free maintenance and repairs to their wheelchair. Apart from carrying out repairs and maintenance, the repairer stocks spare parts; stores wheelchairs for the service; collects and delivers wheelchairs and may also provide a reconditioning service. Although the majority of services have a contract with an outside engineering firm for their repair work, some services have an in-house repair service supplied by the trust engineering department. Arrangements for storage, delivery, collection and reconditioning of equipment may or may not be included, depending on the available facilities.

Specialist services

Additional staff, or a specialist team, may be

available to support the service for adults or children with postural and/or pressure problems or other complex needs which affect their seating and mobility. The team structure will vary depending on local needs, budgets and available expertise.

A seating team comprises all or some of the following members:

- Consultant in rehabilitation medicine responsible for medically examining the user; arranging, if required, referral elsewhere for a further opinion on medication, medical problems, changing orthopaedic or neurological conditions or other relevant care and treatment.
- Senior therapist with additional expertise in posture and mobility who will assess ability in relation to function, consider relevant environmental, social and personal issues taking into account the views and needs of the user and carer in relation to equipment, rehabilitation and life style (see Ch. 6).
- Rehabilitation or clinical engineer who will provide technical advice and expertise to assist prescription of equipment and ensure safety of custom-made seating.

There may also be agreed access to an orthotist, paediatrician, orthopaedic consultant or other persons as appropriate. The degree of involvement by the seating team will vary in different areas. In some cases they act purely in an advisory capacity, providing assessment and recommendation for action. In other centres they will also provide a manufacturing, fitting and follow-up service.

Specialist clinics are seen by many as essential and by others as unnecessary. The DSA strongly recommended the formation of regional or supra-district clinics in order to build up expertise for the small number of all ages of users with complex disabilities. This view was supported by transferring some of the DSA resources into supporting a seating advisory group, together with the provision of seating systems, during 1989/90. The government allocated a further £1m during 1990/91, although this still represented only one-half of the level of expenditure

at that time (Disablement Services Authority 1989–90). A report by the British Society of Rehabilitation Medicine (BSRM 1995) in 1995 further supported this view. Though many services do not have an identified seating team, the majority work closely with an experienced orthotist when faced with challenging postural problems. This does not, however, replace the need for a full medical and physical assessment for those whose postural problems can severely affect other body functions, growth and development. Referral procedures to the seating clinics vary, depending on local policies, but are generally channelled through the wheelchair therapist (see Fig. 1.9 and Ch. 6)

ELIGIBILITY FOR A WHEELCHAIR

Generally speaking there is no 'absolute right' to wheelchair equipment. Lack of clear guidance on this matter frequently causes concern and confusion. Health Service legislation does not specifically refer to equipment but makes general references to provision as part of a wider service. There are minor variations in the legislation covering different parts of the British Isles (Mandelstam 1994), but the NHS Act 1977 s. 3 states: 'there is a duty to provide (to the extent that is considered necessary to meet all reasonable requirements) such facilities for the prevention of illness, care of persons suffering from illness, and after care of persons who have suffered from illness' as are considered appropriate within the terms of the Health Service. Although there has never been any clear criteria for wheelchair provision, guidelines initially produced by the DHSS and reinforced by the McColl report (McColl 1986) state that: 'the general objective of the wheelchair service should be to meet the basic need for short-range mobility of people of all ages who have serious and permanent difficulties in walking'. Based broadly on the above information it is for each service to provide a policy with guidelines and criteria that can meet local needs within the available resources. Wheelchairs for short-term, temporary provision are not generally provided by the wheelchair service. Timely provision of appro-

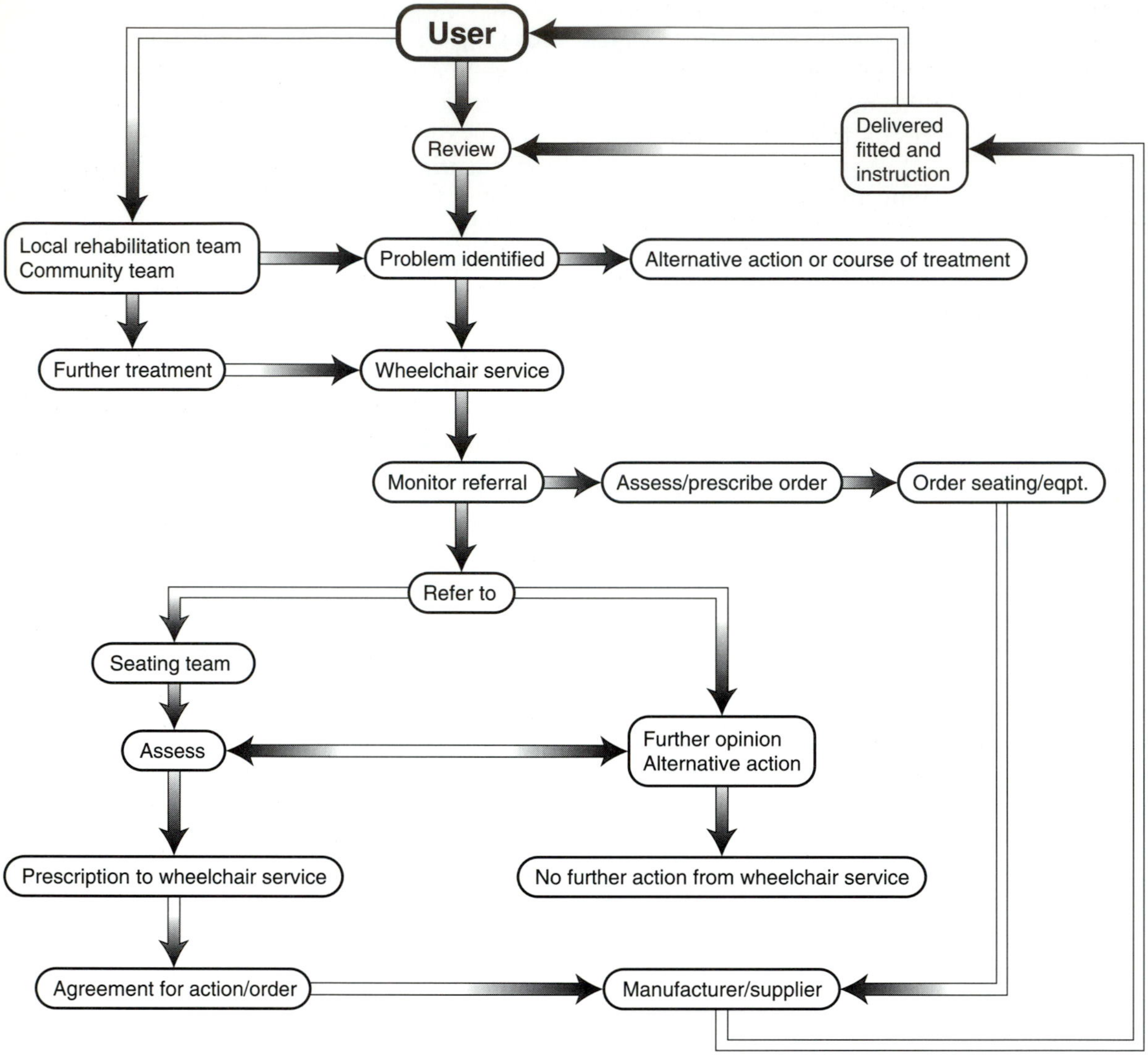

Figure 1.9 Example of common pattern of provision of special seating for NHS wheelchair users.

priate equipment, as part of a total package of care, may enable an individual to remain independent and retain an acceptable quality of life. Whilst minimizing the degree of a disability, equipment cannot fully compensate for any handicap and a wheelchair prescription should not be used to replace proper care or rehabilitation but be part of a comprehensive package aimed at enhancing both mobility and life style.

The particular statutory body with respons-

ibility for funding and providing equipment will depend on the primary purpose or need for the equipment (Mandelstam 1994). Although responsibility for funding is divided between different agencies, such as the Placement Advisory Counselling Team from the Department of Employment (see Glossary) which can provide financial assistance to provide equipment for the work requirements, people have specific needs that cannot be separated in this way. Sometimes the division of resources results in either duplication or a gap in provision of a range of equipment (Morris 1995), when the same piece of equipment is equally appropriate to meet two separate needs; for example, a special wheelchair may provide mobility as well as being appropriate for school use and joint funding should then be considered. Health Service guidelines (EL (94) 79) recommend cooperation between various agencies for these situations (Department of Health 1995a,b). Unfortunately, good practice can be jeopardized by the restrictive practice created when adhering to a budget that is inadequate to meet a growing demand. A degree of goodwill as well as cooperation is required in order to reach a realistic agreement for funding assessment and provision as well as future maintenance or replacement of equipment (National Prosthetic and Wheelchair Services Report 1993–1996). Delay in provision or non-provision of appropriate equipment due to funding disagreements is detrimental to individual care, rehabilitation and quality of life, and should be avoided at all costs.

Referrals for wheelchair assessment are generally accepted from therapists, GPs, primary care teams, consultants and, in some cases, social workers. Self referral is common for review of an existing situation, though further clinical and medical information may be requested. Figure 1.10 illustrates the path of referral and provision.

Providing a wheelchair service that meets the needs of all its users requires a wide range of knowledge, expertise and stamina. The fact that for many users a wheelchair is not simply an aid to mobility, but the key to achieving maximum independence whilst influencing their entire life style, places high demands on assessor and provider who should be sensitive to the views and expectations of each individual, always taking these into account when making decisions that affect personal life style and preferences.

ATTITUDES TO WHEELCHAIR USERS

Although there have been noticeable changes in attitude to disability in recent years, the degree of change is highly debatable. Individual attitudes are very personal and depend on a number of factors such as the age of a person, their relationship with the disabled person, or indeed the nature of the disability. In general there have been many fundamental changes in society, not only as a result of legislation on disability matters such as the introduction of the Disability Discrimination Act (1995), but also due to advances in technology and social changes such as the reduction in the number of long-stay institutions. These changes affect the life style of us all, including those with a disability.

In Britain the National Health Service and Community Care Act (1990), together with the accompanying White Paper, 'Caring for People: Community Care in the Next Decade and Beyond' (Department of Health 1989), introduced a government policy which aimed at minimizing disability and enabling all individuals to have the opportunity to live a life of independence and dignity 'in their own homes or in a homely setting' whenever feasible and sensible. This signified a radical shift away from the traditional 'medical model' to the 'social model' of care, with power and decision making being transferred from the professional to the disabled person or their representative. Enabling people to have greater control over their own lives with opportunity to make choices, increases the necessity for accurate assessment by professionals who will consequently carry greater responsibility for providing the relevant information to equip each individual to make a well-informed decision on their own care and life style. In spite of changed methods of practice, disabled people continue to remain disadvantaged as there are insufficient resources to meet all their needs and expectations (Smith & Goddard 1994). Moreover, the division of responsibility for funding essential equipment frequently falls between different agencies of health, social services, education and sometimes employment (Department of Health 1995a,b, Mandelstam 1994, Stewart 1995). Rather than enabling an individual, this division can create a barrier to independence.

Disabled people themselves are taking a lead-

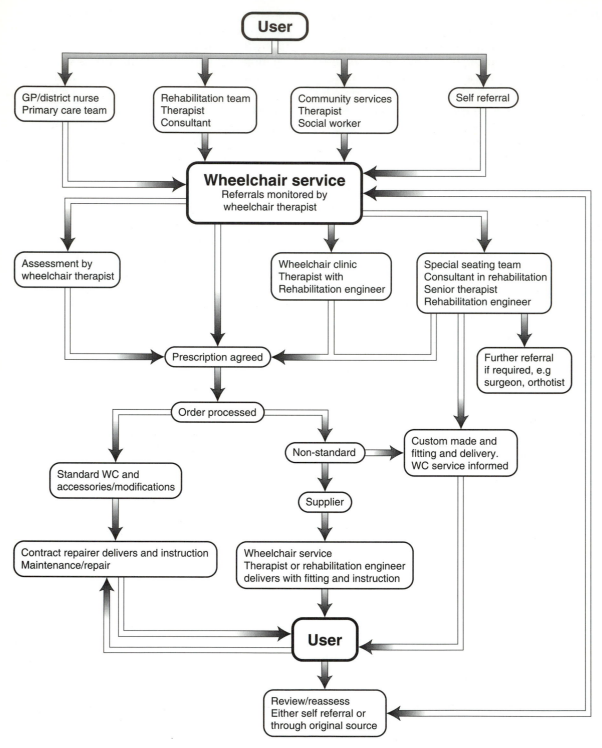

Figure 1.10 Referral to delivery process.

ing role in changing public attitudes and thinking. In 1985 the Prince of Wales' Advisory Group on Disability convened a working party made up of representatives from over 30 voluntary organizations and individuals from statutory bodies to formulate guidelines for planning services for people with severe disabilities. The resulting 'Living Options' publication emphasized the point that disabled people are people first and disabled second. Like others, they have individual attitudes, ideas, concerns, abilities and expectations. Whilst they may require help in certain areas, they also wish to have the opportunity to live in the same way as others (Stewart 1995). This is worth bearing in mind when providing any service, including the provision of mobility equipment.

USER INVOLVEMENT

The value of users and carers as a source of expertise is now widely recognized and their views are being sought in a number of ways (Department of Health 1996a–c). The Patients' Charter (Department of Health 1992), which is the NHS supplement to the Citizens' Charter, clearly recommends user and carer involvement when planning service strategy and setting local guidelines.

Since devolvement of the wheelchair services in 1991, many health authorities have explored various ways of accessing users and encouraging involvement in the decision-making process. A number of disability forums and user groups now address a wide range of relevant matters, including wheelchair issues, access, education, housing, advocacy and all aspects of local life and needs for anyone with a disability (Living Options 1995, National Prosthetic and Wheelchair Services Report 1993–1996). Alternatively, some wheelchair services have established a more local user group who discuss matters directly affecting their local service. Topics discussed may include anything from the local policy for provision to the range of wheelchairs available, access to the service or the standard of the facilities provided. Ideally, users will have the opportunity to discuss these matters directly

with policy makers. As with all committees, it is difficult to organize a well-balanced representation of users interested and willing to meet on equal terms with policy makers. Many active users are in employment whilst elderly people, who are used to accepting a service without complaint, find it difficult to participate in this type of forum. To encourage successful user involvement and contribution to the service, consideration needs to be given to access and transport arrangements, including the refunding of any out of pocket expenses for user representatives. It is equally important that those chosen as a representative have broad views on disability matters and an interest in the whole spectrum of users' needs rather than focusing on their own personal requirements. An open door policy which offers users direct access to staff members at specified times or days is available at many centres and will encourage improved communication and understanding, whilst helping to diffuse potentially sensitive situations between users and service providers. Centres able to establish an active user group quickly appreciate the advantages and find it provides a unique opportunity to develop a progressive and forward-looking service based on mutual ideas and open debate.

COMPLAINTS PROCEDURES

Even when the majority of users express satisfaction with their service, a number of complaints may still be received. Dissatisfaction with wheelchairs is not unique to the health service and is equally common in Sweden where the very latest wheelchair technology is available (Hunter & Walker 1993). The Patients' Charter clearly advocates that any individual using the NHS is entitled to expect a simple and effective complaints procedure. A further document, 'Acting on Complaints' (EL (95) 37), outlines new guidelines for this purpose. A National Association of Health Authorities and Trusts briefing (1995) provides information and guidelines on the complaints procedure which is intended to provide a simplified speedy and open procedure, with common features for complaints about any services provided as part of the NHS with fairness and ease of access for both staff and complainants alike

It recommends that there should be improvements in the quality of service based upon any lessons learned from a complaint, and for the first time complaints regarding clinical judgement are included in this procedure.

STANDARDS AND QUALITY ASSURANCE

Standards and quality of care and equipment are very much part of the present day service, with an increasing number of EU regulations and guidelines which can affect both prescription and client care (Department of Health 1996).

Setting standards and monitoring the effectiveness of wheelchair provision is the combined responsibility of purchaser and provider. It is important for service users, including professionals, to be aware of service criteria and standards in order to avoid either misunderstanding or to have unrealistic expectations when using the service. Carrying out a service or clinical audit may be seen as an unwelcome task by many managers, though it will help identify good as well as bad practice and, providing action is taken on the findings, will contribute to a quality service. Such is the importance given to this area at the present time, that there is a wealth of information available which can be appropriately adapted for reviewing all aspects of a service whether in the form of a user satisfaction survey (Burn, Lawrence & White 1994) or a clinical audit (McCreadie & James 1995).

RESOURCES

As indicated earlier, funding levels in the wheelchair service are generally considered to be inadequate to meet growing demand in both numbers of users and the expectations of both users and professionals. Carrying out an efficient audit can be beneficial and used as evidence when seeking improved resources, though money alone is not necessarily the answer to some of the existing difficulties being experienced world wide. Staffing numbers and the level of both clinical and clerical expertise is variable in the UK. The importance of appropriate training for both users and professionals is discussed in Chapter 14. If disappointments are to be avoided it is important that users should feel confident in the level of assessment provided. The introduction of the National Health Service and Community Care Act (1990), the rapid increase in the range of wheelchair and seating equipment now available and, more recently in England, the announcement of two new schemes for the provision of indoor/outdoor powered wheelchairs and a voucher system, have raised expectations and placed increasing pressure and demands on prescribers. This makes it essential for there to be suitable training programmes available, not only for those working in the wheelchair service but also for social service therapists responsible for the adaptations in the home and indeed for others involved with wheelchair users in education or employment settings.

If the philosophy of choice, access and independence for wheelchair users is to become a reality, then improved knowledge and understanding is essential for putting these ideas into practice.

REFERENCES

Badley E M, Wood P H N 1988 The epidemiology of disablement. In: Goodwill C J, Chamberlain M A (eds) Rehabilitation of the physically disabled adult. Croom Helm/Sheridan Medical, London, ch 2, p 12

Baughan S 1992 The Wheelchair Service in Yorkshire: present and future. Yorkshire RHA

Bar C A 1993 Rationalisation and reorganisation of the Welsh wheelchair service. Welsh Health Common Services Authority, Wales

Bennett-Wilson A Jr 1986 Wheelchairs. A prescription guide. Rehabilitation Press, Charlottesville, USA

Bennett-Wilson A Jr 1995 The evolution of wheelchairs. Topics in Spinal Cord Injury Rehabilitation 1(1): 42–53

British Society for Rehabilitation Medicine 1995 Seating needs for complex disabilities. BSRM Royal College of Physicians, London

Burn A, Lawrence A, White E 1994 Wheelchair prescription. An outcome audit. Greenwich and Canterbury & Thanet

Healthcare Trusts, South East Thames Regional Health Authority (SETRA)

Department of Health 1989 Caring for people: community care in the next decade and beyond. HMSO, London

Department of Health 1992 The Patients' Charter. HMSO, London

Department of Health 1994–95 Wheelchairs and artificial limbs. Government Statistical Service, London

Department of Health 1995a Practical guidance on joint commissioning for project leaders. Department of Health, Wetherby, Yorks

Department of Health 1995b Child health in the community: a guide to good practice. Department of Health, Wetherby, Yorks

Department of Health 1991 Wheelchair training resource pack. Centre of Information for Department of Health, London

Department of Health 1996 Wheelchair training resource pack (revised DoH 1991 publication). College of Occupational Therapists, London

Department of Health 1996a User involvement. Community service users as consultants and trainers. Guidelines for service purchasers on the experiences of the National User and Carer Group. Department of Health, Wetherby, Yorks

Department of Health 1996b Encouraging user involvement in commissioning. A resource for commissioners. Guidelines for service purchasers on the experiences of the National User and Carer Group. Department of Health, Wetherby, Yorks

Department of Health 1996c Consultation counts. Guidelines for service purchasers on the experiences of the National User and Carer Group. Department of Health, Wetherby, Yorks

Disability Discrimination Act 1995. HMSO, London

Disablement Services Authority 1989–90 Annual report of the DSA. DSA, London

Disablement Services Authority 1990 Report on the indoor/outdoor electric wheelchair pilot study. DSA, Blackpool

Dolfus P 1988 The need for wheelchairs. User's perspective. Extract from paper presented at Dundee '88

Fenwick D 1977 Wheelchairs and their users. Office of Population Censuses and Surveys for the Department of Health and Social Security, London

Gall R P, Rebholtz N, Hotchkiss R D, Pfaelzer P F 1997 Wheelchair rider injuries: causes and consequences for wheelchair design and selection. Journal of Rehabilitation, Research and Development 34(1): 58–71

Health Service Guidelines 1996a HSG(96) 34. Powered indoor/outdoor wheelchairs for severely disabled people. Department of Health, Wetherby, Yorks

Health Service Guidelines 1996b HSG(96) 53. The Wheelchair Voucher Scheme. Department of Health, Wetherby, Yorks

Hunter J, Walker J 1993 How should the wheelchair service develop in the 90s? Scottish Home & Health Office Report

Jarvis S 1985 Wheelchair clinics for children. Physiotherapy 71(3): 132–134

Kamenetz H L 1969 The Wheelchair Book. Charles C Thomas, Springfield, IL

Kerridge A 1993 Batteries not included: the campaign for state funding for indoor/outdoor powered wheelchairs. Muscular Dystrophy Group, London

Kettle M, Rowley C 1990 Report on Wheelchair Survey. DSA (90) 18. Disablement Services Authority, London

Lee P 1996 Contracting in the NHS. In: Wheelchair training resource pack. College of Occupational Therapists, London

Living Options 1995 Guidelines for those planning services for people with severe physical disabilities. Prince of Wales Advisory Group on Disability, Kings Fund Centre, London

McColl I 1986 Review of artifical limb and appliance centre services, vol II. HMSO, London

McCreadie M J, James R 1995 An audit of wheelchair service provision in three regions. British Journal of Therapy and Rehabilitation 12(9): 465–472

Mandelstam M 1994 How to get equipment for disability, 3rd edn. For Disabled Living Foundation by Jessica Kingsley & Kogan Page, London

Morris J 1995 The power to change. Commissioning health and social services with disabled people. Living Options partnership. King's Fund Centre, London

National Association of Health Authorities and Trusts 1995 NAHAT briefing: Interim guidance on implementing the new NHS complaints procedure. No. 91 December 1995

National Audit Office 1992 Health services for physically disabled people aged 16 to 64. HMSO, London

National Health Service and Community Care Act 1990. HMSO, London

National Prosthetic and Wheelchair Services Report 1993–1996 DOH funded project. College of Occupational Therapists, London

Office of Population Censuses and Surveys (OPCS) 1989 Disabled Adult Services, Transport and Employment Report 4. OPCS, London

Phillips L, Nicosia A 1990 Choosing a wheelchair system. Journal of Rehabilitation Research and Development, Clinical Supplement 2: 1–4

Scottish Office 1992 NHS MEL (1992)67 Indoor/outdoor powered wheelchairs. Scottish Office, Edinburgh

Smith S, Goddard T 1994 Wheelpower? Case studies from users and providers of the NHS wheelchair service. Spastics Society (Scope), London

Stewart C 1992 Wheelchair evaluation and prescription. Nursing Standard 7(1): 27–29

Stewart M 1995 Introduction. In: Bumphrey E (ed) Community practice. A text for occupational therapists and others involved in community care. Prentice Hall/Harvester Wheatsheaf, Hemel Hempstead, UK, ch 1, p 1

Walmsley W 1996 A brief history of the wheelchair service. In: Wheelchair training resource pack. College of Occupational Therapists, London

World Health Organization 1990 The international classification of impairments, disabilities and handicaps – a manual of classification relating to the consequences of disease. WHO, Geneva

2

Posture: Implications for seating and wheelchair mobility

INTRODUCTION

Knowledge of anatomical terminology, normal function and ideal posture is a prerequisite to analysing and assessing impaired function and posture. In order to record details regarding changes and progress in the user's condition, to establish the effectiveness of a prescription or to share information with others, it is necessary to use recognized terminology. For the majority of wheelchair users, any change or improvement recorded is based on general observation and discussion rather than measurement, but there will be times when it is necessary to use more formal measuring techniques (see Ch. 6), particularly with children and severely disabled users who, due to neurological dysfunction, surgical intervention or orthopaedic conditions have functional or postural impairment. Recognized systems and tools for measuring functional ability, muscle power and range of movement are also referred to later in this chapter.

ANATOMICAL TERMINOLOGY

Although many therapists will be familiar with this terminology, others may not, and as a starting point for communication it is desirable to be accurate.

Planes of the body (Fig. 2.1)

Body movement occurs in three planes which lie perpendicular to one another and intersect

23

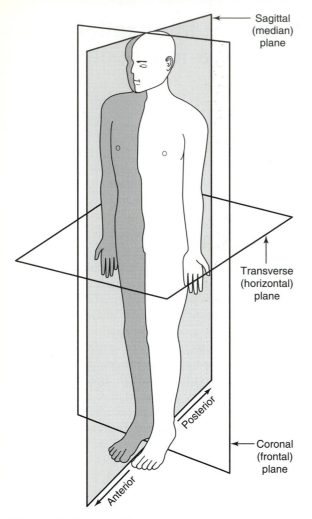

Figure 2.1   Planes of the body.

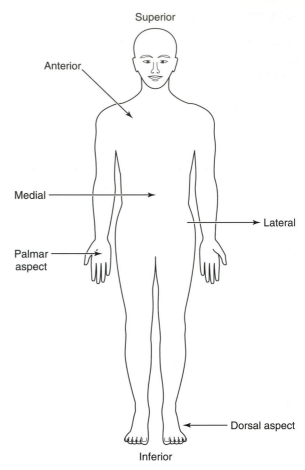

Figure 2.2   The anatomical position.

at the centre of gravity. These can be used as referral points when describing body movement and position.

The sagittal or median plane

This is a vertical plane which runs from front to back parallel to the long axis of the body, dividing it into left and right sides.

The coronal or frontal plane

This is a vertical plane which runs at right angles to the sagittal plane and which divides the body into an anterior and posterior section.

The transverse or horizontal plane

This plane runs at a right angle to both the sagittal and coronal planes and divides the body into an upper and a lower section.

Anatomical position (Fig. 2.2)

Terms of position and direction describe the relationship of one part of the body in relation to another. These terms assume the body to be in the standard anatomical position with the body erect, limbs extended and the palms of the hands facing forwards or the body in the supine position with the palms of the hand facing upwards.

Medial and lateral

In relation to the sagittal plane, the positions closer to the midline are termed medial and those distant from the midline are termed lateral. The little finger is on the medial side of the hand, the thumb is on the lateral side.

Anterior and posterior

In relation to the coronal plane, the positions to the front of the body are termed anterior and those further back are termed posterior.

It should be noted that the feet and the hands have additional terms describing position and also movement, as will be seen later.

The upper surface of the foot is termed dorsal and the lower surface plantar. The back of the hand is dorsal and the front palmar.

Proximal and distal

In relation to the transverse plane a structure closer to the plane is known as proximal, further away is known as distal. These terms are used only in relation to the limbs. In the upper limb, the upper arm is proximal whereas the hand is distal to the body.

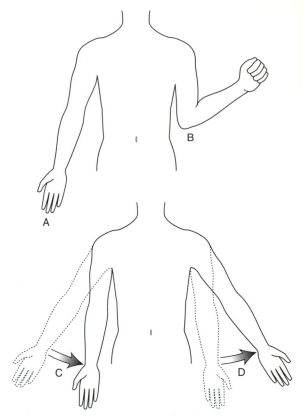

Figure 2.3   Diagram illustrating some terms of movement: **A** extension; **B** flexion; **C** adduction; **D** abduction.

Superior and inferior

These terms relate to the upper and lower end of the body respectively. The head is superior the feet are inferior.

Superficial and deep

These are terms used in relation to the skin and are therefore more commonly used when describing pressure sores or skin adhesions. Superficial is close to the surface of the skin whereas deep is further from the skin surface and nearer to the skeletal frame.

Terms of movement (Fig. 2.3)

Movement of bones occurs at joints. Terms of movement are therefore applicable to joints, not bones. Range of movement is limited by the bony structure of a joint, the ligaments and the muscles crossing the joint. Directions of movement are described in relation to the anatomical position.

Extension

Extension of a joint is generally to straighten it. In the anatomical position most joints are in a relaxed extension. Extreme extension is known as hyperextension. At the ankle joint, extension is termed plantarflexion and occurs when the toe is pointed to the ground (Fig. 2.3).

Flexion

Flexion of a joint is to bend or decrease the angle between the bones of the joint. Flexion of the ankle joint is known as dorsiflexion, which is when the toes of the foot are pulled up towards the lower leg.

Flexion and extension occur in the sagittal plane.

Lateral flexion, which is the sideways bending of the trunk, occurs in the coronal plane.

Abduction

This is movement of a limb away from the midline of the body, or the hand or foot with fingers and toes.

Although one talks of abduction and adduction of the fingers and toes, the similar movement of the ankle joint is generally described as external and internal rotation.

Adduction

This is movement of a limb towards the midline of the body or, in the case of the fingers and toes, movement towards the midline of the hand or foot. Tightness of the hip adductors is common in children with cerebral palsy and results in the scissor gait which is sometimes demonstrated by those with this condition (Fig. 2.3).

Abduction and adduction occur in the coronal plane.

Rotation

Rotation takes place in the transverse plane and is either internal or medial rotation towards the body, or external or lateral rotation turning away from the body.

Rotation also occurs in the spine and is present in scoliosis when the vertebral bodies rotate around the central axis.

Supination. Supination is the external rotation of the radiohumeral joint.

Pronation. Pronation is the internal rotation of the same joint. In the anatomical position, the arm is held in supination with the palm facing forwards, or upwards if the body is in the lying position.

The terms supination and pronation can also be used as alternatives to external rotation and internal rotation at the ankle joint.

Inversion

Inversion describes turning the plantar surface or sole of the foot inwards, elevating the medial border of the foot.

Eversion

Eversion is the reverse movement when the plantar surface or sole of the foot turns outwards, elevating the lateral border.

These movements take place in the coronal plane and occur at the subtalar and transverse tarsal joints.

Deviation

At the wrist joint the term *radial deviation* is the movement of the hand towards the midline and *ulnar deviation* is the movement of the hand away from the midline.

IDEAL POSTURE AND NORMAL FUNCTION

Introduction

What do we mean by the words 'ideal' or 'normal', or indeed other terms used in connection with posture, such as 'good' and 'bad'? What we tend to describe as ideal or good posture is when the body is placed in a symmetrical and well-balanced position. In general, this position, whether lying, sitting or standing, may look ideal, but firstly it is difficult to maintain for any period of time and, secondly, it is not necessarily a good basis for movement (Green, Mulcahy & Pountney 1992).

Posture can be defined as the position of one or many body segments in relation to one another and their orientation in space. Although described as ideal in normal subjects, in fact our posture is constantly changing as we move from one task to another. Generally we have an asymmetrical and ever changing, though balanced posture. This is achieved through integrated muscle activity working against gravity and helping us to keep our body sufficiently balanced to carry out the task in hand. Postural control can also be influenced by extrinsic factors in the form of support surfaces. The degree of external support provided will affect the amount of muscular activity and effort required to maintain a balanced posture. The level of support required will also depend on our individual bony structure, body shape, muscle ability, the type of activity being undertaken and the immediate environment.

Sitting

An optimal sitting position is said to be upright, symmetrical, with the pelvis anteriorly tilted and the iliac crests in alignment and level in the lateral plane. The hips, knees and ankles are all placed at 90 degrees of flexion. In this position the pelvis provides a stable base forming a foundation on which to support the rest of the body. The position of the spine is dictated by the position of the pelvis and ideally will be erect with the intervertebral joints held somewhere in mid range due to a balance of muscle activity between the anterior and posterior spinal muscles. When the pelvis is in the anteriorly tilted position this promotes a mild lumbar lordosis of the spine and the centre of gravity will generally fall anterior to the ischial tuberosities. Normally this upright position cannot be tolerated for any length of time and a good seat design will allow for postural adjustments to take place. As previously indicated, there is no one ideal posture and on the whole we tend to adopt poor postures for a good deal of the normal day, though this is seen as acceptable in people who are able to constantly change their position. A good posture is in fact one that allows maximum efficiency with minimum effort to perform the task in hand. In the case of someone who has a degree of postural deformity or abnormal patterns of movement, abnormal postures may be used as the only means of being independent in daily activities. Providing these postures are not damaging body tissues, systems and joints,

there is no reason to correct or try to 'normalize' posture unless the change results in a marked improvement in energy saving and efficiency. The degree of muscle activity used to maintain a posture can be reduced by providing external support. However, any excessive external support may restrict function and the degree of support used should relate to a specific activity. For example, when playing an instrument, a musician will sit on a stool or chair with limited back support and without arm rests or head support. This allows the freedom of movement to perform without restriction. A typist will select a seat with an upright back and shaped lumbar curve to encourage an upright posture which is well balanced, and will provide adequate support and minimize tension and backache. When one is relaxing, it is common to choose a high backed armchair with a degree of recline, padded arm rests and soft seat for comfort. In this situation muscle activity is reduced, the pelvis rotates posteriorly, resulting in a slight curvature of the lumbar spine, whilst the centre of gravity falls behind the ischial tuberosities. Additional pressure may be placed over the sacral area including the coccyx, though this depends partly on the density of the chair content and covering. An armchair covered with vinyl will increase pressure over the sacrum compared to one covered with a velvet- or cotton-type fabric. Without the additional back support, when relaxed, the sitter will either fall backwards or muscle activity will increase to maintain a more upright though possibly slumped position. This slumped posture is typical of that adopted by many wheelchair users and is aggravated by a sling seat, unstable base and sling back canvas (Fig. 2.4). It is also known to be a major cause of low back pain and can result in shear over the sacral area.

The head position in relation to the spine is of major importance and has a direct effect not only on posture, but also on eating, swallowing, eye contact, communication and respiratory function as well as upper limb function. Loss of head control can quickly affect the rest of the body position. This can be illustrated by the posture of someone who nods off to sleep when attending a

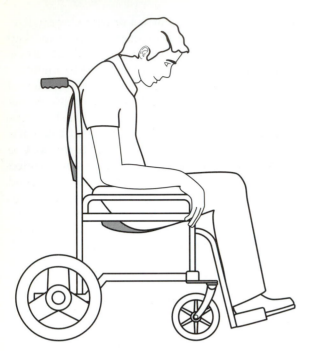

Figure 2.4 A slumped posture – typical of many wheelchair users.

concert. The head falls forwards or sideways and the trunk follows either until it reaches something firm that will provide additional support or, in the extreme, until balance is lost, though generally a sudden jerk reaction will wake the sleeper who will then adjust his or her position.

The choice of support system will depend to a degree on the task to be done and should be appropriate in height and angle for the user to obtain maximum function with minimum energy. Any tilting of a seat or recline of the backrest will have an effect on upper limb function and eye contact and will also influence the spinal posture (see Ch. 3).

Ideal posture, because of the apparent lack of movement, is sometimes mistakenly described as 'static', though in fact there is constant neuromuscular activity being used to maintain body balance.

Standing

The upright posture is generally considered to be the 'ideal' with feet facing forward and slightly apart to form a stable base. Gravity then falls in the midline, passing slightly in front of the shoulder joints, behind the hip joints, in front of the knee joints to a point in front of the ankle joints. The position of the feet will influence both stability and comfort. The distance between the feet, the direction of the feet and, in the sitting position, the height of the foot support, will affect balance and pressure areas. In the standing position, the pelvis is tilted anteriorly and with mild lordosis of the lumbar spine.

The vertebral column depends for its stability on the supporting musculature and although standing may require extensive activity of the antigravity muscles to maintain an upright position (Edwards 1996), only slight or moderate muscular activity is required to maintain this position providing the curvatures of the spine are in correct alignment (Oliver & Middleditch 1991). Rather than standing in one position for any length of time, most people are constantly shifting their balance from one leg to the other or may use a prop, for example, a walking stick, shop counter or kitchen sink, as a support.

Standing improves postural stability and muscle strength. It helps to reduce or delay the development of scoliosis where there is unequal tone in the spinal muscles and allows freedom of movement for function, facilitates respiration, bowel and bladder function and improves peripheral circulation to the lower limbs.

Lying

When lying, the position assumed by the spine will depend on the shape and density of the support surface and the weight and shape of the individual. As long periods of time are spent lying down, control of posture in lying is essential for people with neuromuscular disorders and should always be considered as part of a 24-hour postural management programme (see Ch. 9) for wheelchair users with potential postural problems (Fearn et al 1992, Goldsmith et al 1992, Pope 1996).

Physiological factors

Correct posture is not only important in preventing skeletal deformities but can also improve function of the internal organs. Sitting in a slumped position can restrict respiration and affect digestion as well as bladder and bowel function. The efficiency of a gastrostomy, tracheotomy or a catheter can be reduced by poor positioning. Maintaining a good head position is important not only for swallowing but also for speaking, coughing and swallowing. Asymmetrical sitting for long periods of time without adequate suppport or opportunity to change position, can result not only in discomfort but also development of pressure sores and, in the long term, postural deformity. Long distance lorry drivers, keyboard operators and others who have sedentary jobs are known to develop skeletal deformities related to their working position.

Good general health encouraged by a sensible and balanced diet is important for several reasons. It will promote healthy muscle tissue and good circulation, thus reducing the dangers of tissue breakdown caused by weight loss, decrease in muscle fibre as well as oedema resulting from inactivity and sitting for long periods of time (Bardsley 1993, Engstrom 1993, Stewart 1991). Maintaining a stable weight appropriate to the body build of the individual is essential, as overweight can cause major difficulties for both the wheelchair user and carers. Additional body weight places stress on the cardiorespiratory system when self propelling or transferring, whilst carers are at risk of experiencing back strain when pushing, lifting and transferring a heavy and disabled person. Obesity can cause practical problems with normal daily activities and may well restrict life style due to the additional effort demanded from carers. The choice of wheelchair models available will also be reduced for overweight users (see Ch. 11).

NORMAL DEVELOPMENT

Knowledge of normal development is essential in order to use as a baseline when assessing, monitoring and recording development and the needs of a child with a neurological disorder or developmental delay (Fearn et al 1992). This knowledge is equally essential for the assessment of all age groups of wheelchair users. Normal motor development depends on the state of the nervous system. The effects of any neurological disorder will depend on the location and severity of the lesion. When there is some form of cerebral lesion muscle tone will be variable and consequently interfere with posture and movement. Reflexes (involuntary responses present at birth and which normally are gradually suppressed or integrated as higher control centres mature) may remain and are then described as primitive or primary reflexes. Those most commonly seen and of significance to postural ability and function are as follows.

Asymmetrical tonic neck reflex (ATNR) (Fig. 2.5)

This is elicited when the head is turned. There is an increased extensor tone on the side to which the head is turned and increased flexor tone on the opposite side. In individuals with athetosis the side affected will change depending on the position of the head, though in those with spasticity ATNR will be stronger on one side. This can lead to deformity such as scoliosis of the spine, so should always be carefully monitored. In most

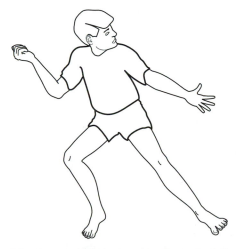

Figure 2.5   Asymmetrical tonic neck reflex to the left showing the arm and leg on the face side in extension whilst the limbs on the opposite side are in flexion.

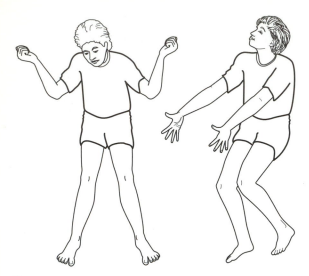

Figure 2.6 Symmetrical tonic neck reflex. When the neck is flexed there is flexion in the upper limbs and extension in the lower limbs. When the neck is extended there is extension of the upper limbs with flexion of the lower limbs.

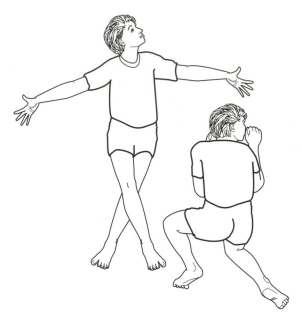

Figure 2.7 Tonic labyrinthine reflex. Change of position of the head in space will elicit this reflex. If the head is posterior to the upright or neutral position (extended), extensor tone dominates; if the head is forward of the upright position (flexed), flexor tone dominates.

cases this reflex is considered to be abnormal after the age of 6 months.

Symmetrical tonic neck reflex (STNR) (Fig. 2.6)

When the neck is flexed the upper limbs flex and the lower limbs extend, whereas if the chin is lifted (neck extension) the reverse occurs and the arms extend whilst the legs are pulled up into flexion. This can interfere with upper limb function, for as the head position changes either up or down, there is change in muscle tone in the limbs. This response is normally integrated between the age of 6 and 12 months.

Tonic labyrinthine reflex (Fig. 2.7)

When elicited in the supine position or with the head in extension, there is an increase in extension throughout the body. In the prone position or when the head is forward of the upright position there is an increase in flexion. Positioning the head in a neutral position will help to reduce the effect of these reflexes. Particular care should be taken when reclining the backrest of a wheelchair.

The positive supporting reaction (Fig. 2.8)

When supported under the shoulders and held upright with feet flat on the floor, there is strong extension of the lower limbs. Normally this response disappears as the infant learns to bear weight through the feet and stand independently, but when retained, and stimuli is applied to the intrinsic muscles of the feet, for example when pushing on a footplate, this will elicit an extensor thrust, with increased extensor tone throughout both trunk and limbs. This can result in development of extension contractures of the hips and lead to sacral sitting.

Moro reflex (Fig. 2.9)

The Moro reflex is elicited by extending the head backwards, resulting in an extension pattern of the body with the arms extended, abducted and externally rotated followed by a flexion or 'embrace' posture. If the Moro reflex remains active, it decreases sitting balance as the child

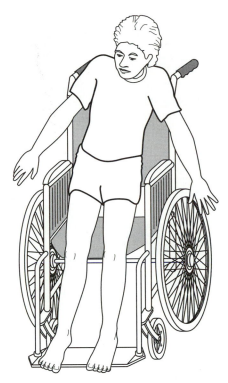

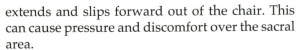

Figure 2.8 The positive supporting reaction. Pressure on the ball of the foot causes a strong extensor pattern or an extensor thrust which can force the individual out of their seated position.

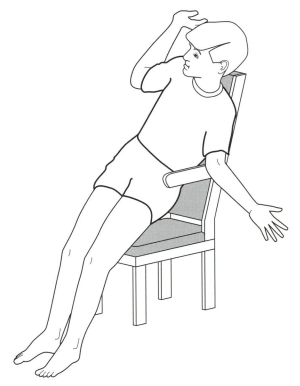

Figure 2.9 The Moro reflex. A downward movement of the head, a sudden noise or suddenly reclining backrest will result in extension, abduction and external rotation of arms with extended fingers. This response is followed by adduction and flexion of the arms over the trunk.

extends and slips forward out of the chair. This can cause pressure and discomfort over the sacral area.

As a child develops and the earlier reflexes are integrated, automatic reflexes or postural responses and reactions begin to develop. Normal postural tone enables an individual to maintain an upright posture against the forces of gravity and to initiate change of position for carrying out functional skills.

Righting reactions

These are automatic responses which help to keep the body aligned and balanced by maintaining the head, trunk, arms and legs in proper relationship one to another. Development of the righting response also allows the infant to acquire head control (Otto Bock 1989). Equilib-

rium reactions are part of postural control and help to maintain or restore balance in different postures. They are assumed to be organized at cortical level and are necessary before sitting balance can be achieved.

Movement outside the centre of gravity is part of everyday life and the body is constantly and automatically making adjustments to maintain balance.

Development of head control has a major part to play in achieving balance and controlling the righting reactions. In normal development the infant will show signs of head extension in the prone position from about 10 weeks. When pulling an infant by their hands, from the supine into the sitting position, signs of head control will be seen at about 5 or 6 months. A child with normal development learns the ability to lie before progressing to sitting, crawling, standing and walking. The relationship between the levels of ability in the different positions of sitting, standing and lying have been demonstrated in work carried out at Chailey Heritage (Green, Mulcahy & Pountney 1992), when it was found that until a child achieved level 4 lying ability, they were unable to sit independently at level 3. This was true of normal children as well as those with cerebral palsy (See Appendix 1).

Some children naturally develop more quickly than others, but understanding the order of normal development and the relationship between the levels of postural ability in the normal child will help in planning treatment, setting realistic targets and providing appropriate seating and support for those with developmental problems.

MEASURING FUNCTIONAL ABILITY AND DEFORMITY

Measuring the effectiveness of equipment and the improvement or changes that result from provision of either seating or postural support and other accessories, is frequently based on general observation, discussion and, in many cases, the comments of the individual and their carer. These tend to be subjective and relate to improvements in ease of care and behaviour as well as the general ability and perceived comfort of the user.

It is important to find an objective method of assessing and monitoring changes in all aspects of life. A number of recognized measurement scales are available (Green, Mulcahy & Pountney 1992, Reed 1991). Undertaking regular measuring and recording of progress is generally the task of the therapist seeing the individual from day to day, whereas measuring changes in range of joint movement for individuals with complex postural problems can also be the responsibility of the seating team. Certainly in the case of many adolescents and adults who are seen in the wheelchair services, there is no formal or regular objective measuring of change. To assess sitting ability, the individual should always be removed from the wheelchair and placed in a free sitting position on the side of an adjustable height

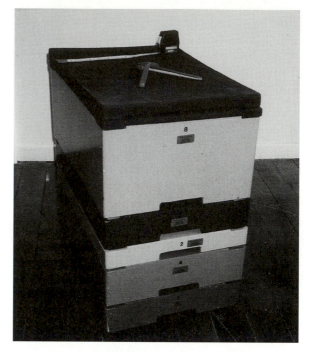

Figure 2.10 Essential equipment for assessment will include a steel measuring tape, a goniometer and several sizes of sitting boxes.

plinth, with feet placed on the floor or on seating boxes of the correct dimensions and a non-slip seating pad such as evazote. When necessary, minimal support should be provided by a helper. Spinal deformities, such as increasing scoliosis, are measured from X-rays by the orthopaedic surgeon (see Ch. 3), but free sitting allows the assessor to identify areas of general concern when observing the individual in an unsupported position. Joint changes and limitations in range of movement can be measured by a therapist using a goniometer (Fig. 2.10). A multi-adjustable assessment chair will enable the assessor to establish how different positions and any joint limitations will affect overall posture. Adjusting the seating position will also help to identify the optimum position for the comfort and function of each user (Fig. 2.11). A method for measuring changes in windswept hips was initially developed to use with children (Goldsmith et al 1992), though this can equally be applied to other age groups. The weight of

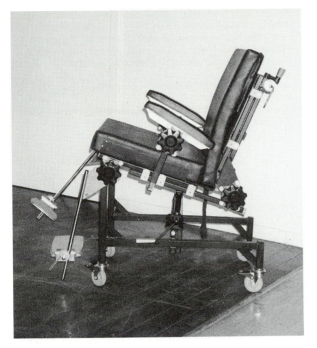

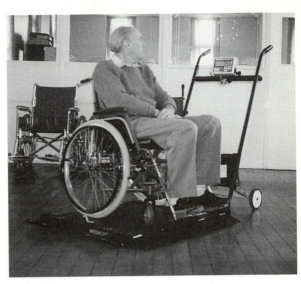

Figure 2.12 Suitable weighing equipment is required if the weight of each user is to be accurately recorded.

Figure 2.11 An adjustable assessment chair will help to establish the optimum position that can be achieved by each individual.

the wheelchair user should also be accurately recorded, as this will influence the range of chairs available and strength of materials used in the final prescription (Fig. 2.12). Assessors should always be aware of and adhere to the weight limit given by the manufacturer on each model. Whatever the method adopted for measurement of ability or deformity, it is important that there should be consistency in the way the measurements are made and compared. Without establishing some baseline for measuring change and progress, it is not possible to monitor accurately the effectiveness of equipment. However, it is

unlikely that a wheelchair or postural support is the only form of intervention with a wheelchair user and all other factors must be taken into account when assessing improvements or change in a condition.

An understanding of normal posture and function assists the clinician to understand the wide range of limitations and difficulties experienced by disabled people. Without the knowledge of normal posture and function incorrect assumptions may be made and certain limitations overlooked or disregarded during assessment for a wheelchair or seating.

REFERENCES

Bardsley G 1993 Seating. In: Bowker P, Condie D N, Bader D L, Pratt D J (eds) Biomechanical basis of orthotic management. Butterworth Heinemann, Oxford, ch 14, p 253

Edwards S 1996 An analysis of normal movement as the basis for the development of treatment techniques. In: Edwards S (ed) Neurological physiotherapy. A problem

solving approach. Churchill Livingstone, London, ch 2, p 15

Engstrom B 1993 Ergonomics. Wheelchairs and positioning. Posturalis, Sweden

Fearn T A, Green E M, Jones M, Mulcahy C M, Nelham R L, Pountney T E 1992 Postural management. In: McCarthy G (ed) Physical disability in children. An interdisciplinary approach to management. Churchill Livingstone, London, ch 25, p 401

Goldsmith E, Golding R M, Garstang R A, MacRae A W 1992 A technique to measure windswept deformity; a technical evaluation. Physiotherapy 78(4): 235–242

Green E M, Mulcahy C M, Pountney T E 1992 Postural management. Theory and practice. Active Design, Birmingham

Oliver J, Middleditch A 1991 Functional anatomy of the spine. Butterworth Heinemann, Oxford

Otto Bock 1989 Seating in review. Current trends for the disabled. Otto Bock, Canada

Pope P 1996 Postural management and special seating. In: Edwards S (ed) Neurological physiotherapy. A problem solving approach. Churchill Livingstone, London, ch 7, p 135

Reed K L 1991 Quick reference to occupational therapy. Aspen, Maryland

Stewart C P U S 1991 Physiological considerations in seating. Prosthetics and Orthotics International 15: 193–198

3

Biomechanics

Mechanics is simply the study of motion and describes the forces that create motion or alternatively prevent it by maintaining a static equilibrium. Biomechanics, therefore, involves applying the science of mechanics to the human body (Bowker 1993).

This chapter will cover some of the basic terminology and concepts of mechanics and explain how they are applied to both the wheelchair user and the wheelchair.

BASIC TERMS AND CONCEPTS

Force

A force is something that makes an object move, stop moving or change shape. A force has both magnitude and direction and is, therefore, a vector quantity. Forces can be compressive, tensile or shear, depending on their direction (Fig. 3.1). In order to define and understand a force it is important to know its magnitude, its direction of application and its point of application.

Buckling

If a compressive load or force is applied to a column there is a possibility the column will fail if the stresses (force per unit area) generated in the column exceed the failure stress of the material.

It is possible for a relatively slender column to become unstable by buckling when subjected to a

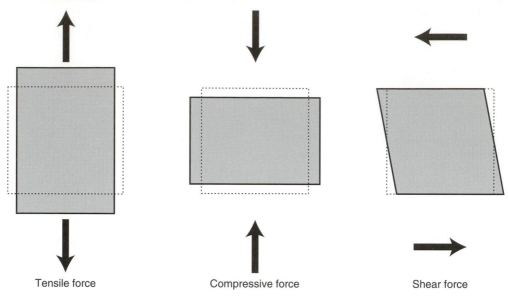

Tensile force　　　　Compressive force　　　　Shear force

Figure 3.1　Examples of tensile, compressive and shear forces.

compressive load which is significantly less than the failure load. The theory of this type of instability was studied and described by the Swiss mathematician Euler in the eighteenth century. A column subjected to a concentric compressive load is regarded as unstable (in the Euler sense) and buckles if the column does not return to its original shape after it is perturbed (Crisco & Panjabi 1992). This type of theory has been used in the study of deformities of the spine discussed later in this chapter.

Moment

As well as tending to make an object deform or move in a straight line, forces can also turn or rotate an object. For example, when climbing a kerb a downward force on the wheelchair push handles or tipping levers helps to tilt the wheel-chair turning it about the rear wheels. The turning effect of this type of force is known as a moment (or torque) and its turning ability is related to both the magnitude of the force and the perpendicular distance from the pivot to the line of action of the force.

$$\text{Moment} = \text{Force} \times \text{Distance}$$

A moment will be greater if the force is increased, or alternatively if the distance of the line of action of the force from the pivot point is increased. The harder you push or the longer the tipping levers, the easier it is to tilt the wheelchair.

Figure 3.2A shows how a force applied to the push handles of an attendant-propelled wheel-chair can apply a turning moment about the axle of the rear wheels of the wheelchair. At the same time the weight of the wheelchair user (U) and the weight of the wheelchair (W) apply a turning moment about the rear wheels in the opposite direction. In order to simplify and calculate the turning moments created by the weight of the user and wheelchair, it can be assumed that the respective weights are represented as forces (U and W) acting vertically down from points at the centre of gravity of the wheelchair user and wheelchair (Fig. 3.2B).

Newton's laws

Newton's third law states that if one object exerts a force on a second object then the second object exerts an equal and opposite reaction force on the

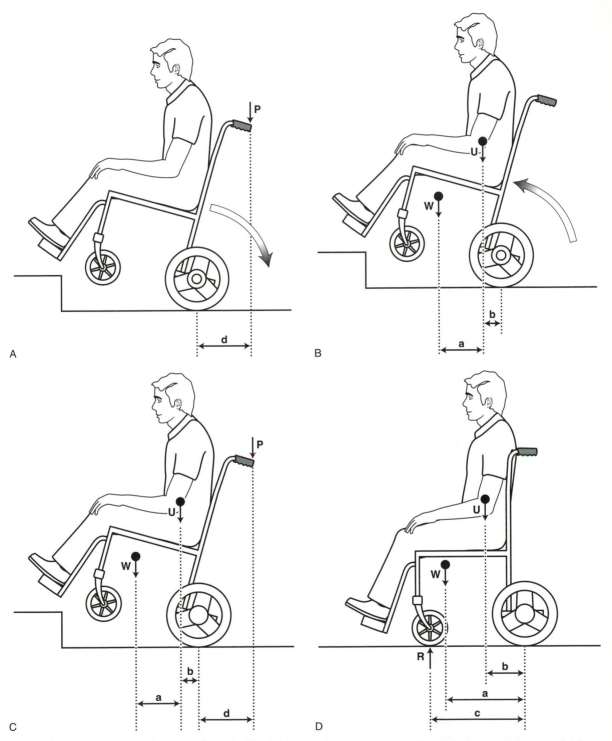

Figure 3.2 Attendant-propelled wheelchair climbing a kerb. (A) Turning moments acting clockwise about the rear wheel = (P × d). (B) Turning moments acting anti-clockwise about the rear wheel = (U × b) + (W × a). (C) In order to tip the wheelchair: (P × d) acting clockwise would need to be greater than (U × b) + (W × a) acting anti-clockwise. (D) For static equilibrium: (R × c) acting clockwise would need to be equal to (U × b) + (W × a) acting anti-clockwise.

first object. For example, a wheelchair user will apply a force down due to the effects of gravity acting on their mass and unless the user is falling or floating in space the seat will apply an equal and opposite force back on the individual. Similarly, if a force is applied to a part of the body by a support, the body will apply an equal force back on the support.

The study of objects at rest is known as statics and relies on one of the fundamental concepts of mechanics: Newton's first law. This law states that an object remains at rest or in uniform motion until acted upon by an unbalanced set of forces.

Static equilibrium

For an object to be truly stationary or in static equilibrium, therefore, there must be no resultant force or moment acting on it. This can be achieved if all the individual forces and turning moments acting on the object cancel each other out, i.e. the sum of all the forces or moments acting in one direction equals the sum of the forces acting in the opposite direction. This principle is particularly relevant to a wheelchair user if the user's posture in the wheelchair, and the wheelchair itself, are to be stable.

Returning to the example in Fig. 3.2C, in order to tip the attendant-propelled wheelchair to negotiate the kerb, the clockwise turning moments about the rear wheel must exceed the anti-clockwise turning moments (Fig. 3.2C). In this case the wheelchair and occupant would be unstable and the desired turning motion would be achieved.

Once back on level ground the attendant would gradually reduce the downward force P on the push handles. If the anti-clockwise turning moments about the rear wheels now exceed the clockwise turning moments, there will be turning motion in the opposite direction. Once the front castors are in contact with the ground a proportion of the weight of the wheelchair and occupant will be applied to the ground through the front castors. The reaction to this force R will be applied from the ground to wheelchair via the front castors. R will apply a clockwise turning

moment about the rear wheels which should equal the anti-clockwise turning moment, hence restoring stability (Fig. 3.2D).

The weight taken through the rear wheels and the corresponding ground reaction force can be disregarded, as this force passes through the rear axle and point of contact of the rear wheels with the ground and therefore does not apply a turning moment about the rear wheels.

BASIC WHEELCHAIR STABILITY
Wheel position

Figure 3.3A shows a wheelchair user in a wheelchair on a gentle slope with the brakes applied. In this situation the centres of gravity of the wheelchair and user both fall in front of the point of contact of the rear wheel with the ground. U and W apply turning moments in a clockwise direction which are counteracted by the turning moment generated by the reaction force through the front castors of the wheelchair and hence the user and wheelchair are stable.

The same wheelchair user is on a steeper gradient in Figure 3.3B. This time the centre of gravity of the user falls behind the point of contact between the rear wheel and the ground. Although the weight of the wheelchair (W) is still applying a clockwise turning moment about the rear wheels, the weight of the user (U) is now applying an anti-clockwise turning moment. At the limit of stability the anti-clockwise turning moment due to the weight of the user equals the clockwise turning moment due to the weight of the wheelchair. The front castors will barely be in contact with the ground and so there will be no weight taken through the front castors and all the weight of the user and wheelchair will be taken through the rear wheels.

If the user was on a similar slope and had a bag hanging from the push handles of the wheelchair, there would be an additional turning moment acting in an anti-clockwise direction (Fig. 3.3C). In this case if the sum of the anti-clockwise turning moments exceeds the clockwise turning moments, the wheelchair and user will topple backwards.

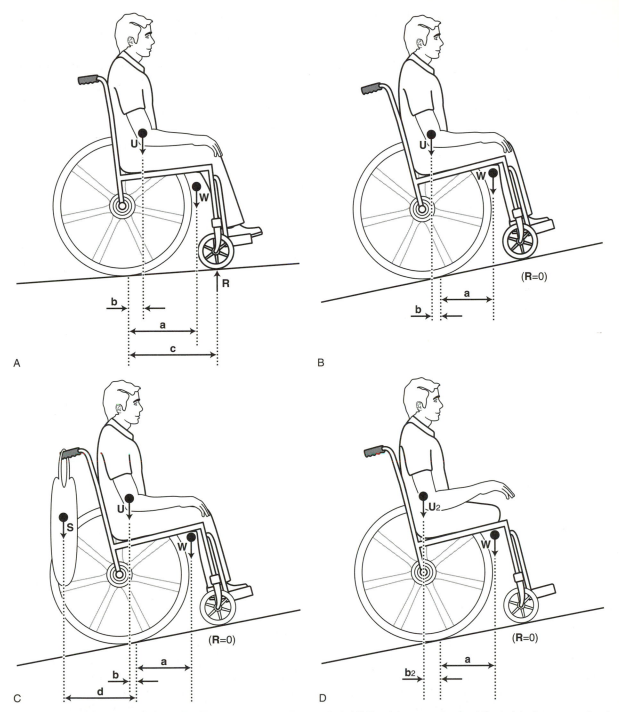

Figure 3.3   Self-propelled wheelchair on a slope with brakes applied: (A) Turning moments about the point where rear wheel is in contact with the ground resulting in stability: $(U \times b)$ clockwise + $(W \times a)$ clockwise = $(R \times c)$ anti-clockwise. (B) Turning moments about the point where the rear wheel is in contact with the ground at limit of stability: $(U \times b)$ anti-clockwise = $(W \times a)$ clockwise. (C) Turning moments about the point where the rear wheel is in contact with the ground resulting in instability causing the wheelchair to tip backwards: $(U \times b)$ anti-clockwise + $(S \times d)$ anti-clockwise > $(W \times a)$ clockwise. (D) Turning moments about the point where the rear wheel is in contact with the ground resulting in instability causing the wheelchair to tip backwards: $(U2 \times b2)$ anti-clockwise > $(W \times a)$ clockwise.

Alternatively, if the occupant of the wheelchair was a double amputee it is probable that their centre of gravity would be displaced significantly posteriorly when sitting. Referring to Figure 3.3D, this would have the effect of increasing the turning moment anti-clockwise because b2 is greater than b in Figure 3.3B. Once again this is likely to result in instability if the anti-clockwise turning moments exceed the clockwise turning moments.

In the examples shown in Figures 3.3C and D, if the rear wheels were set further back then the anti-clockwise turning moments tending to tip the wheelchair and user backwards would be reduced and stability might then be achieved. Similarly, if forward stability was in question, perhaps due to the user's centre of gravity being displaced anteriorly in the wheelchair by the seat system, then moving the front castors forward would help to reduce any turning moments likely to encourage the wheelchair to rotate about the front castors (Fig. 3.4).

Generally the stability of a wheelchair will be increased by moving the front and rear wheels as far apart as possible. The negative effects of this in terms of manoeuvrability and propulsion

efficiency are discussed later in this chapter. Stability can also be improved generally by ensuring that the mass of the user and wheelchair is as low to the ground as possible.

Rear wheel camber

When the plane of the wheel is angled in relation to the vertical it is said to be cambered. The use of a camber on the rear wheels increases the width between the points where the wheels are in contact with the ground – this is known as the track width (Fig. 3.5). This will increase the lateral stability of the wheelchair. However, it will also increase the overall width of the wheelchair, which may cause problems when negotiating doorways of limited width. The top of the wheels will be closer to the wheelchair user due to the camber, which may be beneficial in terms of the ergonomics of propulsion and will help to ensure clearance between the user's hands and the door frame.

There is some debate as to whether rear wheel camber can help with maintaining a straight line on a lateral incline (i.e. a surface that slopes across the direction of propulsion). Brubaker et al

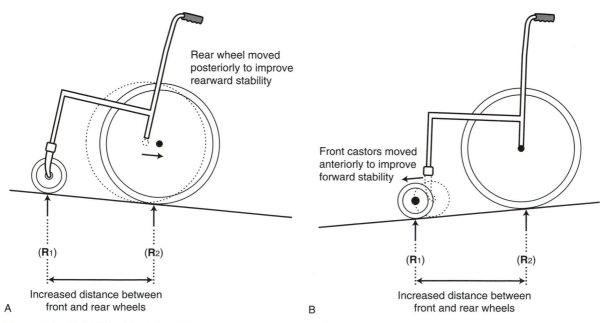

Figure 3.4 (A, B) Wheel base in relation to wheelchair stability on a slope.

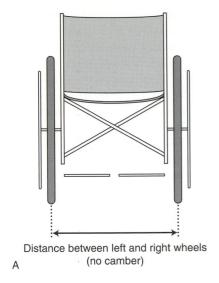

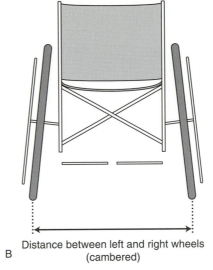

A   Distance between left and right wheels
(no camber)

B   Distance between left and right wheels
(cambered)

Figure 3.5   (A, B) Normal and cambered wheel configuration.

(1985, 1986) and Veeger et al (1989) suggest that it does, whereas Major (1990) thinks that the perceived improvement is due entirely to the increase in track width and is not a direct effect of the camber of the wheels.

WHEELCHAIR PROPULSION EFFICIENCY AND MANOEUVRABILITY

Wheelchair weight

Contrary to the common belief, on flat surfaces the weight of the wheelchair has very little effect on the mechanical efficiency of propulsion (Brubaker 1990). Instead it is the rolling resistance, straight line performance, manoeuvrability and ergonomic efficiency of propulsion mainly associated with the geometry of the wheelchair that are significant. The weight does become more significant, however, if the wheelchair is used on a slope or if the user needs to lift it into a vehicle.

Rolling resistance

Rolling resistance gives an indication of how much energy is lost during propulsion and is proportional to the combined weight of the

wheelchair and user and inversely proportional to the diameter of the wheel in contact with the ground (McLaurin & Brubaker 1991). A larger diameter wheel will therefore result in a lower rolling resistance.

The position of the rear wheels in relation to the wheelchair user is important in determining the distribution of weight through the smaller front castors and larger rear wheels, which thus helps to define the overall rolling resistance of the wheelchair (Disabled Living Foundation 1993).

A standard wheelchair configuration will result in approximately 60% of the combined weight of the wheelchair and user passing through the rear wheels and approximately 40% through the front wheels (Fig. 3.6). By moving the rear wheels anteriorly in relation to the user, this distribution can be changed to 70%/30% or even 75%/25%. The more weight taken through the rear wheels which have a lower rolling resistance, the lower the overall rolling resistance. Brubaker (1986) suggests that by moving the rear wheels forward 2.5 inches (5 cm) in relation to the user, the overall rolling resistance can be reduced by up to 6%, which may be highly significant for a user with limited ability to propel or for any user over a long distance.

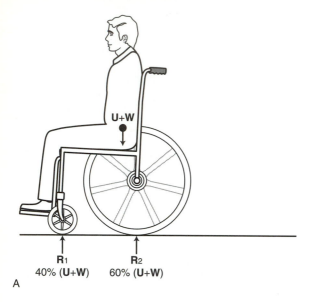

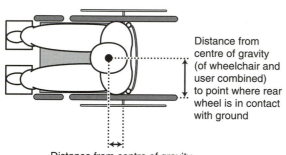

Figure 3.6 (A, B) Position of centre of gravity of wheelchair and user combined in relation to wheel base.

Straight line motion

Equal force to both propelling wheels should result in motion in a straight line if the surface is level. On a lateral slope (e.g. on a pavement sloped to allow rainwater to drain into the gutter), however, there will be a tendency for the wheelchair to turn down the slope. This is due to the effects of gravity acting on the mass of the wheelchair and user, and since the centre of gravity of the wheelchair and user are in front of the rear wheels this produces a turning moment acting on the rear wheels.

In order to keep the wheelchair going in a straight line under these circumstances, it is necessary to propel harder on the downhill side resulting in significantly increased energy expenditure. Brubaker et al (1985) suggested that in a conventional wheelchair, twice as much energy was required to maintain a straight path on a 2 degree lateral slope compared to a level surface.

Moving the rear wheels anteriorly in relation to the user reduces the horizontal distance between the combined (wheelchair and user) centre of gravity and the rear wheel (Fig. 3.6). The turning moment about the rear wheels, tending to make the wheelchair veer down the slope, is therefore reduced. Taken to the extreme, if the user was able to balance on the rear wheels the total combined weight would be over the rear wheels and there would be no turning moment about the rear wheels.

Another influence on the ability of the wheelchair and user to maintain motion in a straight line on a lateral slope is the angle of the front castors. A castor is designed so that the point where it is in contact with the ground automatically trails behind the pivot axis of the castor. Although helpful on a level surface, this feature exacerbates the drifting down the hill on a lateral slope: this experience will be recognized by anyone trying to push a supermarket trolley on a lateral slope (Major 1990).

If the castor is mounted at an angle then the height of the wheelchair will depend on the direction of the castor, and when the castor is in one particular direction the wheelchair will be at its lowest. The effect of gravity on the combined weight of the wheelchair and user will encourage the wheelchair to return to the situation where it is at its lowest. If the castor angle is such that the wheelchair is at its lowest when the wheelchair castors are in the position associated with forward movement, then it will be easier to maintain straight line motion but at the same time turning will be more difficult.

Manoeuvrability

The manoeuvrability of the wheelchair is related to the distance between the front and rear wheels.

As the wheelbase is shortened the turning circle of the wheelchair is reduced, making it easier to turn. Shortening the wheelbase can make it more difficult to negotiate kerbs, however.

The ease of turning when moving is related to the distance from the rear wheels to the centre of gravity of the wheelchair and user combined (Fig. 3.6). The magnitude of the combined mass of the wheelchair and user and these distances define the polar moment of inertia, which can be regarded loosely as the resistance to change in direction of motion. This resistance to change in direction of motion can be reduced by moving the rear wheels anteriorly with respect to the user.

Rear wheel balance

Many wheelchair users find the ability to balance the wheelchair on the rear wheels, with the front wheels clear of the ground, very useful when negotiating kerbs and obstacles. The 'wheelie' is achieved by accelerating and transferring weight rearward. The inertial effect of the body mass above the rear wheel resisting the sudden acceleration causes a turning moment about the axle of the rear wheel, tending to lift the front wheels clear of the ground. If the centre of gravity of the wheelchair and user is maintained vertically above the rear axle then balance can be achieved (Fig. 3.7). Any slight movement of the centre of gravity of the wheelchair and user combined, in relation to the rear axle, will require a small corrective force to move the wheelchair to restore balance. This situation is a case of unstable equilibrium and is only achievable if the user can exercise good dynamic control (Major 1990).

The ease of achieving rear wheel balance is improved by moving the rear wheels forward in relation to the user, thus transferring more weight to the rear wheels and making the wheelchair less stable. Thus the amount of weight transfer required is reduced if the front castors already carry a smaller proportion of the total load. Conversely, a high seat back can limit the range of trunk movement and can make it more difficult to perform a 'wheelie'.

Veeger et al (1989) reported that rolling resis-

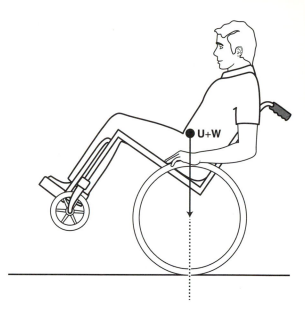

Figure 3.7 Rear wheel balance ('wheelie'). Centre of gravity of wheelchair and user combined balanced over rear wheels.

tance increases when performing a 'wheelie' if the rear wheels are cambered. This would suggest it is easier to maintain rear wheel balance if the rear wheels have a camber.

ERGONOMIC CONSIDERATIONS

Optimizing the ergonomic efficiency of propulsion usually depends on achieving the best position for the user in relation to the propelling wheel. Efficiency can be optimized by minimizing energy consumption in the recovery phase of the propelling cycle. If the wheel is too far posteriorly, then the user must internally rotate, extend and elevate his or her shoulder in order to grip the push rim behind their body for the beginning of the next stroke (Brubaker 1990). With the wheels moved anteriorly, with respect to the user, then recovery is assisted by gravity acting on the upper limbs and little muscle activity is required.

Compromise wheel position

Stability is an area where prescribers understandably tend to be cautious for fear of injury to the user in case the wheelchair tips. Many users, however, might benefit significantly from a less stable wheelchair with rear wheels moved anteriorly for the reasons covered above. Although moving the rear wheels anteriorly reduces the stability, it can be argued that this makes it easier to recover from an unstable position (Brubaker 1990).

Many wheelchairs now offer an adjustable wheel position facility and there will inevitably be a configuration that allows a suitable compromise between various objectives for each wheelchair user. In order to reach the optimum position therefore, the health care professional working in the wheelchair service needs to have an understanding of the effects of changing wheel position. Although there are rules on the minimum stability acceptable when providing wheelchairs, there is a strong argument that these rules should be relaxed where the user wishes the wheelchair to be less stable but understands the risks.

The wheelchairs with adjustable wheel position tend to be associated with more active users; however, the benefits of establishing an optimum wheel position for people of 'marginal propelling ability' can be significant (Perks et al 1994).

POSTURAL SUPPORT

Postural support is typically provided to oppose or slow down the deterioration of posture, improve stability, encourage ability, distribute pressure and provide comfort. Ideally the postural support should complement the user's overall postural management objectives (Fearn et al 1992). When applying postural support within a seating system, it is important to analyse and understand the forces that are being applied to the user's body.

Static equilibrium is necessary in order to achieve a stable posture. As stated earlier, in order for static equilibrium to be achieved the sum of all forces and turning moments acting on an object must be equal to zero. This can be achieved in seating if all the individual forces and turning moments acting on the body in different directions cancel each other out.

Basic sitting stability

The first step to ensuring postural stability is to ensure that a stable sitting base is achieved. With a stable sitting base the user's freedom of movement in the upper body is enhanced. If the sitting base is unstable it is very difficult to balance the upper body, in the same way that it is difficult to build a stack of bricks if the bottom brick is unstable.

In order to balance the trunk over a stable sitting base it is necessary to ensure that the centre of gravity of the upper body is directly over the base of support. Unless the user has a reasonably advanced level of sitting ability and is able to shift body weight, it will be difficult to recover if the centre of gravity falls outside the support base. Stability can be improved by increasing the area of contact between the body and the support surface, thus making the base of support larger. Some postural deformities, however, reduce the area of the support base and therefore decrease stability.

Basic postural support, therefore, is often aimed at assisting the user to achieve a stable pelvic base and positioning the upper body over the base of support in order to compensate for the user's reduced ability to maintain postural alignment (Henderson 1989).

Following chapters will describe specific postural problems associated with users from various diagnostic groups. This chapter will look at some general postural problems and the ways in which support can be provided to oppose them.

Pelvic tilt

When sitting, the base of support is the pelvis and femora. The pelvis is balanced on ischial tuberosities and is therefore inherently unstable (Bardsley 1993). For maximum stability and minimum muscle effort when maintaining an upright posture, the centre of gravity of the upper body should be maintained over the ischial tuberosities (Zacharkow 1988, Fig. 3.8). This reduces the turning moments acting on the pelvis, allowing it to be maintained in a neutral or upright position.

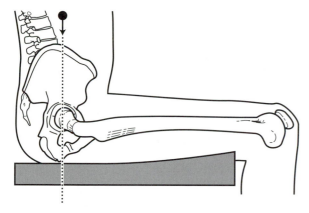

Figure 3.8 Sagittal view of pelvis and femurs. Showing the centre of gravity of the upper body balanced over the ischial tuberosities.

If, however, the centre of gravity of the upper body is situated posteriorly with respect to ischial tuberosities, there will be a turning moment causing the pelvis to tilt posteriorly. The tendency for the pelvis to tilt posteriorly is often reinforced by tension in the hamstrings. If the seat surface is level there is a tendency for the femora to slope down towards the front of the seat, which in the absence of full postural control also contributes to the posterior tilt of the pelvis (Fearn et al 1992). A posteriorly tilted pelvis will flatten the lumbar curvature and encourage a 'slumped' posture. It can also result in significantly increased load bearing and hence pressure over the relatively thin tissue covering the coccyx and end of the sacrum. This, in combination with shearing stresses generated as a result of the pelvis tending to slip anteriorly on the seat surface, can increase the risk of a pressure sore developing.

Some seating systems allow the hips to extend slightly, reducing the tension in the hamstrings to allow an upright pelvis (Pope et al 1988, Stewart & McQuilton 1987).

Another approach is to use a ramped seat base in conjunction with a pelvic belt, sacral pad, kneeblock and appropriate foot support (Fearn et al 1992). The ramped seat base provides a flat platform for the ischial tuberosities and typically a 15 degree ramp to support the thighs and maintain the femora in a horizontal attitude (Mulcahy

& Pountney 1987). The sacral pad applies a force directly to the posterior aspect of the pelvis. Ideally the sacral pad should be curved to follow the contour of the pelvis and ensure that force is transmitted across the width of the pelvis. The sacral pad should not extend higher than L5/S1 to ensure that the force is applied only to the pelvis and sacrum and not the lower lumbar vertebrae (Mulcahy & Pountney 1986).

In order to stop the pelvis slipping anteriorly in the seat and tilting posteriorly from the new position, it is necessary to apply another force to the pelvis in a direction from anterior to posterior. This can be achieved to a limited extent using a pelvic belt but more effectively using a kneeblock pushing along the line of the femora to the hip joint. The combination of the kneeblock force and the reaction force from the sacral pad acting on the posterior iliac spine applies a turning moment to the pelvis to maintain it in a neutral position (Fig. 3.9). The nearer to the upright (neutral) position that the pelvis is, the greater the distance between these two forces and therefore the smaller the force needs to be to produce the same turning moment. In the ideal situation the centre of gravity of the upper body would return to a balanced alignment above the ischial tuberosities of the neutral pelvis, reducing the horizontal components of force to zero.

An added advantage of the above force system is that it anchors the pelvis very effectively and creates a stable base on which the trunk can be

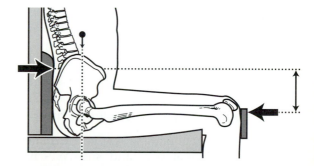

Figure 3.9 Use of kneeblock and sacral pad. Shows the vertical distance between: (i) the force applied along the femur from anterior to posterior by the kneeblock and; (ii) the force applied to the pelvis from posterior to anterior by the sacral pad; resulting in a turning moment to the pelvis opposing the posterior tilt.

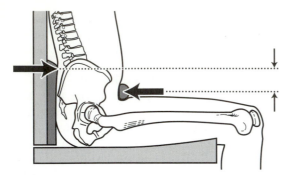

Figure 3.10   Use of sub ASIS padded bar (or belt) to oppose posterior tilt of pelvis. Shows the relatively small vertical distance between: (i) the force applied to the pelvis from anterior to posterior by the sub ASIS bar; (ii) the force applied to the pelvis from posterior to anterior by the sacral pad; resulting in a turning moment to the pelvis opposing the posterior tilt.

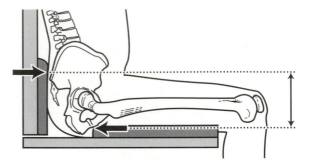

Figure 3.11   Use of cushion with pre-ischial bar anti-thrust blocks. Shows the vertical distance between: (i) the force applied to the ischial tuberosities from anterior to posterior by the pre-ischial bar; (ii) the force applied to the pelvis from posterior to anterior by the sacral pad; resulting in a turning moment to the pelvis opposing the posterior tilt.

balanced more easily. For some users, particularly children with cerebral palsy, this can help to avoid certain secondary postural problems and encourages the development of ability and improved function (Green & Nelham 1991).

Other attempts have been made to prevent the posterior tilt of the pelvis using a firm backrest and either a padded bar/belt acting on the sub ASIS (anterior superior iliac spine) or pre-ischial (anti-thrust) blocks acting on the ischial tuberosities (Trefler et al 1993). When employing the former method, because the vertical distance between the forces is small, a large force is required to keep the pelvis upright which, when applied to a relatively small area, can generate high pressure (Fig. 3.10). The latter method can apply the same moment with less force due to the longer moment arm, however, it can cause dangerous shear stresses and it is relatively easy for the pelvis to lift up and slip out of the blocks (Fig. 3.11).

Pelvic rotation and windswept hips

Attempts can be made to prevent pelvic rotation using the pre-ischial bars and sub ASIS bars mentioned above or alternatively using a Y-shaped belt that is designed to trap the ASIS (Trefler et al 1993).

The kneeblock-based system is particularly effective at opposing a tendency towards a wind-

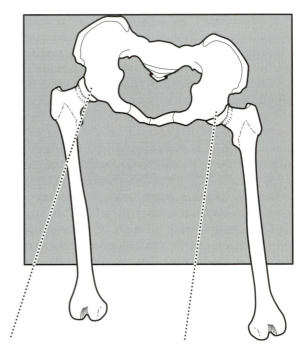

Figure 3.12   Windswept hips.

swept hip posture which will include an element of pelvic rotation (Fig. 3.12). If used properly (Fig. 3.13), the kneeblock should be adjusted so that a force is applied from anterior to posterior, via the abducted femur, to the pelvis on the side that is rotated anteriorly. This in conjunction with the reaction force from the sacral pad will

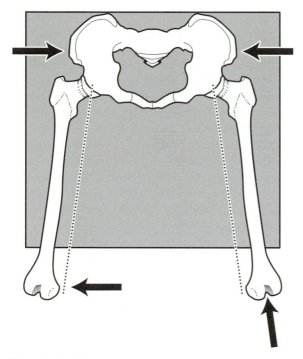

Figure 3.13 Correct use of kneeblock, sacral pad and lateral pelvic supports to oppose a windswept hip position.

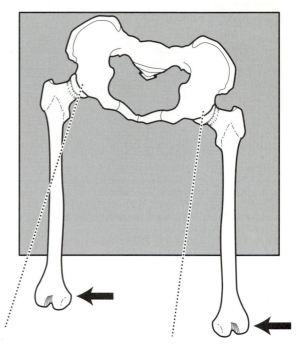

Figure 3.14 Incorrect use of kneeblock – aligning the femurs without correcting the pelvic rotation.

help to de-rotate the pelvis. A force from medial to lateral can then be applied to the medial aspect of the adducted hip in order to provide a turning moment about the hip joint, thus allowing it to be abducted to a neutral position. This should help to reduce the risk of subluxation/dislocation of the hip on the side that was previously adducted. A large support pad will allow the force to be spread over a large area reducing the pressure, and because of the relative length of the femur, a reasonable turning moment about the hip can be generated. Care should be taken to avoid a force from anterior to posterior being applied to a hip that is suspected of being dislocated or not fully covered by the acetabulum (Fearn et al 1992, Green & Nelham 1991). This can be achieved by leaving a small gap between the knee cup and knee on this side. In order to achieve static equilibrium and avoid the risk of the pelvis shifting to the side under the application of the above forces, it is also necessary to apply lateral support forces to the pelvis.

Kneeblocks of fixed shape can be useful when attempting to maintain a relatively normal posture; however, where it is necessary to tackle a windswept deformity it is important that the kneeblock is adjustable in order to achieve the above system of forces. Kneeblocks when used incorrectly may appear to straighten the femora but do not prevent the rotation of the pelvis which in turn may compromise the spine (Fig. 3.14).

Where the windswept hip deformity is so well established that correction is not tolerated, it is perhaps advisable to concentrate on correct pelvic alignment in relation to the trunk and allow the hips to deviate (Fig. 3.15). Attempts to correct the hip joint angles under these circumstances are likely to cause the pelvis to rotate.

Spinal deformity

Back support where there are no existing postural problems normally involves main-

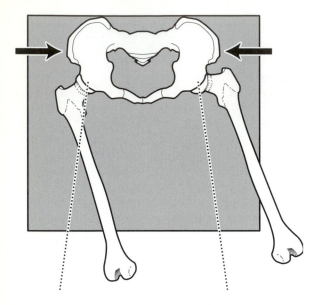

Figure 3.15 Positioning the pelvis and allowing the hips to deviate.

taining the existing physiological curvatures of the spine in the sagittal plane. Where the supporting musculature is weak, the use of lateral supports is often required to maintain a symmetrical alignment in the coronal plane. Supporting the spine becomes more complicated, however, where there are progressive deformities usually associated with a neuromuscular disorder.

Scoliosis

Before employing a biomechanical strategy for intervention it is worth considering the possible mechanism involved in generating a scoliosis. Although the exact causes of the initiation and development of a scoliosis are not fully understood, biomechanical analysis has helped to improve understanding of some of the various theories put forward.

Many believe that the mechanism of progression in scoliosis is due mainly to asymmetrical contraction strength of trunk muscle groups located bilaterally with respect to the vertebral column. Such muscle imbalances may be linked to retention of neonatal reflexes (e.g. asymmetrical tonic neck reflex and Galant response),

abnormal labyrinthine and righting reflexes or exaggerated stretch reflexes in individuals with cerebral palsy (Bernstein & Bernstein 1990). Intuitively it might be expected that the spine would be pulled to the stronger side; however, the concavity of a lateral curve of a paralytic scoliosis often lies to the weaker side of the back. Noone et al (1991) were able to simulate this phenomena using a simple model of the spine as a curved non-linear column to which muscle forces were applied. After an initial asymmetrical rectus abdominus contraction as the primary cause of the scoliosis, the model predicted a curve concave toward the stronger side. With a compensatory contraction from the psoas, perhaps as a reflex action to ensure that the centre of gravity of the upper body is maintained over the pelvic base, the model predicted a double curve with a significant curvature at lower thoracic and lumbar level in the opposite direction.

Several attempts have been made to investigate the development of scoliosis and to predict the forces necessary to cause buckling of the ligamentous spine using Euler buckling theory (Beltschko et al 1973, Crisco & Panjabi 1992, Lindbeck 1985, Lucas and Bresler 1961, Stokes & Gardner-Morse 1991). Stokes & Gardner-Morse (1991) calculated the forces necessary to produce a double curve scoliosis corresponding to a Cobb angle of 10 degrees in a model of a ligamentous spine. They noted that it was unlikely that any anatomical structures could generate forces of the magnitude predicted. It was concluded, therefore, that scoliosis deformity could not be explained purely in terms of forces acting on the spine and that full understanding of the causes of scoliosis would need to take into account other possible mechanisms, such as asymmetrical thoracic growth or asymmetrical vertebral development.

It is widely accepted that poor positioning and posture can contribute to the development of secondary deformities (Scrutton 1989) and that good positioning and posture is fundamental to the control of spasticity and effective management of severe disability (Pope 1992). For example, pelvic obliquity (or lateral pelvic tilt) and scoliotic posture are often observed secondary to a unilateral hip extension contracture (Carlson et al 1986). The hip extension contracture, if not accommodated, is likely to cause the pelvis to be raised on the side of the contracture. The pelvic obliquity may well in turn result in a compensatory scoliosis convex to the opposite side in order to maintain the head over the pelvic base.

Carlson et al (1986) emphasized the importance of maintaining the pelvis in a level and stable position from a biomechanical point of view. Using Euler theory applied to a simple model of the spine as an elastic beam, it can be shown that the beam will support almost twice as much load before buckling with the end 'built in' or constrained compared to the situation where the end of the beam behaves like a flexible joint. This infers that the spine should be able to support significantly more load when the pelvis is maintained in a stable position. If the pelvis

is free to tilt laterally and adopt an oblique position, as is more likely to happen on an unstable cushion or 'hammocking' seat canvas for example, the spine will buckle under lower loading (Carlson et al 1986).

Observations have also shown that axial rotation of the vertebra in the spine is linked to lateral deviation, with the spinous processes usually rotated towards the concavity of the scoliosis (Stokes & Gardner-Morse 1991). The magnitude of vertebral axial rotation correlates with the lateral deviation of vertebrae from the spinal axis and the rotation is greatest near the apex of the curve (Stokes et al 1988). Therefore, it would seem reasonable to suspect that, as well as pelvic obliquity, rotation of the pelvis may also contribute to the initiation and progression of a scoliosis.

Supporting a scoliosis. Figure 3.16A shows a very simplified representation of a posterior view of the head supported over a pelvis by

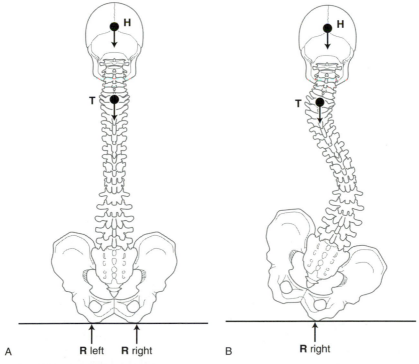

A **R** left **R** right

B **R** right

Figure 3.16 Head supported over the pelvis by the vertebral column (posterior view in coronal plane) with: (A) a straight spine and neutral pelvis; (B) an S-shaped scoliosis (convex to the right) and fixed pelvic obliquity (down on the right).

the vertebral column. For static equilibrium the combined weight of the head (H) and trunk including upper limbs (T) will equal the sum of reaction forces (R LEFT and R RIGHT) taken through the ischial tuberosities. Assuming symmetry the weight taken through each ischial tuberosity will be equal (i.e. R LEFT = R RIGHT).

Figure 3.16B shows a similar representation of a significantly scoliotic spine with the head balanced over an oblique pelvis. All the weight of H and T are now taken through the right ischial tuberosity. If R LEFT is reduced to zero then R RIGHT is likely to be doubled.

Assuming that the scoliosis is fixed, rather than flexible, then it will not be possible to regain a neutral position for the pelvis without throwing the trunk and head over to the left. Besides causing the individual to view the world at a strange angle, this will result in an unstable situation where the weight of the head and trunk fall outside the pelvic base to the left resulting in an unbalanced anti-clockwise turning moment about the left ischial tuberosity (Fig. 3.17).

In order to support the trunk and head in a

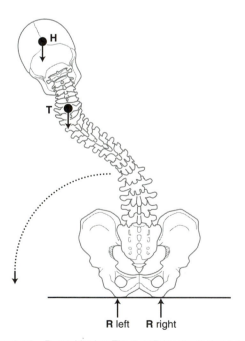

Figure 3.17 Repositioning Fig. 3.16B by displacing head and trunk to the left in order to achieve a level pelvis – static equilibrium is not achieved.

reasonably acceptable upright position, it will be necessary to oppose the turning moment which is causing the upper body to fall to the left. An obvious approach which is often employed is to provide lateral thoracic support on one side, in this case the left side (Fig. 3.18A). The use of a lateral thoracic support on only one side, however, does little to oppose the curvature of the spine and will result in a situation where the forces and turning moments are not balanced and hence static equilibrium is not achieved. In Figure 3.18A the effect of the weight of both the head (H) and trunk (T), reaction force (R RIGHT) and left thoracic support force (T LEFT) is an unbalanced force from left to right and/or a clockwise turning moment about the right ischial tuberosity. The clockwise turning moment is likely to result in a tendency for the trunk to fall to the right. The force from left to right will cause the pelvis to slip laterally, or if opposed by friction between the user and the seat will cause shearing of the skin tissue.

Figure 3.18B shows the use of bilateral thoracic supports. The left lateral thoracic support is preventing the trunk from falling to the left while the right lateral thoracic support is pushing on the convex side at the apex of the spinal curvature. However, in this situation, static equilibrium still has not been achieved. A turning moment exists as a result of the vertical separation between the two horizontal forces (R LEFT and R RIGHT) which are acting in opposing directions. The turning moment is attempting to rotate the trunk in a clockwise direction.

At least three points of support are necessary for stability and static equilibrium. Figure 3.18C shows how the addition of a lateral pelvic support on the left side allows the horizontal and vertical forces as well as the clockwise and anti-clockwise turning moments to be balanced. This type of three-point loading is more effective at opposing the deterioration of the lateral curvature of the spine.

The effect of gravity on head, upper limbs and trunk produces a downward force which is transmitted through the spine. With an opposing reaction force generated at the pelvis the spine is under compression and there may be a buckling

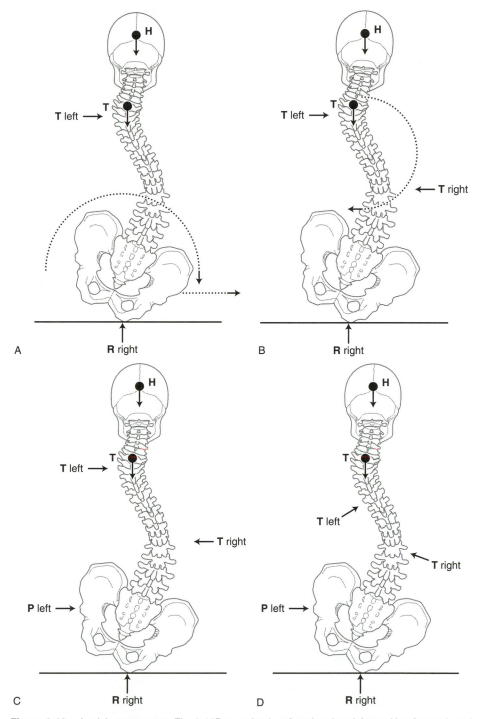

Figure 3.18 Applying support to Fig. 3.16B to maintain a functional upright position for trunk and head. (A) Use of left lateral thoracic support – static equilibrium not achieved. (B) Use of right and left lateral thoracic support – static equilibrium still not achieved. (C) Use of three-point force system (left lateral pelvic support in addition to right and left lateral thoracic support) – static equilibrium is now achieved. (D) Effectiveness of three-point force system improved by angling the support surfaces.

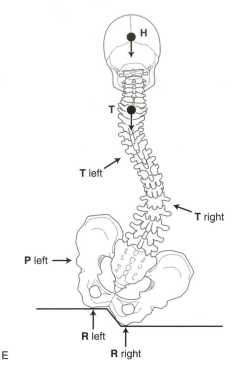

E

Figure 3.18   Applying support to Fig. 3.16B to maintain a functional upright position for trunk and head. (E) Seat raised under left ischial tuberosity in order to achieve better distribution of load and reduce pressure under right ischial tuberosity.

below the apex of the curve on the convex side of the spine, thus lifting the spine away from the anterior superior iliac spine of the pelvis on this side. The opposing supportive force should also be angled upward slightly to help support the weight of the upper body (Fig. 3.18D).

In Figure 3.18E it can be seen that due to the fixed pelvic obliquity the weight of the user is still being taken on the right side, resulting in increased pressure under the right ischial tuberosity. Building up under the left ischial tuberosity will help to balance the loading taken through each of the ischial tuberosities and will help to achieve a more even distribution of pressure.

If the pelvic obliquity is flexible, as opposed to being fixed, it may be possible to apply the supportive forces described above while maintaining the pelvis in a neutral position, i.e. without any obliquity (Fig. 3.19). Alternatively some clinicians attempt to build up under the side of the pelvis which is lower, in order to counteract a flexible pelvic obliquity. If this is attempted, care should be taken to monitor the

effect. The straighter the spine the more efficient it is at supporting the weight. Also, with the spine straighter, the vertical separation between the pelvic and thoracic support pads is increased, thus increasing the moment arm of the lateral forces applied to the trunk. The greater the moment arm the less the force required to provide the same corrective moment. Conversely, for a significant scoliosis the lateral supports will have less vertical separation, reducing the moment arm and necessitating a larger force to maintain the same corrective moment (Trefler et al 1993).

The uneven pressure distribution caused by a support surface that does not conform to the surface anatomy is likely to cause discomfort and could also cause tissue trauma. When supporting the spine the support forces are more effective if they are applied along the line of the ribs to the spine. Ideally, therefore, the lateral thoracic supports should be angled to push in and up just

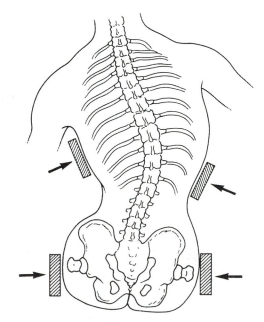

Figure 3.19   Application of system of forces to support the trunk and spine and maintain a neutral pelvis in the case where the pelvic obliquity is flexible (M'Carthy 1992, with permission).

effects of the interface pressure acting on the ischial tuberosity on the side of the build up.

Tilting the seat posteriorly while maintaining the hips near to 90 degrees may help to reduce the buckling effect caused by gravity acting on the upper body by allowing a component of this weight to be taken through the backrest (Pope et al 1988, Trefler & Taylor 1991). The advantages of tilting, however, should be weighed against the potential loss of functional ability that can be caused (Bardsley 1993).

Kyphosis and lordosis

Tight hamstrings are one of the major factors in causing a kyphosis. Tension in the hamstrings causes the pelvis to tilt posteriorly, resulting in loss of lumbar lordosis and increased kyphosis (Bernstein & Bernstein 1990). This can be exacerbated by attempts to extend the knee in order to position the feet on the wheelchair footrests.

An alternative cause may be the presence of pathological reflexes such as the retention of neonatal reflexes and abnormal labyrinthine reflexes (Bernstein & Bernstein 1990).

Supporting a kyphosis. Achieving and maintaining an upright pelvis (discussed earlier in this chapter) is an important step in deterring the development of a kyphosis.

Theoretically a three-point loading system, involving forces acting from anterior to posterior at the pelvis and at the shoulders, in addition to a posterior to anterior force acting at the apex of the kyphotic spine, would be required to oppose an established but flexible kyphosis. It is difficult, however, to achieve such a loading in a way that is both practical and comfortable using conventional seating. In practice this type of loading is commonly attempted using a pelvic restraint in conjunction with a custom contoured backrest and anterior support (often either a harness or pad). As discussed above in the section on scoliosis, the effects of gravity acting on the upper body and subjecting the spine to compressive loading can be reduced slightly if the complete seat is tilted posteriorly (Pope et al 1988, Trefler & Taylor 1991).

An alternative approach aimed at providing support and stability for the spine is to anteriorly tilt the user while providing anterior chest support and also support for the upper limbs. Pope et al (1988) described seating that brings the user's trunk forward over an anteriorly tilted saddle type seat in conjunction with a custom contoured chest support, handle bar and foot support which are all mounted on a mobile platform.

Although there is no doubt that seating has an important role in the management of spinal deformity, it is often necessary to use it in conjunction with other forms of biomechanical intervention, for example the use of an orthosis or even fixation of the spine through surgery.

The aetiology and management of a scoliosis and kyphosis are also covered in Chapter 8.

Encouraging lumbar curvature

A lumbar support is often used to try to encourage a lumbar lordosis. Ideally the lumbar pad should not be used on its own to attempt to enforce a lumbar lordosis where the pelvis is posteriorly tilted, as this is likely to impose a large shear force on the lumbar vertebrae and specifically the vulnerable L5/S1 joint (Bardsley 1993, Green & Nelham 1991).

Care should also be taken in using a lumbar support with a young child who has an immature posture and hence an underdeveloped lordosis. In this situation it is likely that the lumbar support will result in the child being pushed into a flexed position or pushed anteriorly in the seat and it is possible that the child will use the lumbar support to extend against (Green & Nelham 1991). A better way of achieving the desired spinal curvature is to apply the force directly to the pelvis, as discussed above in the section on pelvic tilt.

CONCLUSION

An understanding of biomechanics is essential when providing postural support. It is not sufficient just to know what piece of equipment should be used for a particular problem, as appropriate equipment can easily be used inappropriately resulting in the original problem being compounded or shifted to another area. Instead it is essential that careful thought is given to the cause of the problem and the biomechanical application of any supportive forces.

It should be remembered that realistically the forces acting on a body at any one time are complex. It is tempting to regard the body as a simplistic passive mechanical structure made up of a number of segments which react when subjected to gravity, muscle action, tension in passive tissues and intracavity pressures. The neurophysiological response of the body to any intervention is a complex matter that is far less easy to predict. Therefore, although it may help understanding to regard a part of the body, such as the spine, as a simplistic model, it is dangerous to forget the simplifying assumptions made when forming a conclusion or instigating a particular course of intervention.

REFERENCES

Bardsley G 1993 Seating. In: Bowker P, Condie D N, Bader D L, Pratt D J (eds) Biomechanical basis of orthotic management. Butterworth Heinemann, Oxford, ch 14, pp 253–280

Belytschko T, Andriacchi T, Schultz A, Galante J 1973 Analog studies of forces in the human spine: computational techniques. Journal of Biomechanics 6: 361–372

Bernstein S M, Bernstein L 1990 Spinal deformity in the patient with cerebral palsy. Spine: state of the art reviews 14(1): 147–160

Bowker P 1993 An update in essential mechanics. In: Bowker P, Condie D N, Bader D L, Pratt D J (eds) Biomechanical basis of orthotic management. Butterworth Heinemann, Oxford, ch 2, pp 5–26

Brubaker C E 1990 Ergonometric considerations. Journal of Rehabilitation Research and Development (Clinical Supplement 2): 37–48

Brubaker C E 1986 Wheelchair prescription: an analysis of factors that affect mobility and performance. Journal of Rehabilitation Research and Development 23(4): 19–25

Brubaker C E, McLaurin C A, McClay I S 1985 Effects of sideslope of wheelchair performance. In: Proceedings of the 8th Annual Conference on Rehabilitation Technology, vol 5, pp 81–85

Carlson J M, Lonstein J, Beck K O, Wilkie D C 1986 Seating for children and young adults with cerebral palsy. Clinical Prosthetics and Orthotics 10(4): 137–158

Crisco J J, Panjabi M M 1992 Euler stability of the human ligamentous lumbar spine. Part 1: Theory. Clinical Biomechanics 7: 19–26

Disabled Living Foundation 1993 Adult manual wheelchairs. In: Wheelchair information. Disabled Living Foundation, London, pp 13–44

Fearn T A, Green E M, Jones M, Mulcahy C M, Nelham R L, Pountney T E 1992 Postural management. In: McCarthy G T (ed) Physical disability in childhood. An interdisciplinary approach to management. Churchill Livingstone, Edinburgh, ch 25, pp 401–450

Green E M, Nelham R L 1991 Development of sitting ability, assessment of children with a motor handicap and prescription of appropriate seating systems. Prosthetics and Orthotics International 15(3): 203–216

Henderson E (ed) 1989 Biomechanical considerations in seating the disabled. In: Seating in review – current trends for the disabled. Otto Bock Orthopaedic Industry of Canada Ltd, Winnipeg, MB, pp 10–19

Lindbeck L 1985 Analysis of functional scoliosis by means of an anisotropic beam model of the human spine. Journal of Biomechanical Engineering 107: 281–285

Lucas D B, Bresler B 1961 Stability of the ligamentous spine. Technical report esr. 11 No 40. Biomechanics Laboratory, University of California, San Francisco

Major R E 1990 Some aspects of wheel geometry relating to manually propelled wheelchairs. Physiotherapy 76(10): 663–665

M'Carthy (ed) 1992 Physical disability in childhood – an interdisciplinary approach to management. Churchill Livingstone, Edinburgh, p 433

McLaurin C A, Brubaker C E 1991 Biomechanics and the wheelchair. Prosthetics and Orthotics International 15: 24–37

Mulcahy C M, Pountney T E 1986 The sacral pad – description of its clinical use in seating. Physiotherapy 72(9): 473–474

Mulcahy C M, Pountney T E 1987 Ramped cushion. British Journal of Occupational Therapy 50(3): 97

Noone G P, Mazumdar J, Ghista D N 1991 Developmental and corrective biomechanics for scoliosis. IEEE Engineering in Medicine and Biology 1991 June: 37–41

Perks B, Mackintosh R, Stewart C P U, Bardsley G 1994 A survey of marginal wheelchair users. Journal of Rehabilitation Research and Development 31(4): 297–302

Pope P M 1992 Management of physical condition in patients with chronic and severe neurological pathologies. Physiotherapy 78(12): 896–903

Pope P M, Booth E, Gosling G 1988 The development of alternative seating and mobility systems. Physiotherapy Practice 4: 78–93

Scrutton D 1989 The early management of hips in cerebral palsy. Developmental Medicine and Child Neurology 31: 108–116

Stewart P C, McQuilton G 1987 Straddle seating for the cerebral palsied child. British Journal of Occupational Therapy 50(4): 136–138; and Physiotherapy 73(4): 204–206

Stokes I A F, Armstrong J G, Moreland M S 1988 Spinal deformity and back surface asymmetry in idiopathic scoliosis. Journal of Orthopaedic Research 6: 129–137

Stokes I A F, Gardner-Morse M 1991 Analysis of the interaction between vertebral lateral deviation and axial rotation in scoliosis. Journal of Biomechanics 24(8): 753–759

Trefler E, Taylor S J 1991 Prescription and positioning: evaluating the physically disabled individual for wheelchair seating. Prosthetics and Orthotics International 15: 217–224

Trefler E, Hobson D A, Taylor, Nonahan L C, Shaw C G 1993 Biomechanics. In: Trefler E, Hobson D A, Taylor, Nonahan L C, Shaw C G (eds) Seating & mobility.

Therapy Skills Builders, University of Tennessee, Memphis, pp 45–64

Veeger D H E J, Van der Woude L H V, Rozendahl R H 1989 The effect of rear wheel camber in manual wheelchair propulsion. Journal of Rehabilitation Research and Development 53(3): 37–46

Zacharkow D 1988 Posture, sitting, standing, chair design and exercise. Thomas, Illinois

4

Clinical features affecting wheelchair users with postural problems

INTRODUCTION

Many of the clinical factors that need to be considered during assessment of posture and mobility are common to a number of disorders. In some cases these features may be present but unattached to a specific diagnosis, possibly as the cause has not been identified or indeed secondary to another problem including the side effects of medication which can result in movement disorders; for example, dyskinesia, associated with the drug levadopa prescribed for Parkinson's disease.

Assessment of posture and advice on correct positioning with or without equipment should be based on sound knowledge of normal movement patterns and joint range (see Ch. 2), together with an understanding of the cause and effect of abnormal patterns. Anyone responsible for positioning a disabled person needs to be aware of the factors affecting optimal development and stressors on the musculoskeletal system (Burgman 1994). Incorrect positioning can result in the development of spinal asymmetries and increase loading of spinal structures (Jenkins 1991), with additional damage to tissue.

This chapter looks at general anatomical and neurological classifications as well as the terminology used in describing postural ability and problems that are common to wheelchair users of all ages.

Neurological disorders can be classified either according to the area of the body affected by the lesion, i.e. anatomical classification, or according

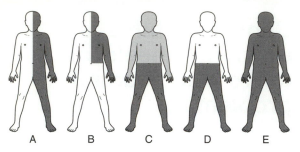

Figure 4.1 Anatomical classification: (A) hemiplegia; (B) monoplegia; (C) diplegia (D) paraplegia; (E) quadraplegia.

to the movement demonstrated, i.e. neurological classification.

ANATOMICAL CLASSIFICATION (Fig. 4.1)

Hemiplegia

This is paralysis or weakness of one side of the body. Where there is less involvement of either an upper or lower limb this can be described as monoplegia.

Diplegia

When paralysis or weakness affects the whole body but the lower part of the body, including the pelvis and lower limbs, is more noticeably weakened than the upper part of the body, this is termed diplegia. Where the upper limbs are minimally or indeed not involved, the condition is then described as paraplegia.

Paraplegia

In this condition paralysis is confined to the abdomen and both lower limbs. The level of the lesion in the spinal cord will determine the severity and areas affected (Fig. 4.2).

Quadraplegia or tetraplegia

These terms describe partial or complete paralysis with involvement of the head, neck and all four limbs. With spastic quadraplegia, the lower

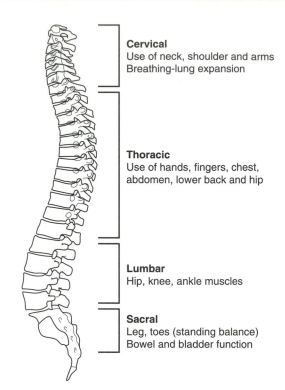

Figure 4.2 Diagram indicating areas of the body affected in relation to a lesion of the spinal cord with damage to the spinal nerves.

limbs are generally more involved than the upper limbs.

NEUROLOGICAL CLASSIFICATION

Muscle tone

Muscle tone refers to the force with which a muscle resists being lengthened (Gordon & Ghez 1991). It has been defined as resistance to passive elongation or stretch (Harris 1991). Normal tone in a muscle will assist in maintaining posture and enabling function. Abnormal tone is the result of damage to or destruction of the nerve cells either in the brain or spinal cord. The severity and degree of interference with tone is determined by the site and extent of a lesion (Fig. 4.3). Spasticity, dyskinesia which includes athetosis, chorea and ataxia are terms used to describe the effects of disturbance to different areas of the nervous system which interfere with muscle tone and reflexes.

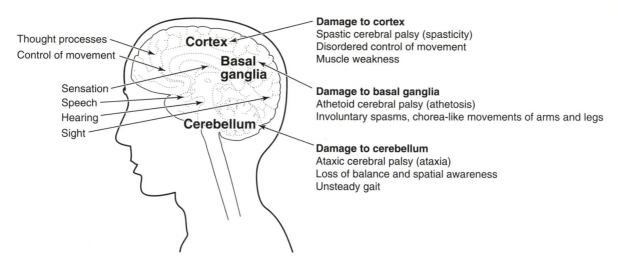

Thought processes
Control of movement
Sensation
Speech
Hearing
Sight

Cortex
Basal ganglia
Cerebellum

Damage to cortex
Spastic cerebral palsy (spasticity)
Disordered control of movement
Muscle weakness

Damage to basal ganglia
Athetoid cerebral palsy (athetosis)
Involuntary spasms, chorea-like movements of arms and legs

Damage to cerebellum
Ataxic cerebral palsy (ataxia)
Loss of balance and spatial awareness
Unsteady gait

Figure 4.3 Diagram of the brain showing the effects of damage on the three main areas (adapted from SCOPE information leaflet, with permission).

Spasticity

Spasm or spasticity is a state of increased tension (hypertonia) or contraction of the muscles. Spasticity is due to damage of the cerebral motor cortex and is responsible for the most common type of cerebral palsy. It is said to be present in 60% of people with this disorder (Haskell & Barrett 1989). It is also seen in many other neurological disorders such as multiple sclerosis and spinal cord injury (see Ch. 7) where there is damage to the nerve cells in either the brain or spinal cord. Spasticity is characterized by increased tendon jerks with an increase in muscle tone and deep tendon reflexes, particularly in the flexors in the arms and extensors in the legs. Increased muscle tone, with an imbalance between the agonist and antagonist muscle groups, can increase the risk of scoliosis and rotation of spinal segments (Tredwell & Roxburgh 1991). Muscle shortening is also associated with the development of spasticity and can eventually lead to contractures, which in turn increase spasticity (Nash, Neilson & O'Dwyer 1989). A range of therapies are available for dealing with spasticity. These include physiotherapy, orthotics, plaster immobilization, tendon releases and bone surgery, selective dorsal rhizotomy, the use of drugs (most commonly baclofen),

botulinum injections and nerve blocks. In recent studies on the loading and unloading of muscles (Lin, Brown & Walsh 1994), it was found that muscle unloading resulted in fast twitchy muscle and increased reflex excitability and clonus, thus indicating the inappropriate use of some of the above methods of treatment. On the other hand, muscle loading was shown to produce the opposite effect and found to be 'antispastic', reducing clonus whilst also slowing the speed of muscle relaxation. The authors of this work concluded that strengthening and slowing muscle action is essentially antispastic.

Preserving muscle length and maintaining joint range is commonly achieved through one of three methods (Green, Mulcahy & Pountney 1992), which are:

● passive movement
● stretching
● long-term positioning.

On the whole, methods used for treating spasticity tend to be selected on a trial and error basis and involve a number of different approaches. Those carrying out treatment need to establish a suitable means of recording the method(s) used and measuring progress to ensure that there is long-term benefit to the recipient.

Dyskinesia

This term refers to abnormal or impaired movement and is used to describe a group of involuntary movements that include athetosis and chorea, both of which are caused by damage to the basal ganglia.

Athetosis

This term describes frequent involuntary movements caused by fluctuation and constant alternating between very high and very low muscle tone. This results in slow or fast movements; jerky or writhing responses or unpatterned movements, all of which interfere with normal body activities. The constant change in muscle tone upsets postural balance and stability but rarely results in any postural deformity. These uncontrollable and sudden movements can cause extreme frustration, particularly when speech is affected. Athetoid movements are increased by excitement and also effort when trying to make a voluntary movement. Factors that decrease athetosis are fatigue, fever, lying prone or intense concentration (Levitt 1982). Supportive seating that provides stability by securing the pelvis in a good position whilst allowing freedom of upper limb movement can help to reduce the effects that athetoid movements will have on function. Even though postural patterns may be abnormal they can also be used in a positive manner and help maintain independent function. Careful assessment and discussion with the individual concerned will establish the degree of compromise that needs to be made in order to obtain the balance between function, independence and acceptable posture. Early intervention and advice can prevent development of bad habits and later problems.

Chorea

Strong disorganized movement that may be present on its own or may be accompanied by athetoid movements is known as chorea. When both the writhing and jerky involuntary movements are present together, these are termed 'chorea athetosis' and are typically seen in Huntington's chorea (see Ch. 7). Chorea-like movements are wide ranging, uncontrolled and tend to affect the shoulders, hips and face, making it extremely difficult to position the person, particularly in a wheelchair. Deep and angled armchairs, such as the Kirton HD armchair (Fig. 4.4), designed specifically for people with Huntington's chorea, the Symmetrikit and others with similar design and soft padded surfaces, are the most appropriate for providing comfort and preventing injury to anyone with gross chorea-like movements. Dyskinesia can also be observed as one of the more common side effects found in people taking levodopa in the treatment of parkinsonism (McLellan 1988).

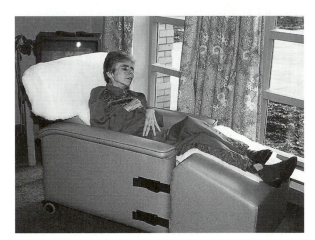

Figure 4.4   Selection of an appropriate armchair is essential for both comfort and correct positioning. The Kirton HD armchair is designed specifically for people with gross chorea-type movement such as those with Huntington's chorea who, in the later stages of their illness, are at risk when seated in a wheelchair (photograph courtesy of Kirton Healthcare).

Ataxia

Damage to the cerebellum results in ataxia which is characterized by poor coordination, sudden excessive and inaccurate movements with unreliable reactions to any loss of balance and an unsteady gait. Ataxia can be associated with athetosis or spasticity. The child with ataxic cerebral palsy is said to have a three times higher incidence of scoliosis than the child with spastic diplegia or hemiplegia cerebral palsy. The majority of children in this group with scoliosis have a right thoracic curve (Bleck 1987).

Hypotonia

When muscle tone is reduced, hypotonia, there is an inability to counteract the force of gravity resulting in a floppy posture often associated with lack of postural reactions in children with cerebral palsy (Levitt 1982). Decreased muscle tone can result in development of a kyphosis or lordosis (Letts 1991) with increased hip flexion or, alternatively, deformities such as scoliosis, hyperextended knees as well as valgus knees and feet (Levitt 1982). In muscular dystrophy (see Ch. 7) progressive weakness of the spinal muscles is aggravated by the downward force of gravity, resulting in spinal collapse leading to kyphosis and scoliosis. There is also likelihood of the development of contractures in the lower limbs due to muscle imbalance between agonist and antagonist muscle groups (Hsu 1990). For people with hypotonic spinal muscles who need to sit in a wheelchair all day, spinal collapse is hastened as the musculature supporting the spine is unable to counteract the burden of gravity. When there is rapid collapse of the spine, fitting a spinal jacket is also contraindicated as this has been shown to restrict chest movement and adversely affect respiration. In these cases, pain and discomfort make sitting in the upright position intolerable. Tilting a wheelchair (Fig. 4.5) will reduce downward pressure from gravity but limits upper limb function and consequently restricts independence which is important to retain, however limited. Provision of a shaped tray which supports under the forearms at a comfortable height, can be used as forward support for short periods of relaxation during the day and also help to maintain a straight spine. Improvements in modern powered wheelchairs, some of which now have a user-operated tilt and recline, will have noticeable benefits for people needing to reduce downward pressure on the spine whilst maintaining independence. When treating or caring for anyone with hypotonic muscles, care must be taken not to overstretch the joint tissues or damage joint surfaces (Green, Mulcahy & Pountney 1992).

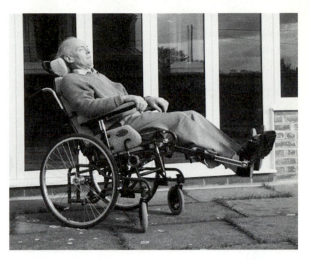

Figure 4.5 Tilting a wheelchair reduces downward pressure on a collapsing spine but reduces upper limb function and eye contact.

It is important to determine whether a person is hypotonic, hypertonic, athetoid, spastic, ataxic or has a mixture of tonal disturbance. A person who is diagnosed as having spastic quadraplegia can demonstrate hypertonic extremities with hypotonic trunk muscles (Johnson Taylor 1997). It is also important to decide which deformities are correctable and which are fixed and therefore require accommodating. The aim with seating and mobility should always be to minimize the effects of abnormal tone and reflexes, to accommodate or delay development or progression of orthopaedic deformities and to increase functional skills whilst providing comfort and ease of care. This on its own is a major challenge, even before other factors such as environmental issues and user preferences have been addressed.

PRIMITIVE REFLEXES

Evaluating tone will involve assessment of the presence of primitive postural reflexes and will focus on their effect on function when prescribing seating. Failure to recognize the presence of a primitive reflex can create difficulties for an individual as incorrect positioning may aggravate the situation, whereas correct positioning can reduce the impact of certain reflex patterns. Four commonly observed primitive reflexes are outlined below. These are discussed in more detail in Chapter 2.

Asymmetrical tonic neck reflex (ATNR)

In this reflex there is increased extensor tone on the side of the body toward which the head is turned, with increased flexor tone on the opposite side. Imbalance in tone can result in spinal deformity if not carefully monitored.

Symmetrical tonic neck reflexes (STNR)

When the neck is flexed the upper limbs flex and the lower limbs extend, whilst the reverse happens when the neck is extended. The position of the head is important if both these responses are to be controlled.

The tonic labyrinthine reflex

This reflex occurs when the person experiences increased extension when placed in the supine position, whilst there is an increase in flexor tone when placed in the prone position. In the upright sitting position, the head should be maintained in neutral to reduce this response. The effect of this should be borne in mind if a tilting or reclining facility is built into a seating system.

The positive supporting reaction

This reaction occurs when the balls of the feet are placed either on the floor or on a footplate, resulting in a strong extensor thrust which is capable of jerking the individual out of their wheelchair. There are differing views on the positioning, and indeed the role, of a footboard for someone who demonstrates a positive supporting reflex. Placing the feet in dorsiflexion may reduce this response, or in some cases it is considered appropriate to remove all foot support, though care must be taken not to place pressure under the thighs.

CLASSIFICATIONS OF SITTING ABILITY

Although there are no universally agreed definitions relating to sitting ability, attempts have been made to define the degrees of postural ability and also to identify levels of sitting, standing and lying ability. The descriptions commonly used are listed below and, in the absence of agreed definitions, can be used as a basis for recording changes measured and observed when assessing and prescribing postural support and seating. Further information on measurement techniques for joint range and functional ability are referred to in Chapters 2 and 6.

Levels of postural and functional ability

Work carried out over a period of years at Chailey Heritage, a centre in England for children with physical disabilities, resulted in the publication of levels of postural ability linked to stages of normal development in children (see Appendix 1). The study demonstrated that there is a recognized sequence of development whereby one level of postural ability cannot be achieved until a lower level is reached. For example, it was found that it was not possible for any child to sit independently (level 3 on the Chailey scale) until at least level 4 lying ability had been achieved (Green, Mulcahy & Pountney 1992). These levels of ability are of value when working with children who have developmental delay affecting their postural ability. It also enables the therapist to understand the normal pattern of development of postural skills and realistically plan and measure progress for each individual. It should be remembered that the levels of ability identified by Chailey were established for child development and are not therefore necessarily appropriate for use with adults who have acquired postural deficits though they can be adapted to suit this purpose. This has been demonstrated by Pope (1996) who, whilst finding the seating levels useful to measure postural competence, has extended the chart to include quality of posture (Table 4.1).

Table 4.1 Physical ability scale – measurement of quality and quantity. (Adapted from Pope 1996; based upon Mulcahy et al 1988)

	Quantity	Quality
Level 1	Unplaceable in sitting	Trunk symmetrical
Level 2	Placeable with support	Head midline
Level 3	Can balance not move	Arms resting by side
Level 4	Can move forwards within base, cannot reach sideways	Knees mid-position
Level 5	Can sit independently, move arms freely and reach sideways	Feet flat on floor
Level 6	Can transfer across surface, cannot gain sitting position	Weight evenly distributed
Level 7	Can move into and out of sitting position	Score number of ticks

Box 4.1 Classification of sitting ability. (Based on Otto Bock (1989) and Bar (1992))

Hands free sitter	Able to sit without additional support. Generally independent mobility in wheelchair
Hands dependent sitter	Require trunk support to free hands for function. Modular seating systems providing a stable base, pelvic and thoracic support are generally suitable
Propped sitter	Sitting is impossible without custom-made support to provide close body contact over a large area to accommodate deformities

Other definitions which have been found to be useful classify either according to postural stability or general ability and level of support required. Those given in Boxes 4.1 and 4.2 are used by some centres and have been taken from several sources.

Propelling ability

As with sitting ability there are no recognized levels of propelling ability, though it is useful to have some form of classification to identify the needs of each individual. Guidelines produced for purchasers and providers of NHS wheelchair services were published in a report following a project on the national wheelchair service in England (Department of Health 1996). These provided definitions of users based on ability and are summarized in Table 4.2.

The types of wheelchair users seen in everyday life are many and varied and consequently people do not fall easily into a particular category. Terminology can be misleading even between professionals and over the years there has been constant discussion regarding the terms occasional user, casual user or social user. The former term indicates that a wheelchair is not used on a regular basis, whereas the latter signifies that the wheelchair enables someone to go out and about visiting friends or shopping. In either case, this group tend to be treated as non-essential and low-priority users. The term marginal user has been adopted to identify those who are part-time users due to a fluctuating condition such as multiple sclerosis, where a

Box 4.2 Classification based on support and level of disability. (Based on British Society of Rehabilitation Medicine (1995) and Department of Health (1996))

Minimum support Mild disability	Good head control. Good to fair trunk control. May be unstable when sitting unsupported. Good functional ability when seated on stable base with minimum support
Medium support Moderate disability	Variable head control. Poor trunk control. Requires support to maintain stable position. Limited hand function. Modular system supporting hip and trunk with adjustability to meet changing needs
Maximum support Severe disability	Poor head and trunk control. Unable to sit without support. Limited upper limb function. Possibly spinal curvature and joint contractures. Custom-made seating required to provide maximum support

Table 4.2 Definition of wheelchair users. (Adapted from Department of Health 1996 with permission)

Wheelchair user	Description
Full-time user	
High activity	Independent mobility and life style. Self propelling
Restricted activity	Independent mobility with powered wheelchair. Degree of daily living independence
Low activity	Limited independence for all daily living activities and mobility. Limited ability to self propel
Part-time user (long term)	
Marginal user	Fluctuating condition. Generally independent mobility and life style
Occasional user	Regular part-time need. Independent walking short distance and semi-independent life style
Part-time user (short term)	
Temporary need	Loss of independence in mobility for limited period due to illness, operation or accident

wheelchair is essential if they are to continue to lead a normal life at times when their condition deteriorates, or to conserve energy for essential daily activities. Although there is some consensus on these terms they are neither nationally nor universally recognized at present but they are an attempt to move away from describing users according to the type of wheelchair used and to focus on individual need or ability and level of independence.

COMMON POSTURAL PROBLEMS

Pelvic misalignments

Good positioning depends predominantly on the stability and positioning of the pelvis. As the lumbar spine articulates directly with the sacrum, asymmetry of the pelvis, whether in the sagittal or coronal plane, directly affects the level of activity of the trunk musculature (Hobson & Tooms 1992). Any attempts to maintain a level pelvis must always consider the resulting affect on the spine and the comfort of the individual. Attempts to contain the pelvis may exacerbate spinal asymmetries through compensation whilst compromising joint structures and ligaments when there are fixed deformities. In a well-balanced sitting position, the pelvis balances on the ischial tuberosities and weight is evenly distributed under the thighs. This stability is maintained by the activity of the muscles of the hip and trunk. The degree of muscle activity

required to maintain the upright posture can be reduced if external pelvic support is provided. If adequate support is not provided, a wheelchair user will find ways to stabilize themselves (Zacharkow 1988). Change of position when sitting will move the centre of gravity anteriorly or posteriorly from the ischial tuberosities (Bardsley 1993). Also, when there is some form of deficit in the area of the hip due to subluxation, dislocation, amputation or other intervention, maintaining a level and balanced pelvis may not be a realistic option and it may be necessary to accept a degree of lateral tilt where the ischial crest on one side lies lower than on the other. This is frequently associated with windswept hips (Fig. 4.6), a term used when a person presents with an asymmetrical deformity associated with pelvic obliquity and scoliosis where the legs fall to one side when sitting or lying. As the windswept deformity develops, the hip joints and structures around the hip joints and pelvis adapt to accommodate the preferred position (Goldsmith et al 1992). The pelvis rotates in the transverse plane, posteriorly to the windward side and anteriorly to the leeward side. This is associated with rotation and scoliosis of the spine. This problem is commonly seen in children with cerebral palsy but also in adults with neurological lesions, in particular those with multiple sclerosis and also Alzheimer's disease, when no attention has been paid to correct positioning in all postures and, in particular, lying in bed. Side lying during the night with

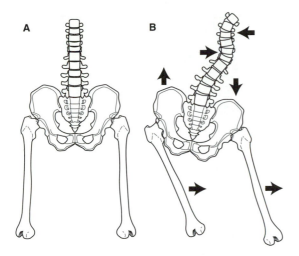

Figure 4.6 Diagram showing the position of the pelvis and spine in the development of windswept hips. (A) Before deformity develops. (B) Windswept position: the arrows indicate direction of change.

the hips and knees in a flexed position is one of the common factors contributing to deformity and windsweeping of the hips. Absence of adequate support under the femora when sitting in a wheelchair, for example when the footplates are too high, will also increase windsweeping.

Restriction in flexion at the hip joint may be due to one of many causes, including disarticulation, joint pain and stiffness or shortening of the hamstrings. Inability to achieve 90 degrees hip flexion will need to be accommodated by opening the back to seat angle when sitting. If the seat is kept in the horizontal position whilst reclining the backrest, the pelvis will rotate posteriorly, causing the sitter to sacrally sit and slide forward in the chair. Ramping the seat whilst using a pelvic strap will help to overcome the forward slide and secure the pelvis, providing the correct angle is achieved between the backrest and the seat. There can, however, be other factors that need to be considered as an additional seat ramp and tilt can interfere with functional activities and independence such as standing to transfer or using a urine bottle and can also cause backflow in a catheter tube. Emphasis on maintenance of postural symmetry and correction of asymmetry is essential if defor-

mity is to be delayed or controlled. Failure to address this at an early stage can create long-term problems for both the health and care of an individual. Crossing the legs at the knees when sitting is a commonly observed posture adopted by able as well as disabled people and is a method used to balance the body in the absence of adequate external support. In someone with a neurological deficiency, tightness of the hip adductors will encourage this position, but in the long term this can result in major problems and make a person unseatable if left uncorrected (Fig. 4.7). Whilst the use of a kneeblock may be acceptable in correcting this posture and maintaining alignment at the hip joint with a child whose deformity is still correctable (see Ch. 3 and Ch. 9), it is rarely suitable with an adult when an abductor pad or Putney leg dividers may be more acceptable though provide a less positive point of fixation and lower limb alignment.

Spinal deformities (see Ch. 3)

Spinal deformities are generally due to muscle imbalance. Descriptions of these deformities follow.

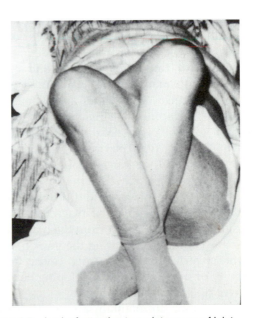

Figure 4.7 Lack of attention to maintenance of joint alignment can result in fixed deformities which make the person unseatable and cause major care and hygiene problems, as seen with this lady with multiple sclerosis.

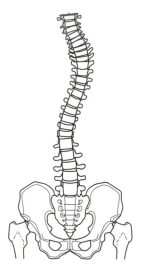

Figure 4.8 Diagram of spinal deformity showing scoliosis (anterior view).

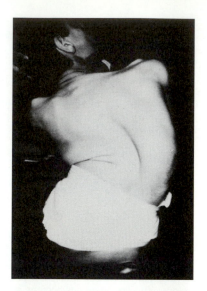

A

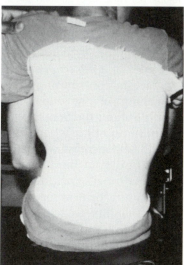

B

Figure 4.9 (A) Lack of sitting balance due to marked pelvic obliquity with rotation of the spine and scoliosis. (B) Correction of scoliosis with a well fitting spinal jacket can improve sitting balance.

Scoliosis (Fig. 4.8)

This is a lateral curvature commonly involving the lumbar and thoracic area of the spine. Scoliosis can be either postural with no fixed deformity usually secondary to a condition outside the spine such as a short leg, or structural where there is muscular imbalance with additional abnormalities of the vertebrae and ribs. In the latter case a secondary curve may develop to compensate for the primary curve and consequently help to maintain the head in a central position. Structural scoliosis is associated with rotation of the spine. As the vertebral bodies rotate, the spinous processes deviate towards the concavity of the curve. The ribs on the concentric side are crowded together and pushed forward resulting in a rib hump. In time the lower edge of the rib cage twists forwards and down, coming into close proximity with the iliac crest on the same side (Fig. 4.9A). Apart from the major difficulties this causes with seating the person, there is severe restriction in the lung cavity and a possibility of pressure sores developing between the lower rib cage and iliac crest.

Early attention to maintain a correct position at all times can reduce or delay the problems resulting from a severe scoliosis. Apart from providing suitable seating and postural support, fitting a spinal jacket (Fig. 4.9B) may be an alternative option in some cases, though it is unlikely to be effective if the spinal curvature is over 40 degrees as measured on X-ray (Cobb's angle). Spinal surgery may also be an option that should be carefully discussed with all concerned. As surgery carries certain risks, particularly when respiration is restricted, a thorough presurgery assessment will be carried out by the surgeon.

Whilst keeping the spine upright and stable, a spinal jacket, as with surgery, will limit lateral movement and may interfere with upper limb function. Independent feeding can be affected and it may be necessary to assess for feeding aids including making adjustment to work surfaces following either the fitting of a spinal jacket or surgical intervention. On the whole, the benefits of fitting a jacket at an early stage usually outweigh the difficulties, and provide the opportunity to delay surgery until a child is fully grown. This is generally a preferred choice as early intervention will restrict the normal growth rate.

Kyphosis (Fig. 4.10)

This is the general term used to define an excessive posterior curvature of the spinal column which is present in sacral sitting when the pelvis is tilted posteriorly. In time this results in the 'C' shaped spinal curve and slumped posture frequently seen in wheelchair users and aggravated by a sling seat and back support. Structural kyphosis can be due to osteoporosis of the spine, ankylosing spondylitis or fracture of the spine, as well as muscle weakness and low tone in the trunk (see Ch. 8). An acute kyphus or gibbus is

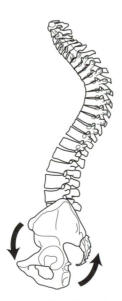

Figure 4.10 Diagram of spinal deformity showing kyphosis (lateral view).

where there is a sharp posterior angulation. Early kyphosis occurs in children with cerebral palsy who demonstrate extensor spasticity in the lower extremeties with tight hamstrings. In time the spine becomes permanently 'C' shaped with increasing restriction of hip flexion. When there is a fixed and severe kyphosis affecting the full length of the spine, the chin drops on to the chest as the head falls forward. Lifting the head does not reduce the kyphosis but results in chin poking. This makes both drinking and eating difficult, affects horizontal vision and eye contact and eventually interferes with breathing as gravitational forces continue to increase the curvature. Tilting the wheelchair may be the only way to deal with this problem once the spine becomes fixed, though the degree of tilt required may not be acceptable, or indeed even adequate to deal with the problem. When there are indications of a kyphus developing, provision of a well-shaped tray to support forward leaning, or fitting a grab rail on the wheelchair or buggy, will help to encourage use of the extensors of the spine and an upright position. This can be further encouraged by positioning the individual in the prone lying position for sleeping. Recent, though controversial research is said to link cot deaths with sleeping in the prone position and may therefore be resisted by parents of small children.

Lordosis

Lordosis is an excessive anterior curvature of the lumbar or sometimes cervical spine. A mild lumbar lordosis is encouraged in the sitting position as it enables the pelvis to tilt anteriorly and assists in maintaining an upright balanced position, evenly distributing body weight over the buttocks. In general a lumbar lordosis does not cause a problem with sitting, though there are conditions when there is an exaggeration of lumbar lordosis as seen in people who have multiple sclerosis and spasm of erector spinae muscles. With age there is generally a loss of the lumbar lordosis and this should be taken into consideration when providing seating for the those in the upper age group (see Ch. 11). Once the ability to achieve a lumbar curve has been lost, it is unwise and inappropriate to provide a lumbar roll as this will cause discomfort and push the sitter forward in their chair. Unfortunately it is common for chairs provided for the elderly to not only have a built in lumbar roll, but also to be firm and covered in stiff vinyl fabric. This can cause severe discomfort to elderly people and tends to increase the kyphotic shape of the spine due to the firmness of the back support.

Common deformities of the lower limb

Lower limb deformities can occur at any joint, though problems around the pelvis and hip joint tend to be the most common (see Ch. 3).

Maintaining a full range of movement at all joints and constantly monitoring positioning is vital if function is to be maintained and secondary problems do not develop. Knee flexion deformities when severe, generally as a result of shortening of the hamstring muscles, will result in an individual becoming unseatable. In extreme cases, the heels become fixed close to the buttocks and there is no choice for the individual but to remain in a semi-recumbent position.

Ankle deformities

These are less common, but nonetheless should always be avoided. Allowing the development of valgus or possibly varus at the ankle with foot drop (plantarflexion) will prevent standing and walking, whilst also affecting weight distribution in the seated position. A continued opportunity to stand each day delays the development of scoliosis and is an important part of postural management. Night splints and positioning equipment, including seating, when appropriately prescribed, play an essential role but have little effect unless backed up by regular physiotherapy and maintenance of joint range. Unfortunately, physiotherapy is not always available and few adults with neurological disabilities will be seen by a therapist on a regular basis. Equally, work being carried out with new drugs to reduce spasm, such as the botulinum toxin, can not be effective in practice unless the need for regular exercise is also recognized and provided on a long-term basis (see 'Twenty-four-hour postural management' in Ch. 9).

ADDITIONAL CONSIDERATIONS

The fact that the vestibular system is one of the most important tools in controlling posture is often overlooked (Horak & Shupert 1992). Information from the vestibular system and other sensory systems, visual and proprioceptive, provide information which the central nervous system uses to maintain body alignment and stability. Absence of, or interference with, normal sensory responses will affect posture, as is often demonstrated by adults with acquired disabilities such as multiple sclerosis.

Physiological factors, though less commonly recognized as a source of difficulty, should always be considered and addressed in the clinic. Pain, constipation, urinary infection, siting of catheters, gastrostomy tubes and such like, must be considered in a final prescription for seating and postural support, as discomfort or malfunction due to lack of consideration can adversely affect the success of the final result.

REFERENCES

Bar C A 1992 Seating for the disabled. In: Educational, training and teaching manuals. Bencraft, Birmingham, section A, p 5

Bleck E E 1987 Orthopaedic management in cerebral palsy. Lavenham Press, Suffolk

Bock Otto 1989 Seating review. Current trends for the disabled. Otto Bock, Canada, p 2

British Society of Rehabilitation Medicine 1995 Seating needs for complex disabilities. A working party report of the British Society of Rehabilitation Medicine (Chairman K Andrews), vol 2. BSRM, London, p 3

Burgman I 1994 The trunk/spine complex and wheelchair seating for children: a literature review. Australian Occupational Therapy Journal 41: 123–132

Department of Health 1996 Guidelines for purchasers and providers based on categories of users. DoH funded project. College of Occupational Therapists, London

Fearn T A, Green E M, Jones M, Mulcahy C M, Nelham R L, Pountney T E 1992 Postural management. In: McCarthy G (ed) Physical disability in childhood. Churchill Livingstone, Edinburgh, pp 401–450

Goldsmith E, Golding R M, Garstang R A, MacRae A W 1992 A technique to measure windswept deformity, a technical evaluation. Physiotherapy 78(4): 235–242

Gordon J, Ghez C 1991 Muscle receptors and spinal reflexes: the stretch reflex. In: Kandel E R, Schwartz J H, Jessell T M (eds) Principles of neural science. Elsevier, New York, pp 564–580

Green E M, Mulcahy C M, Pountney T E 1992 Postural management. Theory and practice. Active Design, Birmingham

Harris S R 1991 Movement analysis. An aid to early diagnosis of cerebral palsy. Physiotherapy 71: 215–221

Haskell S H, Barrett E K 1989 The education of children with motor and neurological disabilities, 2nd edn. Chapman and Hall, London

Hobson D A, Tooms R E 1992 Seated lumbar/pelvic alignment: a comparison between spinal-cord injured and non injured groups. Spine 17: 293–298

Horak F B, Shupert C 1992 Role of the vestibular system in postural control. In: Herndon S J, Borello-France D F, Whitney S L (eds) Vestibular rehabilitation. F A Davis, Philadelphia

Hsu J D 1990 Spine care of the patient with Duchenne muscular dystrophy. Spine: State of the Arts Review 4(1): 161–172

Illingworth R S (ed) 1983 The diagnosis of cerebral palsy. In: The development of the infant and young child. Normal and abnormal, 8th edn. Churchill Livingstone, Edinburgh, pp 266–285

Jenkins D B 1991 Hollinshead's functional anatomy of the limbs and back, 6th edn. W B Saunders, Philadelphia

Johnson Taylor S 1987 Evaluating clients with physical disabilities for wheelchair seating. American Journal of Occupational Therapy 41(11): 711–716

Letts R M 1991 General principles of seating. In: Letts R M (ed) Principles of seating the disabled. CRC Press, London

Levitt S 1982 Treatment of cerebral palsy and motor delay, 2nd edn. Blackwell Scientific, Oxford

Lin J P, Brown J K, Walsh E G 1994 Physiological maturation of muscles in childhood. Lancet 343: 1386–1389

McLellan L 1988 Parkinson's disease. In: Goodwill C J, Chamberlain M A (eds) Rehabilitation of the physically disabled adult. Croom Helm, London, pp 342–363

Mulcahy C M, Pountney T, Nelham R L, Green E M, Billington G D 1988 Adaptive seating for motor handicap: problems, a solution, assessment and prescription. British Journal of Occupational Therapy 51(10): 347–352

Nash J, Neilson P D, O'Dwyer N J 1989 Reducing spasticity to control muscle contracture of children with cerebral palsy. Developmental Medicine and Child Neurology 31: 471–480

Pope P 1996 Postural management and special seating. In: Edwards S (ed) Neurological physiotherapy: a problem solving approach. Churchill Livingstone, London, pp 135–160

Tredwell S, Roxburgh L 1991 Cerebral palsy in seating. In: Letts R M (ed) Principles of seating the disabled. CRC Press, London, pp 151–168

Zacharkow D 1988 Posture: sitting, standing, chair design and exercise. Charles C Thomas, Springfield, IL

5

Biopsychosocial aspects of disability

INTRODUCTION

A handbook about wheelchairs and associated seating that simply covers the anatomy, physiology, biomechanical principles of seating and practical solutions to physical problems, would be incomplete without including some of the findings from the psychological literature and the social aspects of disability, however briefly.

Approximately 8% of the population in the UK has a physical disability. Special care is needed for four out of every 1000 of these disabled people, and of these, one in four are aged under 65 years. So in each average health authority with a population of 250 000, there will be approximately 250 under 65 years who are severely disabled and require special care. These individuals will generally be well known to the local wheelchair service and this figure does not include those many elderly people who are requesting wheelchairs to increase their mobility and quality of life. When mechanical or bioelectric aids become a necessary part of a disabled individual's life style, alienation is sometimes felt more towards the inanimate assistive equipment than towards the body requiring assistance (Pulton 1984). This can therefore apply to the wheelchair.

The impairment, disability and handicap may have profound effects on these individuals concerned and their families, affecting both their material, social and psychological well being (Wilkinson 1989).

THE BIOMEDICAL VERSUS THE BIOPSYCHOSOCIAL MODEL OF HEALTH CARE

There is much discussion about health care in relation to the biomedical or psychosocial models of delivery. The dominant paradigm (the mental model or framework of how science is to be conducted which identifies questions that can be studied and determines the research methods that may be used (Kuhn 1962)) of the twentieth century, has been the *biomedical* model. This model defines mind and body as separate substances, the body as a machine and the mind as a spiritual entity. The discovery of external agents of disease, such as bacteria, viruses, vitamin deficiencies and chemicals, strengthened this model in modern medicine. The social, psychological and behavioural dimensions of health fall outside its narrow framework (Sheridan & Radmacher 1992). The biomedical model is said to promote specialisms and does not promote prevention, health enhancement or individual responsibility for health (Gordon & Fadiman 1984).

The biomedical model has more recently been expanded to become the *biopsychosocial* model, with the addition of social and psychological influences on today's health problems. It is a more realistic model accepting that social and psychological factors influence biological functioning and play a role in health and illness (Sheridan & Radmacher 1992). An example of the importance of life style in 20th century disease is seen in the fact that behavioural factors are implicated in seven out of the ten major causes of death in the USA (Raub 1989). Smoking, obesity, drug addiction, alcoholism and lack of exercise are common examples.

The reaction to impairment or disability can be just as important for the individual as the original biological deficit, and this has been recognized in a model which incorporates the social reaction (Fig. 5.1).

The traditional medical model encompasses the specific physical impairment and its preceding causes if these are known. The physical impairment has two consequences. First it leads to functional limitation and activity restriction, which are labelled together as disability, and then through the changes in self-perception and expectation of others, it creates social handicap which in turn may affect and exacerbate the underlying physical impairment (World Health

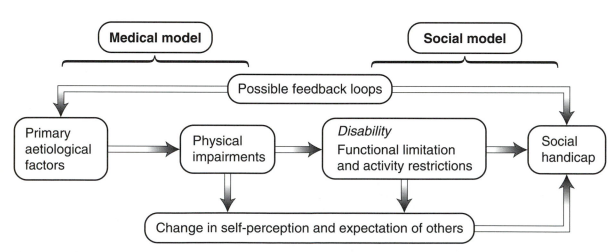

Figure 5.1 A model of impairment, disability and handicap. (Armstrong 1989, after WHO 1980, with permission from Butterworth Heinemann)

Organization 1980, Armstrong 1989) (see also Ch. 1). So the reaction to loss will include physical loss, loss of function, sexual loss, loss of self-image, loss of self-esteem, losses in society and vocational loss. The individual has tasks to overcome to achieve recovery: accept the reality of the loss, experience the pain of grief, adjust to the environment with the loss, withdraw emotional energy and reinvest it into tasks to be overcome. It is helpful if staff concentrate on the quality of life and the personal meaning of the illness to the particular person rather than a traditional disease-orientated model (Pulton 1984). The biopsychosocial model is very appropriate to apply when dealing with wheelchair users.

COMMUNICATION

Communication is most commonly thought of as verbal but it can also take the form of non-verbal communication including sign language and the written form. The conscious mind is said to communicate verbally and the unconscious mind through non-verbal communication. Problems can arise in communication from both the user's and the health care worker's perspective (Weinman 1987). From the user's perspective these include:

- lack of information
- communication gap
- poor recall
- low empathy
- activity or passivity.

From the health care worker's perspective these are:

- low compliance
- poor information.

Lack of information

A lack of information can lead to increased stress and anxiety levels and poorer recovery rates after surgery. Therefore a lack of information can have direct consequences on how patients feel and respond (Weinman 1987). In the wheelchair service this is commonly due to a lack of written

information and explanation as well as verbal information. Booklets or leaflets should be given with new and reconditioned equipment which explains the service's working methods, for example the criteria for issue.

A communication gap

Health professionals come into their training as lay people and as time goes by they learn professional jargon which can be either meaningless to or is misinterpreted by patients (Boyle 1970, Korsch & Negrete 1972). In studies, patients have been found to be not necessarily dissatisfied, but the understanding of the conversation between the patients and the professionals was obviously different. Commonly misunderstood words included: malignant, secretions, cardiac, tendon, terminal and nerve (Samora, Saunders and Larson 1961). Patients also use jargon and this is increased with ethnicity and where there is an age gap between the two. It is therefore important that health care professionals check the information given and received and that it is clearly understood by both parties. In the wheelchair service, users generally criticize the terms EPIC, EPIOC, jargon regarding battery information and a lack of explanation of medical factors. Language and cultural aspects should also be considered.

Poor recall

Only a limited amount of information can be retained for a fairly short period of time and information to be held for longer needs to be 'encoded' in a form that is meaningful to the individual (Ley & Spelman 1965, 1967). The amount forgotten increases with the number of statements or topics made (Cheadle & Morgan 1975, Ley 1979). If it is essential that a user remembers something then only two statements should be made. Getting users or their carers to write down the instructions or what they have been told, marginally improves unprompted recall and gives the patient a record to refresh their memory at a later stage (Thompson 1984). Age does not affect recall (Ley & Spelman 1965). Recall has been found to be best for diagnoses, which tend to be discussed early in the conversation, and worse for instructions, which tend to be left to the end of the session (Ley & Spelman 1967). Therefore, for the greatest effect, it is important that instructions are given verbally, in writing and personalized by the user or carer. Too much information should not be given at any one time. Ley (1979) found that when longer words and sentences were used, fewer people could understand the pamphlet.

Low empathy

If the professional is unsympathetic, it has been found that this will affect attendance levels, discussions of personal problems and compliance with advice (Weinman 1987). Often wheelchair service staff see users in clinics or at home where time is short and privacy is lacking. Both time and space are important in any interaction.

Activity/passivity

Professionals who adopt a patient-centred rather than a professional-centred approach to interviewing the patient and who use more open-ended rather than closed or directed questions, have been found to be more likely to get to the root of the problems and increase the patient's satisfaction with the interaction. Remembering this in initial and subsequent discussions with users will be helpful but it should be remembered that sometimes the user's medical condition affects the interaction.

Compliance

Poor compliance rates have been reported in a number of studies, notably in connection with medication and attendance rates. Written instructions can only help compliance if they can be easily read by the people to whom they are directed. Ley (1973, 1977) found that when longer words and sentences were used, fewer people could understand the pamphlet. Some wheelchair manufacturers' booklets use jargon and long words that do not take into account the readers, the disabilities commonly seen or those who do not have English as a first language. Many carers are also elderly and find new equipment and instructions daunting.

When listening to the user it is important that the verbal message is interpreted as well as observing and interpreting the non-verbal communication and general appearance through attending (or silent listening) to the user (Egan 1982). A good listener does not interrupt, is accepting, non-judgemental, does not undervalue the problem, gives time, avoids direct advice, gives full attention and clarifies the situation (Brumfitt 1986).

Listening skills with the use of reflection (i.e. reflecting back the emotional content and feelings of the person) and paraphrasing (i.e. reflecting back what the person has said) are basic skills that are vital for the health professional working with those with physical illnesses. Open questions should be used to create space, open up the topic and move the interview forward. Closed questions give 'yes/no' answers and are interrogation-type questions in general. Good listening and reflecting skills help the communication process, the recall, compliance and also overcome the use of jargon.

Non-verbal communication

The verbal channel (language) is used to communicate information about events external to the speaker and the non-verbal channels (facial expression, body posture, autonomic physiological responses, movement and vocal quality) are especially effective at communicating attitudes, feelings and relationships (Argyle et al 1970, Argyle, Alkema & Gilmore 1971). Non-verbal communication channels have a special relationship with affect or feeling because they 'leak' information that may be deliberately concealed in the controllable verbal channels. Such communication includes:

- visual
- posture and gestures
- proximity
- paralinguist cues
- sensitivity/empathy.

Such communication is important for wheelchair service staff to pick up to help with interpretation and behaviour.

Visual

The closer people are together, the tendency is for eye contact to decrease. More eye contact is found with those who are listening than those who are speaking, though speakers look to see if they are being understood. Less eye contact is made with people who are disliked and those who are found to be unattractive. Also topics that the speaker finds difficult to express or are embarrassing are found to produce less eye contact. Prolonged eye contact is seen as a strong emotional response, either affection or anger, and averted eye contact is an indication of guilt, fear or rejection (Kent & Dalgleish 1984, Weinman 1987). Watching eye contact, especially in difficult discussions, may help the therapist to direct the conversation or help the user with their difficulty. But ethnic and cultural aspects should also be taken into consideration, for example Asians avoid direct eye-to-eye contact in conversations (Jayaratnam 1993).

Posture and gestures

Body movements have been found to indicate the intensity of emotion whereas the face identifies the nature of the emotion (Ekman & Friensen 1977).

Therefore the user's body movements indicate the level of tension or relaxation and how someone is coping with their emotional state is seen in detail in the face. For example, slight forward leaning is said to reflect warmth (LaCrosse 1975); closed arms – coldness or rejection; shoulder shrugging – uncertainty; head nods – agreement or disagreement; scratching, picking, rubbing, licking lips – discomfort or tension (Weinman 1987), and moderately open arms – warmth and acceptance (Smith-Hanen 1977). Posture and gestures can therefore alert the therapist to the user's emotional state.

Proximity

The distance between people is termed personal space (Kent & Dalgleish 1984). Hall (1969) categorized proximity into four zones:

- intimate (0–45 cm; 0–18 inches)
- personal (45–130 cm; 18 inches–4 feet)
- social (1–4 m; 4–12 feet).
- public (> 4 m).

People also tolerate more proximity at the side than at the back or the front. Patients have been known to disclose more personal details to nurses while they were performing intimate treatments (Johnson 1965). The position the wheelchair staff take in the discussion and the assessment should therefore be appropriate.

Paralinguist cues

Features such as the tone, rate and fluency of speech can provide useful information about the person's emotional state and intentions. When anxious, people hesitate more often and make errors of speech, when they are anxious and excited they often speak faster and use more body movements. Depressed people speak in a slow, soft and monotonous voice. Observation of this by the therapist should help the therapy interaction or reaction to be appropriate.

Sensitivity/empathy

Noting all the other influences on communication, the health care workers should be sensitive to the behaviour and feelings of users. This involves an awareness of the user's non-verbal behaviour, such as hesitation, restlessness and signs of embarrassment (Kent & Dalgleish 1984). Such awareness should again help the quality of the interaction with the user.

Relationships with health care professionals

Patients usually remember much about the emotional and interpersonal tone of their encounters with health care professionals (Korsch, Gozzi & Francis 1968), as professionals are present at emotionally momentous occasions (both positive and negative) in people's lives.

The practitioners who are most effective interpersonally have been found to be sensitive to each patient's feelings, are warm, empathic, genuine, self-disclosing and use their social influence to find solutions that satisfy the patients and fulfil the requirements of the role of professional healer (Lazare et al 1978). The health care professional is privy to all parts of the patient's body and the most intimate details of their lives (Dimatteo & Dinicola 1982) and so the social skills of consideration, motivation, impression and rapport are required for successful interpersonal relationships to develop (Strongman 1979). The interpersonal relationship of professional and patient/client may be more empathic if the professional has experienced life 'dramas', which may have been characterized by physical or social change, or changes in thought, content and emotional responsiveness. The integration of these new experiences adds to the professional sources of personal history and so to their maturity (Shepherd 1982). The wheelchair therapist should take note of these factors and should encourage the mature work-returner to move into the area of practice.

User satisfaction

The increase today in a scientific and technological approach to medical care has led to an increase in patients' dissatisfaction (Fitzpatrick 1984). In the past, evaluation of health services had focused on morbidity and mortality but today this is changing and patients' opinion on their care are being sought through clinical audit in all areas of clinical work (Fitzpatrick 1991). Satisfaction with care is reported as having a cognitive and emotional component. Cognitive satisfaction appears to be associated with verbal behaviour and emotional satisfaction is more closely related to non-verbal behaviour (Kent & Dalgleish 1984). Older people tend to be more satisfied with health care than the young and this is thought to be because the young are more aware of the changes in access, charters, etc. and the elderly are less likely to criticize (Raphael 1969, Pope 1978) perhaps because of their awareness of the days before the NHS. Problems of

user satisfaction are commonly seen in the wheelchair services where local criteria do not always meet individual requests or desires. However, good communication channels with information, health reasons and criteria lists and through verbal communication and empathy generally all help satisfy the user.

PSYCHOLOGICAL ASPECTS

In considering the psychological aspects of disability it is necessary to be cautious in making general statements because of factors which may have a specific impact on adjustment. Such factors are:

- The age of the onset. For example, congenital conditions will affect a family differently than diseases of later life. Guilt may persist.
- Insidious conditions compared to traumatic conditions may have a different psychological impact.
- The stability of the condition and its prognosis will influence the person's perception of future disabilities, life style or reduced life expectancy.
- The severity of the disability and the degree of dependency will place different burdens on carers and vary the degree of restriction placed on the individual.
- Intellectual functioning and personality change.
- The presence or absence of pain and the frequency of periods of associated illnesses (Wilkinson 1989).

Stages of psychological adjustment

An individual negotiates and progresses through the normal and expectable stages of adaptation at a time of physical trauma and disability. The five stages outlined below are usually present in some form in the healthy adaptation of psychological adjustment to physical disability. They are not, however, always distinct, neat or progressive. Impediments to emotional rehabilitation usually manifest as difficulty in negotiating one of these stages (Krueger 1984) – a point for staff to remember. The stages can be conceptualized as:

1. Shock, which is the immediate reaction to trauma and can last from moments to several days.
2. Denial, which initially is useful and professionals should recognize that this is a necessary defence mechanism which may last from a few days to several weeks.
3. Depressive reaction in the form of grief and depression which emerges when denial recedes. If it does not occur, professionals should be more alarmed as it indicates that the loss has not been emotionally recognized. Depression, anxiety, anger and grief are to be expected as natural and appropriate and the individual may externalize hostility and blame for the disability.
4. Reaction against independence is especially seen in patients who are about to be discharged from hospital and personality traits may be exaggerated at this time of stress (Krueger 1984).
5. Adaptation following disability has been likened to the bereavement process following a death. There is a mourning for the function, body image and the loss of the future expectations due to the loss of function both by the individual and family and carers.

Wheelchair staff, although aware of these variations, may not have thought all the factors and stages through when trying to understand the user.

Psychological care

The psychological care of the individual includes:

- emotional care
- informational care
- counselling, monitoring the situation and referring on and promoting independence.

Emotional care

Physical illness generates changes in emotions and behaviour. The health professional can assist by providing emotional care also. That is, an understanding that coping strategies and emotional responses are a normal part of illness. Staff should be aware of the skills which are necessary, which include:

- making the situation safe or non-threatening
- enabling the individual to recognize their own feelings
- facilitating the expression of feelings
- communicating understanding and acceptance
- giving time and support (Nicholls 1984).

Time should be made available in the clinic setting or at home for this to take place.

Informational care

The individual's psychological state may reduce their capacity to receive and process information. The information should be given, whenever possible, in both the verbal and written form. The professional should remember that anxiety and urgency alter listening, recall and general responses. It is essential that the therapist regularly checks what the user knows, identifies the gaps and repeats the information if it is necessary. Remember the following:

- appropriate language
- the user's intelligence
- avoid jargon
- vocabulary differences
- the quantity of information given
- the use of 'unit' or 'department' answers when necessary
- the family's involvement.

Counselling

Although the basic skills of counselling of empathy, acceptance and genuineness are within the reach of all health care workers, true counselling should only be carried out by a qualified person.

'True counselling' has been defined as:

when a person, occupying regularly or temporarily the role of 'counsellor', offers or agrees explicitly to give time, attention or respect to another person or persons temporarily in the role of 'client'. The task of counselling is to give the 'client' an opportunity to explore, define and discover ways of living more satisfactorily and resourcefully within the social grouping with which he identifies (British Association for Counselling 1979).

Counselling is therefore a different, specific and a special kind of helping or caring relationship and one that is also regarded as a psychological process (Nelson–Jones 1990, Stewart 1985). The relationship between the two people, the counsellor and the client, is important and the other factors that are also regarded as essential from the counsellor as a person are, for example, his/her attitudes, approach, self-awareness and self-knowledge and also his/her specific skills in treating the client holistically (Egan 1982). As well as possessing self-awareness and self-knowledge, counsellors are also required to have some specific technical skills. These include the skills of listening, attending, observing, goal setting or plans of action, awareness, know-how, assertiveness, appropriate verbal communication, responding skills, empathy, and challenging, confrontation and decision-making skills (Egan 1982).

Personality

Personality can be defined as:

> the characteristic patterns of thought, emotion and behaviour that define an individual's personal style and influence his or her interaction with the environment (Atkinson et al 1985).

Early in a child's development, mood-related characteristics or temperaments are seen, which suggest there is a genetic factor to personality, but other influences also act to develop the child's personality. These are the environmental influences and the individual's reaction to them. For example, different individuals will react in different ways to the same environment in which they live. Different individuals will also provoke different responses from others they meet daily and each individual will choose different environments in which to interact and spend time during their life.

Environmental factors are especially important in shaping personalities in the young rather than the adult. Parents will react to their children in different ways, provoking different responses in their offspring which will influence personality shaping. Personalities also continue to change throughout life. Intellectual performance, extroversion, emotional stability and impulsive control remain strong factors in the continuity of a personality, whereas measures of self-opinion, for example, are not so strong (Atkinson et al 1985).

The personality of the individual with an impairment will therefore affect their reaction to their disability and subsequently their social handicap.

Personality theories

A number of psychologists have tried to define personality and these can be broadly categorized into five areas:

- personality types
- personality traits
- the psychoanalytic approach
- the social learning/behaviour theories
- the cognitive approach.

Personality types. Personality types were discussed as early as 400 BC but more recently Sheldon described three physical types:

- endomorphs who are soft and round, relaxed and sociable
- mesomorphs who are muscular and athletic, assertive and energetic
- ectomorphs who are tall and thin, introverted and fearful.

Personality traits. Trait theories describe variables that differ from one individual to another. Such variables are discussed by the general public and include the following terms: aggressive, cautious, excitable, intelligent or anxious. In 1953 Eysenck described four major personality factors – introversion, extroversion, emotional stability and instability – in terms of nervous system functioning. Although there is disagreement amongst psychologists as to how many trait factors there are, there is a consensus emerging that a five-trait dimension is the best compromise (Atkinson et al 1985). These are as follows, with descriptions of the extremes of the traits given:

- neuroticism (hardy–vulnerable, secure–insecure)
- extroversion (retiring–sociable, quiet–talkative)
- openness (conventional–original)
- agreeableness (irritable–good natured)
- conscientiousness (unreliable–reliable) (McCrae & Costa 1987).

Neuroticism has many consequences for health and illness. It is the extent to which people worry or respond emotionally and is related to the body's nervous system. Placebos, for example, produce different responses from individual to individual and in the same person at different times depending upon the situation in which the placebo is administered. People who are anxious are likely to seek help and drug tolerance is greater in introverts whereas extroverts are more sensitive (Weinman 1987). The reverse is seen in anxious patients.

Personality traits will normally be exaggerated at times of stress or massive insult. Some traits are adaptive for the patient in a dependent role and some more adaptive for rehabilitation. Antisocial personalities may make the adjustment more difficult and may for example neglect the tedious self-care needed following a spinal injury. Dependent personalities may, in illness, find social justification for living a dependent life and the masochistic, through injury, may have visible proof of their suffering. The paranoid will intensify their belief that others are there to harm them and the schizoid avoidant personality may find illness or disability disrupts their isolated life which becomes threatening and anxiety provoking (Servoss 1984).

Individuals who are highly anxious have been found to experience more pain at surgery (Chapman & Cox 1977). Eysenck hypothesized that personality traits are associated with cardiovascular disease and cancer and that they are at opposite ends of personality dimensions and that extroverts correlated negatively with cardiovascular disease and positively with cancer.

Furham & Brewin (1990) reported a positive correlation between happiness and neuroticism. Argyle & Lu (1990) reported that extroverts' happiness could be explained by greater participation in social activities – such social activities and social support help to keep people healthy at times of stress (Kobasa 1979, 1982).

Psychoanalytic approach. The creator of this approach was Freud, who built a structure of three items: the 'id', which consists of the basic biological drives, the 'ego', which develops as the child regulates these drives and needs in relation to the environment, and the 'superego', the individual's conscience which judges whether the action is right or wrong in society. Freud also described psychosexual phases throughout development (Atkinson et al 1985).

The social learning/behaviourist approach. With this approach, the individual's personality is modified by outside factors which may be other individuals' actions or the environment itself. Individuals observe actions and their subsequent consequences which then modify or alter their own behaviour. Psychologists who have worked in this area are Pavlov, who developed the Classical Conditioning Theory, Mischel who developed the Social Learning Theory which focuses on personal variables, Watson, who founded the Behaviourist Movement in the USA, Kobasa and Maddi, who developed the Existential Theory of Personality in 1977 (Kobasa 1979), Skinner, who felt that theories of behaviour are also theories of personality and, finally in 1956, Selye's model of General Adaptive Response (see Ch. 10).

The cognitive approach. These approaches describe how the individual perceives and interprets events they experience in their own world. Such cognitions are thoughts, anticipations, expectations and beliefs (Weinman 1987). The Humanistic approach is the most central and includes the work of Rogers and Maslow. Rogers described the Personal Centred theory and felt each individual wants to fulfil his/her possible potential rather than regress. Each individual has the motivation and ability to change and they are the best person to choose the direction they take. Maslow described the Hierarchy of Needs where the basic needs have to be satisfied in order for self-actualization or the individual's potential to be reached (Atkinson et al 1985). Kelly developed the Personal Construct theory which describes how the individual construes or interprets themselves and their social world. He felt we all try to predict and understand behaviour. Rotter's Health Locus of Control theory describes individual differences in the perceived control over events in people's lives. Some people feel they can influence events, whereas others feel that they have little or no control over things that happen to them, the Internal–External control of reinforcement theory. Seligman's Learned Helplessness theory describes depression in learning about one's own apparent inability to effect environmental change. People who are prone to depression feel that adverse happenings are due to themselves, whereas good events are thought to be due to chance. Many of these approaches can be applied to the individual's reaction to disability.

The individual's personality is complex and is affected by many outside stimuli at different times. The psychological and the physical aspects of illness and health must be taken into account when the individual's disorders are met and analysed alongside sources of illness such as viruses. Different people react to health, illness and the treatment situation in different ways, and knowledge of these theories will help health care professionals understand the individual's attitude to their own health and their reaction to illness.

The effects of life events on illness

Holmes & Rahe (1967) described a life event as being stressful if it causes a change in and demands readjustment of an average person's normal routine. Some individuals are able to cope well and are described as having *hardy personalities* (Kobasa & Maddi 1977). Following a study of executives, looking at high stress and low illness scores compared to high stress and high illness scores, Kobasa concluded that the 'hardiness' way of coping with stress acts as an insulation against illness. Selye's theory suggests that stress produces illness to occur at the weakest system or organ. Mild symptoms of illness may be overlooked by the hardy personality even though pathological changes may be occurring in the body. This can be seen in wheelchair users, some of whom complain little whereas others make heavy weather out of all situations.

The *Health Locus of Control* theory divides into the internal and external personality. The internal personality feels that they are responsible for their health and the external personality believes that powerful other factors are responsible (Wallston & Wallston 1982). Again, some people help themselves while others wait for others to take the initial action.

Coping

Any illness is likely to have both psychological and social functioning effects on the individual (Weinman 1987). Folkman & Lazarus (1988) define coping as the 'cognitive and behavioural efforts to manage specific external and/or internal demands that are appraised as taxing or exceeding the resources of the person'. Antonovsky (1979) proposed that there are three major components:

1. Rationality – the accurate, objective assessment of the situation or the stressor.
2. Flexibility – the availability of a variety of coping strategies to overcome the stressor and the willingness to consider all of them.
3. Farsightedness – the ability to anticipate the consequences of the various coping strategies.

How each person copes with the stresses of physical illness will vary and will take into account the factors illustrated in Figure 5.2 and described further below (Weinman 1987).

The person. The individual's perception of the illness will vary with a variety of factors, including:

- the age of the person
- their previous experience with illness
- their personality
- their psychological state at the time of their illness, which can determine its perceived

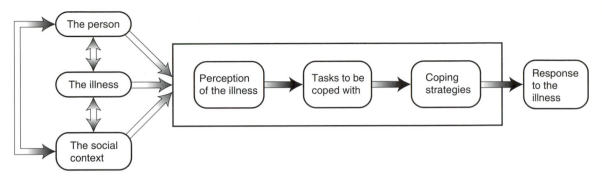

Figure 5.2   A conceptual model for understanding the factors influencing the response to physical illness (Weinman, 1987 with permission from Butterworth Heinemann).

severity, and if they are anxious (Weinman 1987).

The illness. The actual severity of the illness does not appear to correlate strongly with the psychological responses to it, since the individual's own perception of the severity and threat are more crucial factors. The particular part of the body that is affected can also have subsequent consequences for the individual, for example people who are active with sports who are affected with disorders that affect mobility and exercise. It has been suggested that disabling disorders are perceived as more threatening to men and disfiguring conditions for women. Also, the nature of the onset and its duration may determine the person's response. An unexpected and acute onset may initially be quite disruptive but may resolve more quickly than a slow, developing, chronic illness where the psychological reactions may be less dramatic but are likely to be longer lasting because of the long-term disability associated with chronic illnesses (Weinman 1987). Apart from sexual dysfunction, bowel and bladder disturbances may represent one of the more alienating experiences a disabled person will learn to cope with (Pulton 1984). Wheelchair staff should be aware of this.

The social context. Some social circumstances will also affect the impact an illness has for the individual. The illness may, for example, occur at a very unsuitable time in the individual's life, or it may occur at a time when it is almost gratefully accepted as a relief from an adverse social situa-tion. Illness or attention-seeking behaviour may also develop (Chiotakakou-Faliakou, Dave & Forbes 1996).

Tasks to be coped with. A major physical illness will affect an individual and their families in many ways and require different types of adaptation. Some of these demands are unique to illness and others can be applied to other general life stresses. For example, dealing with pain and incapacity and yet retaining a reasonable emotional balance, dealing with alien environments and yet maintaining a self-image and competence, developing relationships with health care staff and maintaining links with family and friends and preparing for an uncertain future (Weinman 1987).

Coping strategies. Two broad categories of coping are applied to the demands of physical illness (Weinman 1987). These are problem focused, attentional strategy or direct coping behaviour where the problem or situation is dealt with directly in order to make it more manageable or tolerable. The person focuses on the distress, confronts the situation, evaluates it, seeks information about the situation, perhaps turns to others and then takes action. This strategy is said to be better in the long run (Ridgeway & Mathews 1982, Suls & Fletcher 1985).

The second is emotion focused, palliative coping or the avoidant strategy which reduces anxiety without dealing with the situation and is concerned with managing the emotions generated by the illness. It is used more for health-related stressors (Lazarus & Folkman 1984). With the avoidant strategy, the patient turns their attention away from aspects of the disease. They are deliberately distracted or unconsciously deny painful aspects of the disorder. This often leads to anger, aggression, apathy, depression and withdrawal. This approach is better under short-term conditions, for example used on the same day. Authors suggest that the coping strategy used may vary with the disease (Cohen & Lazarus 1979) and depends upon experience, intellectual ability and the capacity for self-control. Problems often arise when this avoidant strategy of coping is used with wheelchair users. Parents put off the need to have a wheelchair rather than a buggy for their child, individuals do not accept aids in their homes or postural seating equipment, for example.

The role of the health professional in assisting patients to cope with the psychological aspects of their illness is important and readily possible. For example, there should be give and take between the user and health professional, with the professional confronting the user with realities when it is necessary while understanding the need to keep them at bay at other times. The professional should know about the experience of the disease and about its common psychological effects which are different from the physiological effects. It is well known that being connected to another person or pet has a positive effect on a person's health and recovery from illness (Lynch 1977, 1985). The health professional should be aware of the importance of social support and this should not be underestimated. Other agencies may also need to be introduced and the therapist may be the only professional visiting at that time and therefore he/she may need to alert others. The user's permission to involve others should always be sought. Depending on the coping strategy chosen at a specific time, the need for information to be available and for the professional to give information is important. Written information will be used when the user is ready for it and may be requested at different times in their illness, whereas verbal information may be wasted if the time is not right for the individual. The profes-

sional should also be aware of non-compliance among users and the ways of improving this.

Health-related behaviours

Several theories have been applied to the problem of understanding health-related behaviour in the psychological literature, for example the Health Belief Model, the Reasoned Action Theory and the Self-efficacy Theory.

Health Belief Model. This model was developed in the 1950s to explain variations in health behaviour. Individuals will only take health actions if certain conditions, cues or triggers are present (Weinman 1987). Our health-related behaviour can be predicted by our assessment of:

- the perceived threat of illness or injury
- the costs and benefits of the particular behaviour (Becker & Rosenstock 1984).

Whether we perceive something as a threat depends on a number of demographic and social variables and our answers to the following questions:

- How likely is it that we will develop the particular problem?
- How serious are the consequences of the problem if we develop it or leave it untreated?
- How salient are the cues that remind us of the seriousness of the problem or that we need to take action?

We also take into account the costs and benefits of a particular health-related behaviour. Smoking and overeating are examples that can apply here and some users do not accept postural support as they ignore the seriousness of the problem.

Reasoned Action Theory. This theory states that 'intervention' is the best predictor of behaviour. An intention toward a behaviour is influenced by our attitude toward that behaviour. This attitude is influenced by the strength of belief that the behaviour will result in a certain outcome and the evaluation of the outcome (Fishbein & Ajzen 1975).

Self-efficacy Theory. This is the degree to which we believe we are capable of meeting some particular challenge. According to Bandura (1982), our self-efficacy judgements determine our choice of activities and settings. Self-efficacy also influences how much effort we will expend when we are faced with obstacles. Self-efficacy is determined by:

- our previous successes or failures
- observing the performance of others
- feedback from others about our abilities
- our physiological states.

Questions such as:

- Will tolerating special postural supports result in a better spinal outcome?
- Will wearing an orthosis make a difference?
- Is it worth the trouble?

may be asked by users or carers.

Depression

One of the commonest reported psychological responses to illness is that of depression. This may be mild and transient but it can also be so strong and pervasive that it causes crying, withdrawal and even suicidal feelings (see also Ch. 11).

Pain

Pain is defined as:

> a subjective experience that can be perceived directly only by the sufferer. It is a multidimensional phenomenon that can be described by pain location, intensity, temporal aspects, quality impact and meaning. Pain does not occur in isloation but in a specific human being in psychosocial, economic and cultural contexts that influence the meaning, experience, verbal and non-verbal expression of pain (Spence 1990).

Pain is therefore whatever the individual says it is and exists wherever he/she says it does (McCaffrey 1983). One cannot feel another's pain, only observe it (Niven 1989), and each person's response is unique and affected by many factors. A number of theories have been recorded regarding pain, notably: the specificity theory, the pattern theory, the affect theory, the Gate control theory and the concept of a neuromatrix. Psycho-

logical factors that have been reported as having an effect on pain include: personality, learning behaviour, social conditioning, ethnicity, culture, depression, anxiety, gender, coping strategy, context and the placebo effect. Wheelchair users with the same amount of pain will therefore respond differently and therapists have to treat whatever they meet.

Motivation

Motivation is a term frequently used by health care professionals but because motivation is an internal experience, its existence and nature are inferred from observation and experience and the underlying motives for behaviour are often difficult to define and classify. Regaining independence or personal goals are motivating factors for most people and the health care professional can assist by providing effective feedback about performance related to the person's own goals rather than those of the health care professional.

Children

Children born with disabling diseases such as cerebral palsy or spina bifida affect their families throughout their lives. Healthy siblings may get less than their expected share of parental time as parents attend to the increased physical needs of the affected child with the increased parent–child bond that may follow this (Frank 1989). The physical and emotional bond on the parents in these situations is enormous (Bax et al 1988). Fatigue, social isolation and financial hardship may result in sexual problems, anxiety and depression (Maguire & Morris-Jones 1988). Coping with disability and 'moving on' as the child develops remain a problem for the wheelchair service staff when dealing with paediatric cases (see Ch. 9).

SOCIAL ASPECTS OF DISABILITY
Social class

In the nineteenth century it was observed that certain causes of mortality seemed to be linked to various occupations and occupational groups. In an attempt to encapsulate these wider aspects of occupations, the British Registrar General in the 20th century devised a system of classifying occupation into eight different groups, or social classes, which would convey something of their social standing and skills. The groups were later reduced to five (Armstrong 1989). The wife and family are classified under the father or husband's occupation and this, amongst other aspects, has come under severe criticism recently. Various attempts are underway to develop a new classification system which will still relate to health but will be easier to operate.

These social classes have been shown to have an important relationship to health and illness. For example, infant, childhood and adult mortality is known to be greater in social class V compared to social class I with a gradient between the classes II and IV. Subjective measures of health status suggest worse health for those lower down the social class scale. Social class is correlated with many aspects of modern society, for example income, housing, education, leisure activities, diet, behaviour, so that each of these is also likely to be linked to illness (Armstrong 1989). The illnesses in our community seem to be linked, as in the nineteenth century, with deprivation in its widest sense. Services working in areas of inner city should be aware of these facts and be funded appropriately.

Cultural factors

It is known that different societies, even at the same stage of economic development, have different patterns of disease. An example is given between the USA and Japan. In Japan the major cause of death amongst men is stroke, whereas in the USA it is ischaemic heart disease. Japanese men who emigrate to the USA and become acculturated into the society die more frequently from heart disease. The standards of living of the two countries are the same and so the only solution is thought to be the different ways of life in the two countries, the culture (Marmot et al 1975).

Social support

The World Health Organization defines health as a complete state of physical, social and mental well-being, which includes absence of a disability, freedom from symptoms and a general state of wellness. A number of studies have identified a relationship between social support, coping and physical disability. For example, men with weak social networks were nearly two and a half times more likely to die within a defined period as were men with extensive networks (Berkman & Breslow 1983). Individuals with fewest social ties were found to be at greater risk of mortality (Schoenbach et al 1986). A number of researchers have emphasized the effects of social support as a buffer to life stresses and the chronically ill may have a greater than average need for various forms of social support. Some carers may support the comfortable option, not the treatment option, and therefore show an increased non-compliant behaviour to treatment plans (Kaplan & Toshima 1990) (see also Chs 9–11).

The staff in the wheelchair service see many people for short periods of time only. Other users become better known, either because of their complex needs, because their medical condition is constantly changing or deteriorating or, as with children, they are growing and physically changing, which entails many sessions with the service. The interaction therefore varies in time, frequency and its nature. By having some knowledge of the psychosocial factors that affect these interactions, staff will be able to maximize the interaction, make it as satisfactory as possible and begin to understand the foundations that underpin different users' reactions to their disability.

REFERENCES

Antonovsky A 1979 Health, stress and coping. Jossey Bass, San Francisco

Armstrong D 1989 Social Patterns of Illness: II. In: An outline of sociology as applied to medicine, 3rd edn. Wright, London, pp 39, 47, 51–60, 63–68

Argyle M, Lu L 1990 The happiness of extroverts. Personality and Individual Differences 11(10): 1011–1017

Argyle M, Alkema F, Gilmore R 1971 The communication of friendly and hostile attitudes by verbal and non-verbal signals. European Journal of Social Psychology 1: 385–402

Argyle M, Salter V, Nicholson H, Williams N, Burgess P 1970 The communication of inferior and superior attitudes by verbal and non-verbal signals. British Journal of Social and Clinical Psychology 9: 222–231

Atkinson R L, Atkinson R C, Smith E E, Bem D J, Hilgard E R 1985 Personality through the life course. In: Introduction to psychology, 10th edn. Harcourt Brace Jovanovich, London, pp 474–501

Bandura A 1982 Self efficacy mechanisms in human agency. American Psychologist 37: 122–147

Bax M C O, Smyth D P L, Thomas A P 1988 Health care of physically handicapped young adults. British Medical Journal 296: 1153–1155

Becker M H, Rosenstock I M 1984 Compliance with medical advice. In: Steptoe A, Mathews A (eds) Healthcare and human behaviour. Academic Press, London

Berkman L F, Breslow L 1983 Health and ways of living: findings from the Alameda County study. Oxford University Press, New York

Boyle C M 1970 Difference between patients' and doctors' interpretation of some common medical terms. British Medical Journal 2: 286–289

British Association for Counselling (BAC) (1979) Standards and ethics committee

Brumfitt S 1986 Counselling. Winslow Press, Oxon

Chapman C R, Cox G B 1977 Determination of anxiety in elective surgery patients. In: Spielberger C G, Sarason I G (eds) Stress and anxiety, vol. 4. Hemisphere, Washington

Cheadle A J, Morgan R 1975 The chronic patient's comprehension and recollection of his own review. British Journal of Psychiatry 126: 258–262

Chiotakakou-Faliakou E, Dave U, Forbes A 1996 Wheelchair use: a physical sign in gastroenterological practice. Journal of the Royal Society of Medicine 89: 490–492

Cohen R, Lazarus R S 1979 Coping with the stresses of illness. In: Stone G C, Cohen F, Adler N E (eds) Health psychology: a handbook. Jossey-Bass, San Francisco

Dimatteo R M, Dinicola D D 1982 Achieving patient compliance. Pergamon, New York

Egan G 1982 The skilled helper. Brooks Cole, Monterey, CA

Ekman P, Friesen W V 1977 Non-verbal behaviour. In: Ostward P L (ed) Communication and social interaction. Grune & Stratton, New York

Eysenck H J 1985 Personality, cancer and cardiovascular disease: a causal analysis. Personality and Individual Differences 5: 535–557

Fishbein M, Ajzen I 1975 Belief, attitude, intention and behaviour: an introduction to theory and research. Addison-Wesley, Reading, MA

Fitzpatrick R 1984 Satisfaction with health care. In:

Fitzpatrick R, Hinton J, Newman S, Scambler G, Thompson J (eds) The experience of illness. Tavistock Publications, London

Fitzpatrick R 1991 Surveys of patient satisfaction: important general considerations. British Medical Journal 302: 887–889

Folkman S, Lazarus R S 1988 The relationship between coping and emotion: implications for theory and research. Social Science and Medicine 26: 309–317

Frank A O 1989 The family and disability – some reflections on culture: a discussion paper. Journal of the Royal Society of Medicine 82: 666–668

Furham A, Brewin C R 1990 Personality and happiness. Personality and Individual Differences 11(10): 1093–1096

Gordan J S, Fadiman J 1984 Towards an integral medicine. In: Gordan J S, Jaffe D T, Bresler D E (eds) Mind, body and health human sciences. Human Sciences, New York

Hall E T 1969 The hidden dimension. Bodley Head, London

Holmes T H, Rahe R H 1967 The social readjustment rating scale. Journal of Psychosomatic Research 11: 213–218

Jayaratnam R 1993 The need for cultural awareness. In: Hopkins A, Bahl V (eds) Access to health care for people from black and ethnic minorities. Royal College of Physicians of London, London

Johnson B S 1965 The meaning of touch in nursing. Nursing Outlook 13: 59–60

Kaplan R M, Toshima M T 1990 The functional effects of social relationships on chronic illnesses and disability. In: Sarason B R, Sarason I G, Pierce G R (eds) Social support. John Wiley, Chichester

Kent G, Dalgleish M 1984 The consultation. Reading XVI. In: Murphy J, John M, Brown H (eds) Dialogues and debates in social psychology. Lawrence Erlbaum Associates, Hillsdale, NJ

Kobasa S C 1979 Stressful life events, personality and health. An inquiry into hardiness. Journal of Personality and Social Psychology 37(1): 1–11

Kobasa S C 1982 The hardy personality. In: Sanders G S, Suls J (eds) Social psychology of health and illness. Lawrence Erlbaum Associates, Hillsdale, NJ

Kobasa S C, Maddi S R 1977 Existential personality theory. In: Corsini R (ed) Current personality theories. Irasca, Peacock, Illinois

Kohl S J 1984 Psychological stressors in coping with disability. In: Krueger D W (eds) Rehabilitation Psychology. Aspen, Maryland

Korsch B M, Negrete V F 1972 Doctor–patient communication. Scientific American 227: 66–72

Korshi B M, Gozzi E K, Francis V 1968 Gaps in doctor–patient communication. In: Doctor–patient interaction and patient satisfaction. Paediatrics 42: 855–871

Krueger D W 1984 Psychological rehabilitation of physical trauma and disability. In: Krueger D W (ed) Rehabilitation psychology. Aspen, Maryland

Kuhn T S 1962 The structure of scientific revolutions. University of Chicago Press, Chicago

LaCrosse M D 1975 Non-verbal behaviour and perceived counsellor attractiveness and persuasiveness. Journal of Counselling Psychology 22: 563–566

Lazare A, Eisenthal S, Frank A, Stoekle J 1978 Studies on a

negotiated approach to patienthood. In: Gallagher E B (ed) The doctor–patient relationship in the changing health scene. Washington DC

Lazarus R S, Folkman S 1984 Stress, appraisal and coping. Springer, New York

Ley P 1973 The measurement of comprehensibility. Journal of the Institute of Health Education 11: 17–20

Ley P 1977 Psychological studies of doctor–patient communication. In: Rachman S (ed) Contributions to medical psychology, vol 1. Pergamon, Oxford, pp 9–42

Ley P 1979 Memory for medical information. British Journal of Social and Clinical Psychology 18: 245–256

Ley P, Spelman M S 1965 Communication in an outpatient setting. British Journal of Social and Clinical Psychology 4: 114–116

Ley P, Spelman M S 1967 Communicating with patients. Staple Press, London

Lynch J E 1977 The broken heart: the medical consequences of loneliness. Basic Books, New York

Lynch J E 1985 The language of the heart. Basic Books, New York

McCaffrey M 1983 Nursing the patient in pain. Harper & Row, London

Maguire G P, Morris-Jones P 1988 Helping parents of children with cancer. In: Frank A O, Maguire G P (eds) Disabling diseases – physical, environmental and psychosocial management. Heinemann Medical Books, Oxford

Marmot M G, Syme S L, Kogan A, Kato H, Cohen J B, Belsby J 1975 Epidemiological studies of coronory heart disease and stroke in Japanese men living in Japan, Hawaii and California. American Journal of Epidemiology 102: 514–525

McCrae P R, Costa R T Jr 1987 Validation of the five factor model of personality across instruments and onservers. Journal of Personality and Social Psychology 52: 81–90

Nelson-Jones R 1990 The theory and practice of counselling psychology. Cassell, London

Nicholls K A 1984 Psychological care in physical illness. Croom Helm, London

Niven N 1989 Psychobiological perspective: pain and stress. In: Health psychology. Churchill Livingstone, Edinburgh, pp 107–149

Pope C R 1978 Consumer satisfaction in a health maintenance organisation. Journal of Health and Social Behaviour 19(3): 291–303

Pulton T W 1984 A social-psychological inquiry into alienation and disability. In: Krueger D W (ed) Rehabilitation psychology. Aspen, Maryland, pp 89–97

Raphael W 1969 Patients and their hospitals: a survey of patients' view of life in a general hospital. King Edwards' Hospital Fund, London

Raub W F 1989 High fibre diet may inhibit large bowel neoplasia. Journal of the American Medical Association 262: 2359

Ridgeway V, Mathews A 1982 Psychological preparation for surgery: a comparison of methods. British Journal of Clinical Psychology 21: 271–280

Samora J, Saunders L, Larson M 1961 Medical vocabulary knowledge among hospital patients. Journal of Health and Human Behaviour 2: 83–89

Schoenbach V J, Kaplan B H, Fredman L, Kleinbaum D G 1986 Social ties and mortality in Evans County, Georgia. American Journal of Epidemiology 123: 577–591

Servoss A G 1984 Mobility impairment. In: Krueger D W (ed) Rehabilitation psychology. Aspen, Maryland, pp 249–256

Shepherd E 1982 Coping with the first person singular. In: Shepherd E, Watson J F (eds) Personal meanings. John Wiley, Chichester, pp 33–46

Sheridan C L, Radmacher S A 1992 Health psychology. Challenging the biomedical model. John Wiley, Chichester

Smith-Hanen S 1977 Effects of non verbal behaviour on judged levels of counsellor, warmth and empathy. Journal of Counselling Psychology 24: 87–91

Spence A (Chairman) 1990 Commission on the provision of surgical services. Royal College of Surgeons (Eng). The College of Anaesthetists, London

Stewart W 1985 Philosophy of counselling. In: Counselling in rehabilitation. Croom Helm, London, pp 18–41

Strongman K T 1979 Psychology for the paramedical professions. Croom Helm, London

Suls J, Fletcher E 1985 The relative efficacy of avoidant and non avoidant coping strategies: a meta analaysis. Health Psychology. 4: 249–288

Thompson J 1984 Compliance. In: Fitzpatrick R, Hinton J, Newman S, Scrambler G, Thompson J (eds) The experience of illness. Tavistock Publications, London

Wallston K A, Wallston B S 1982 Who is responsible for your health? The construct of health locus of control. In: Sanders G S, Suls J (eds) Social psychology of health and illness. Erlbaum, Hillsdale, W Jersey

Weinman J 1987 An outline of psychology as applied to medicine. Wright, Bristol

World Health Organization (WHO) 1980 The international classification of impairments, disabilities and handicaps – a manual of classification relating to the consequences of disease. WHO, Geneva

Wilkinson S M 1989 Psychological aspects of physical disability. In: Broome A K (ed) Health psychology. Processes and applications. Chapman and Hall, London, pp 234–254

6

Assessment

Wheelchair services operate in different ways and every wheelchair service has its own method of dealing with referrals and assessments. This will depend not only on the staffing levels within the service, but also the knowledge and expertise of the staff and that of the professionals in the field.

Some wheelchair services work in conjunction with a network of trained assessors who assess the needs of the majority of wheelchair users and refer the remainder, with the more complex problems, to the wheelchair service. Other wheelchair services tend to prefer to see the majority of their users (Nuffield Institute of Health 1995, National Prosthetic and Wheelchair Services Report 1993–1996).

Figure 6.1 shows an example of a service in which equipment can be provided in several ways, following assessment at three different levels.

Level 1

Information provided with a self-referral or referral from a GP would usually be scanned by a clerk or therapist, resulting in the direct provision of a standard item of equipment such as an attendant-pushed wheelchair. Although apparently straightforward on paper, there is a danger that relevant information may be missing from the referral and hence inappropriate equipment provided. Alternatively, some services might arrange for a quick clinic appointment with a wheelchair service therapist, therapist helper or wheelchair coordinator.

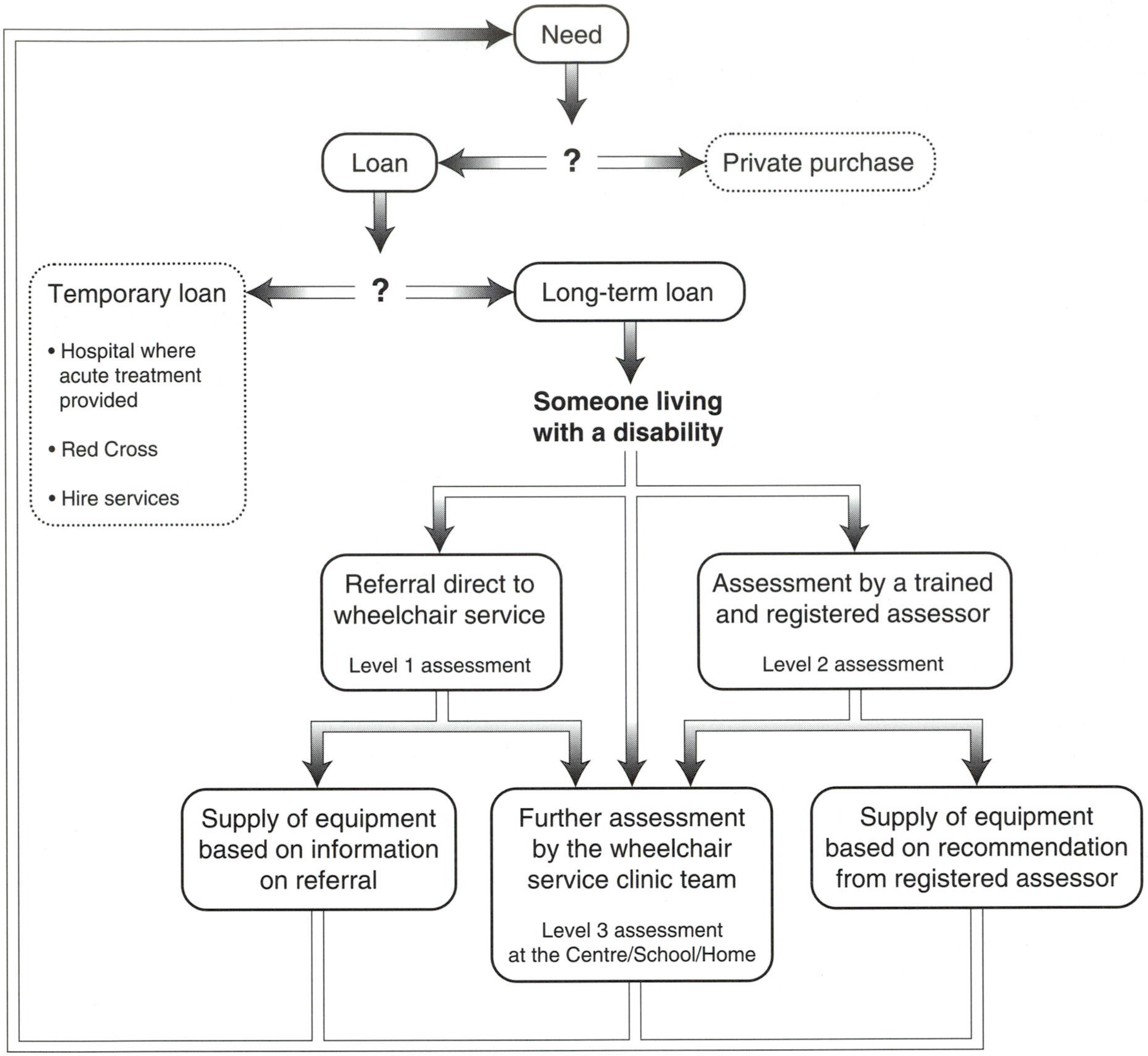

Figure 6.1 Flowchart showing potential routes for provision of equipment. (The wheelchair service is normally funded to provide equipment on a loan basis to people with a long-term disability.)

Level 2

Recommendations are normally accepted for basic models of wheelchair from therapists who are known to the service and who have attended a local training course. The recommendation made by the recognized assessor, on behalf of the wheelchair service, would usually be checked by a wheelchair service therapist or in some services a clerk. If the recommendation made appears to meet the user's needs and complies with the wheelchair service's policy guidelines, then the recommended equipment would be provided directly. Alternatively, an appointment might be made to see the user in order to carry out a more detailed assessment, if anything unacceptable or complicated is noted or if further assessment is requested by the trained assessor.

Action based on assessments at levels 1 and 2 may help to avoid the user having to spend time waiting unnecessarily for an assessment by wheelchair service staff. Most services, however, would prefer to be more involved in the assessment process, if the user's needs appear to be complex or the equipment recommended is outside a defined range.

Level 3

A full assessment by wheelchair clinic staff or joint assessment in conjunction with a specialist service following a tertiary referral.

An example of a referral form, or referral/ recommendation form, for each level is shown in Appendix 2.

REFERRAL

The source of an initial referral is usually a physiotherapist, occupational therapist, consultant or GP. An initial self-referral from the user might be accepted by some services, although the majority of services would require confirmation from the GP. Most services will subsequently accept self-referrals from the user after the initial referral.

Referral forms are usually designed to give essential information about the person being referred and the nature of the problem. If the form is too detailed there is a danger that it will not be completed fully; if it is too vague the wheelchair service clinic team may be unprepared for the specific nature of the problems being presented at a subsequent assessment appointment.

Where equipment is to be provided directly without the user being seen by the wheelchair clinic staff, it is important that basic information about the user should be included on the referral/recommendation form:

1. User details including: full name; date of birth; full address and previous address (if he/she has recently moved); alternative delivery addresses (e.g. school, day centre, etc.); telephone number; and alternative contact person if appropriate.
2. User's disability and secondary conditions.
3. User's GP.
4. User's weight in order to ensure it does not exceed weight limit of wheelchair provided.
5. Basic sitting measurements covered later in this chapter to ensure the wheelchair provided is an appropriate size.
6. Method of transfer which could influence choice of wheelchair, for example a user needing to transfer from the side will require detachable armrests, whereas someone transferring from the front will require swinging or detachable footrests.
7. Any specific information about the user's home, or other places where the wheelchair will be used, which should be taken into consideration when selecting a specific model of wheelchair. Obvious examples include where the doorways are of a limited width or where space for manoeuvring is restricted.
8. Any specific information related to how the wheelchair will be transported. This might include the need for the wheelchair to fold to a compact size to fit into the back of a car, the ease of lifting the wheelchair into the car, the suitability of the wheelchair if the user is to remain sitting in the wheelchair during transportation.
9. Relevant information required to relate to the wheelchair service's policy guidelines on provision, for example the potential level of use of, and dependency on, the wheelchair.

If an assessment by one of the wheelchair service clinic teams is required, the following information may be helpful to the wheelchair service before an assessment appointment is arranged:

1. Basic user details covered in 1–3 above.
2. Confirmation of the other relevant health care professionals and carers who are involved.
3. An indication of who, besides the potential wheelchair user, should attend the

assessment appointment and also how and when they can be contacted.

4. An indication of the preferred location for the assessment appointment.
5. The user's requirements related to how they will be transported to the appointment if it is not at their home.
6. The user's preferred means of transferring and whether special equipment will need to be available at the appointment.
7. An outline of the problem so that appropriate clinic staff, facilities and equipment can be made available.

WHERE SHOULD THE ASSESSMENT TAKE PLACE?

One of the most significant improvements made to the wheelchair service since the devolvement to local level has been to increase the number of assessments carried out at the user's home. Some services now aim to see all users at home, apart from children who are seen at their school, and users with complex needs who are sometimes seen at the wheelchair centre. This is a development which has been welcomed by users.

There can be various advantages and disadvantages associated with seeing each individual user at the wheelchair centre, their home, or elsewhere, and these are detailed below.

At the wheelchair centre

Advantages

● The wheelchair service's demonstration stock of wheelchairs, cushions, seating and accessories will be available so that a reasonable range of equipment can be seen and tried.
● Other equipment which may be needed in the assessment process will be more readily accessible such as a plinth, a set of assessment boxes, a positioning chair, a pressure monitor, a camera, reference literature, tools, etc.
● If appropriate stocks of equipment are kept at the wheelchair service base then equipment can be handed over at the assessment appointment. If certain specialized equipment needs to be adjusted and set up specifically for an individual user, then this can also be done at the assessment appointment and if successful, handed over, avoiding the need for a separate fitting appointment.
● Wheelchair service clinic staff can potentially see more people and therefore it can be a more efficient use of their time.

Disadvantages

● The user may feel anxious or intimidated by unfamiliar surroundings and people.
● The user may have difficulty getting to and from a central clinic and such transport problems may be compounded by their disability.
● Problems with the timing and reliability of ambulance transport can cause distress to the user, create delays and reduce flexibility when scheduling appointments. Sometimes difficulties are also experienced when trying to book transport that will bring the user to the centre with their existing wheelchair.

In the above circumstances the user is not being seen in their typical state and the value of the assessment is undermined.

● It is not possible to see the user's home or daily environment to get a better understanding of the practical needs.
● Non-attendance of appointments can be a problem, resulting in lost clinic time and prolonged waiting lists.

At the user's home

Advantages

● This option is generally welcomed by users and carers.
● The user is likely to be more relaxed in their home environment.
● The assessor can see first hand the home environment in order to get a better picture of the user's practical needs associated with the use of a wheelchair at home.
● It may be easier for relatives and carers to be present.

• Assuming the appropriate equipment is available, the user can have a chance to try it out in their own home environment.

• The rate of non-attendance is likely to be much lower than if appointments are carried out at a central clinic, as non-attendance at a home appointment is rare.

Disadvantages

• If the user has postural problems it can be harder to carry out a detailed level 3 physical assessment if there are no sufficiently firm, stable and accessible surfaces on which the user can lie and sit whilst joint ranges, pelvic position and spinal shape are examined. With children, however, it is relatively easy to take a floor mat and a set of assessment boxes.

• Less equipment will be available to try, unless sufficient information was received with the referral so that the assessor knows in advance what to take. The amount of equipment that can be taken also depends on the type of transport available to the assessor. Some services may have a van available for this purpose.

• It may also be necessary to schedule a number of additional appointments if the assessor has to return with alternative equipment to try or needs to arrange for minor modifications to be carried out to specialized equipment back at base.

• Depending on the area and the density of population covered by the wheelchair service, the number of appointments that can be managed within a finite time may be less due to the time the clinic staff spend travelling between appointments. This will have an effect on waiting times.

For a particular individual the relative advantages of one of the above options may outweigh the disadvantages. Some services offer both options but point out that waiting times might vary between options. In an ideal situation, however, the user should have the choice.

At school, day centre, etc.

An effective compromise can be to see a number of people at a 'satellite' or 'outreach' clinic. This can work well, particularly where the area covered is large, or where there is already a local day centre or specialist centre attended by a number of users. Schools, with a reasonable number of children with disabilities, can also be targeted as specific clinics.

Advantages

• Holding the clinic nearer to the user's home in a district that is relatively large may help to reduce the user's journey. More importantly, special transport will not be required as the user will already be attending the centre.

• The user can be seen in a familiar environment.

• Therapists, teachers, centre staff and carers, are available to be involved in the discussions at the assessment, and at fitting to try handling the equipment. Parents, relatives and other carers can also be invited to the satellite clinic.

• The session can be coordinated by the therapist at the school so that he or she decides the priority order for who should be seen in the time that the wheelchair service staff have dedicated to the clinic. For an adult day centre a therapist, centre manager or key case worker might be available to coordinate a clinic.

• If appointments overrun the child or adult is not kept waiting, assuming they are able to get on with what they would have been doing had they not had an appointment.

• If the clinic is run regularly the subsequent clinic can be used as a target date for a fitting appointment and also regular reviews can be planned.

• Clinic time is not lost travelling between appointments.

• There is an improvement in communication between the wheelchair service and the school, day centre, etc.

Although some of the disadvantages associated with the limited amount of equipment that can be easily transported still exist, it may be possible to base some assessment equipment at the satellite clinic venue if the wheelchair service budget allows. Alternatively, the repairer may be able to deliver and collect the necessary equipment on a set date.

WHO SHOULD BE PRESENT AT THE ASSESSMENT?

The key people are detailed below.

The wheelchair user

The wheelchair user is obviously the most important participant because without the user the appointment cannot proceed.

People associated with the wheelchair user

There will usually be other people who will have a direct interest in the wheelchair and seating needs of the user.

- It is essential that the key carer (e.g. parent, guardian, relative, friend, respite carer or foster carers) should attend the assessment, unless there is a particular reason why they cannot attend, or unless the user has requested to be seen on his or her own. The carer's view must be taken into account as they will often need to handle both the user and the equipment provided.
- It is important to involve the physiotherapist or occupational therapist who is most closely associated with the user in the community, at school or in hospital, who will know the user better than the wheelchair service clinical staff. Furthermore, any postural support provided should complement the overall programme of postural management being employed by this therapist. There is a danger, however, that if more than one such professional is involved this may inadvertently pull the user and wheelchair service in different directions, leading to confusion and wasted resources. Hence there is sometimes a need for a key therapist to be identified who is responsible for the individual's equipment management and who is able to liaise with all relevant services including the wheelchair service.

- There may be a specialist service involved working on the provision of equipment to assist communication, environmental switching or feeding. Posture and positioning in the wheelchair will be important in terms of the user's potential ability to use such equipment. Therefore it is essential to assess jointly at an early stage rather than passing the user back and forth between services.
- It is also possible the user's GP may be invited to attend or a link formed with an existing orthopaedic/paediatric clinic.

It is important that the wheelchair staff has a record of the key people involved with a particular user and is notified when they change.

The wheelchair service clinic team

The following professionals may have a specific role to play within an assessment team:

- physiotherapist
- occupational therapist
- rehabilitation technologist/rehabilitation engineer
- bioengineer/clinical engineer
- technician
- orthotist
- tissue viability nurse/dietician
- consultant in rehabilitation medicine, orthopaedics, neurology, the elderly, or a paediatrician.

Each professional potentially brings a different and complementary set of skills to the assessment team. Realistically, however, a multidisciplinary team of this size clearly would not be practical for all levels of assessment. Too many people in the clinic can be: an inefficient use of limited resources; intimidating for the user; or counterproductive due to a lack of focus. In addition, too many people can make the team less mobile to go out to see the user in their own environment and less flexible in scheduling appointments due to the greater number of diaries involved. Sometimes there is simply insufficient room in the clinic for so many people to work effectively.

Hence there is usually a need for a smaller team made up from varying numbers and combinations of the professionals listed. Different services tend to use different teams depending on the personnel available and the level of assessment required. For an assessment likely to result in the provision of standard equipment, with minor modifications or the addition of accessories, one individual from the above list such as a therapist may be sufficient. Most services employ a rehabilitation engineer who will attend the assessment appointment with a therapist and provide technical advice on how to achieve non-standard prescriptions.

A level 3 assessment team carrying out a full assessment on a user with complex needs will usually include a therapist who may need access to some of the other professionals listed above such as an orthotist, tissue viability nurse, dietician, technician, rehabilitation engineer, etc. Although many services do not have direct access to an identified consultant who has an interest in posture and mobility, there are advantages associated with the input that such a person can offer. Many people with complex postural problems can have a number of medical and orthopaedic problems that can affect the prescription. Alternatively, medication or surgery may be required in addition to appropriate seating. It is therefore useful to form a link with a paediatrician or consultant in rehabilitation medicine, orthopaedics, neurology or the elderly, as appropriate to the need.

There is also arguably a need for more staff with interdisciplinary training, such as a therapist trained in biomechanics or a bioengineer who has undergone training in the clinic environment (a certified clinical engineer) working directly with the user and the user's own therapist.

PHILOSOPHY BEHIND THE ASSESSMENT

In earlier times the wheelchair service remit was linked quite strictly to mobility so that only the mobility aspect of an individual's need was considered. Sometimes this could in fact reduce rather than increase a user's independence: Professor Ted Marsland is recorded in the original Wheelchair Training Pack (Department of Health 1991) as saying that he thought the wheelchair he had been given was designed specifically to keep him in one room. Professor (now Lord) McColl, however, recognized the need for wheelchair prescription to meet daily living needs as well as mobility needs in his report of 1986. The importance of postural support was also recognized officially in 1986 when John Major, the Minister of Health at that time, announced that the provision of wheelchair-based seating should be included in the wheelchair service's role.

The remit has evolved and is now more a case of trying to meet both clinical and practical objectives with the aim of enhancing mobility, comfort, ability, independence and posture. Another important goal is to prevent secondary disabilities from occurring.

Whilst assessment should identify clinical and functional needs, it is also equally important to listen to the user in terms of what he or she wants to achieve, and the fact that it may be necessary to compromise if the user's expectations and preferences do not match the clinical prescription – there is no value in prescribing something that is not going to be used.

It is essential that the assessment procedure is consultative, i.e. involves the wheelchair user and offers choice.

BASIC MEASUREMENTS TO BE TAKEN AT THE ASSESSMENT

Several user measurements will be needed at all levels of assessment so that appropriate wheelchair or seating can be selected. These are shown in Figure 6.2 and listed below.

Seat depth

A measurement from behind the knee (popliteal fossa) to the back of the pelvis/sacrum will help to determine the desirable seat depth. Approximately 2.5–5 cm is removed from the former measurement so that the front of the seat canvas

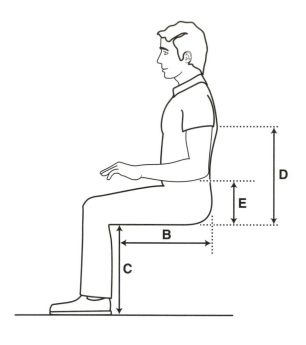
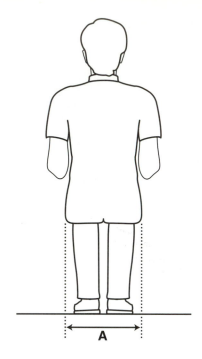

Measurement

(A)	Distance between hips or shoulders (+5cm)	Seat width
(B)	Popliteal fossa to back of buttock (–5cm)	Seat depth
(C)	Leg length – popliteal fossa to heel base	Legrests
(D)	Buttock base to scapula	Backrest height
(E)	Buttock to olecranon with elbows flexed at 90°	Armrest height

Note Use a steel measure
User should be clothed and wearing normal shoes

Figure 6.2 Basic user measurements.

is not directly in contact with the nerves and vessels of the popliteal fossa. If the wheelchair seat is too long the tendency will be for the pelvis to slip anteriorly and tilt posteriorly. This could encourage pressure and shear forces to be applied to the relatively thin tissue covering the sacrum. If the seat depth is too short the thigh will not be fully supported, which is likely to result in increased pressure over the reduced area in contact with the seat.

Seat width

The width across the hips will determine the minimum wheelchair seat width. Clearance of between 1–2.5 cm is left between the user and the skirt guard an each side in order to: avoid pressure being applied to the tissues over the greater trochanter; to allow room for the user to adjust posture and lift to relieve pressure; and to accommodate thicker winter clothing.

Armrest height

The desired height of support for the upper limbs in relation to the seat should be noted. At an appropriate height the upper limbs should be supported without the shoulder being elevated or without the user needing to drop the shoulder to reach the armrest. A seat cushion will obviously raise the user and should be taken into account. The wheelchair armrest height, size or shape may need changing, or a tray might be needed, where more postural support is required. Besides supporting the upper limbs the armrest should ideally be an appropriate height to assist in transferring or lifting to relieve pressure. It can be more difficult for the user to reach the propelling wheels if the armrests are too high.

Backrest height and angle

The ideal backrest height will vary depending on the needs of the user, however, it is often taken as the height from the seat to just beneath the scapula. The height of the backrest might need to be lower for an active user to allow more freedom of arm movement and higher for a user requiring more postural support. The angle of the backrest might need to be varied to suit an individual user if the user wants to be more upright or alternatively is unable to maintain an upright posture. Care should be taken if the backrest is reclined without appropriate measures to prevent the user's pelvis from slipping anteriorly in the seat as this is likely to result in postural instability and dangerous shear forces. In this case it is often better if the seat and backrest are tilted together to maintain a constant angle at the hips.

Footrest height

The leg length or height measured from the popliteal fossa to the heel base can be used to set the wheelchair footrests to an appropriate height. This measurement should be taken with the user wearing the type of shoes that he or she would normally wear. Ideally, the thighs should be in contact with, and supported by, the seat and 25% of the body weight should be taken through the footplates with the remainder through the seat. If the footrests are too high there will be a gap under the anterior part of the thigh and the user will take more weight under the pelvis, increasing the pressure over the ischial tuberosities. If the footrests are too low the user will not be supported under the feet, resulting in more load and greater pressure under the anterior part of the thigh, and the user is less likely to maintain 90 degrees of hip flexion, resulting in an increased tendency for the pelvis to slip anteriorly on the seat.

Seat height

Besides being important for transfers and allowing access to tables, seat height can be important in order to allow some users to propel themselves with one or both feet. They will therefore require the seat to be low enough to the ground for effective propulsion. A hemiplegic user may require a compromise seat height so that the one foot can be comfortably supported on a footplate and the other can reach the ground.

User's weight

The individual's weight will be relevant where there is concern that it may exceed the weight limit of an otherwise appropriate wheelchair.

Box 6.1 lists and summarizes typical problems relating to an ill-fitting wheelchair which can easily result from inaccurate or missing measurement information. Such problems are also demonstrated in Figure 6.3.

Where the user needs to self-propel and there is a choice of position of the propelling wheels, or where seating might affect the position of the user, consideration should be given to the ergonomic factors related to self-propulsion (discussed in Ch. 3). Alternatively, where the wheelchair is to be propelled by the attendant, basic ergonomic factors such as the height of the push handles should be taken into account.

When specialized seating is to be provided, following a level 3 assessment, additional information about the user related to the type of

Box 6.1   Some problems that can result from inappropriate wheelchair prescription. (From Department of Health 1991, with permission)

1. SEAT WIDTH
   a. Too narrow
      — No room for user to adjust sitting position by lifting in the seat or wriggling
      — Undue pressure on bony points and skin may lead to pressure sores
      — Lack of allowance on seat width may lead to difficulty getting out of chair
      — Some extra space will also be needed for thicker and warmer clothes in colder weather, especially if the chair is to be used out of doors.

   b. Too wide
      — More difficulty than necessary manoeuvring chair in confined spaces
      — The pelvis can roll in chair which can lead to poor sitting position and postural deformities
      — More energy required to propel chair.

2. SEAT LENGTH
   a. Too short
      — Part of thigh unsupported with undue pressure on the back of the thigh, which could lead to hindrance of the circulation
      — The user may be unable to sit relaxed and comfortably owing to the lack of sufficient support.

   b. Too long
      — Unable to bend knees to 90 degrees
      — Undue pressure on the back of the calf
      — The pelvis may tilt posteriorly resulting in a rounded back.

3. SEAT HEIGHT
   a. Too low
      — Footplates foul on the ground
      — The hips and knees are overflexed
      — Unnecessary pressure on abdomen and chest, preventing satisfactory functioning of internal organs
      — Anterior part of thigh unsupported and greater load taken through the ischial tuberosities.

   b. Too high
      — The user may have to move body forwards in order to get feet onto the floor to transfer or to rest feet on footrests

      — The feet may not reach footrests, in which case they will be unsupported and that could lead to discomfort, deformity and/or pressure problems

4. ARMRESTS
   a. Too high
      — The user may have to sit with hunched shoulders if resting elbows on armrests, causing poor functioning of the chest and sitting with the chin poking forward
      — Too much pressure on elbows could cause pressure sores
      — There may be difficulty getting near to tables.

   b. Too low
      — User may have to lean forwards or sideways in order to use armrests which will lead to poor sitting posture
      — Having to lean to use armrests can impede breathing
      — With some users there is a great danger of them falling out of the chair if they sit leaning forwards.

5. FOOTRESTS
   a. Too low
      — The feet may drop because they are not supported
      — The user may shuffle body forwards in order to support feet and this leads to poor posture.
      — Pressure on the back of the thigh from lack of support for feet
      — The chair may not run smoothly over a rough surface because there is not sufficient clearance. The minimum clearance should be 2 inches (5 cm)
      — Lack of clearance of obstacles could lead to client being tipped out of chair.

   b. Too high
      — Flexion of hip and knee leading to fixed deformity. Discomfort from pressure on pelvis. Compression of the abdomen perhaps leading to digestive and constipation problems.

seating will be required. For example, in order to position lateral thoracic supports appropriately it would be necessary to know the seat to axilla height and width across the trunk. Ultimately, if a custom-contoured seat is to be made a record of the user's three-dimensional shape, when appropriately supported, would be required. This is usually achieved using a cast or scanning device.

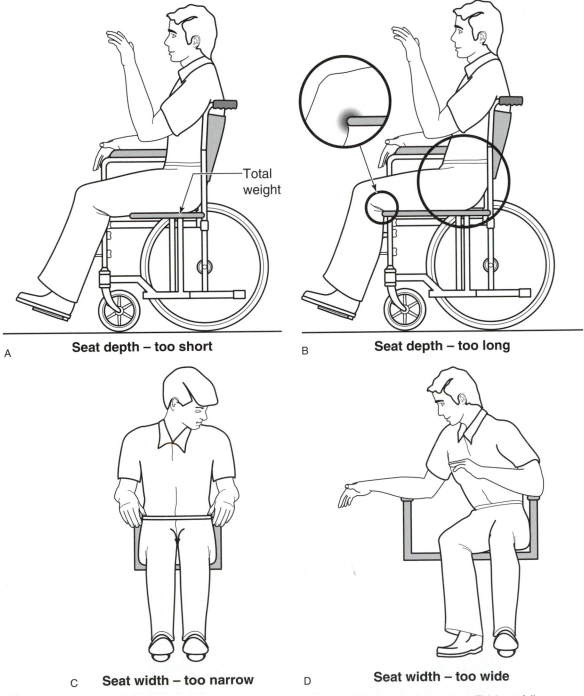

A   **Seat depth – too short**

B   **Seat depth – too long**

Total weight

C   **Seat width – too narrow**

D   **Seat width – too wide**

Figure 6.3A–D   Example of problems caused by an ill-fitting wheelchair. (A) Seat depth too short. Thigh not fully supported, increasing pressure under ischial tuberosities and reducing stability. (B) Seat depth too long. Pressure on nerves and vessels of popliteal fossa and tendency to encourage pelvis to tilt posteriorly leading to sacral sitting. (C) Seat width too narrow. Pressure on greater trochanters and restricted movement, and hence pressure relief, in the wheelchair. (D) Seat width too wide. Sitting stability reduced, self-propulsion more difficult and potential environmental access problems. If seat canvas sags there may be shear stresses generated in the lateral margin of the thigh.

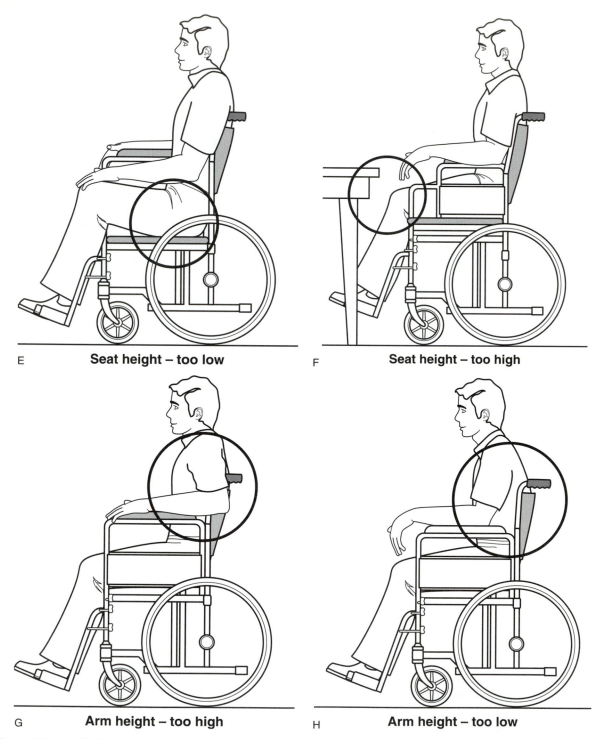

E   **Seat height – too low**   F   **Seat height – too high**

G   **Arm height – too high**   H   **Arm height – too low**

Figure 6.3E–H   (E) Seat height too low. At the correct footrest height the footplates may foul on the ground, kerbs, etc. and if as a result the footrests are raised there will be increased pressure under ischial tuberosities. (F) Seat height too high. Potential problems reaching propelling wheels and with knees not fitting under tables. (G) Armrest too high. More difficult for user to reach propelling wheels and shoulders elevated, causing poor posture and muscle fatigue. If armrest not used then potential for instability. (H) Armrest too low. User has to 'stoop' to put arms on armrests leading to 'slumped' kyphotic posture.

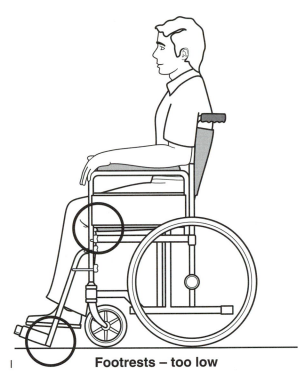

Footrests – too low

Figure 6.3 (I) Footrests too low. Feet unsupported and greater loading and pressure under anterior part of thigh. Potential for footrest to foul on ground, kerbs, etc. (A–I from Department of Health, 1991, with permission)

RELEVANT FACTORS

A first step may be to provide the new user with a checklist to run through before they have an assessment appointment. This may help them to think about the things they want to do, where they want to go, what space they have, etc., and also to think about priorities.

As an assessor, it is easy to react to a first impression of a problem. Correcting a problem in one area, however, can sometimes create a new problem somewhere else. For example, fitting lateral pelvic supports, an abductor build up and adductor wedges to a seat cushion might improve positioning of the pelvis and hips but it might also prevent that person carrying out sliding transfers on which he or she relies for independence. It is therefore worth taking a step back so that you can consider the overall situation from both a clinical and practical point of view.

It often helps to have an assessment form to work through so that the assessor is prompted to ask about factors that may be relevant. Not all the questions on a detailed assessment form will be relevant for everyone but it is better to skip over sections that are not relevant for a particular individual rather than leaving them off the form and consequently failing to cover a particular subject matter with someone for whom that subject is particularly relevant. On the other hand, no matter how detailed the assessment form there may well be other factors, not specifically referred to on the form, which may be relevant for a particular individual. Therefore scope should be left for general questions which may allow the user to volunteer the relevant information.

There are many different types of assessment form currently in use with many services developing their own. It is up to the individual assessor or wheelchair service to decide which type of form they are most comfortable working with. A number of factors that may be relevant for a particular individual are listed below. They are taken from an assessment form developed at the Dundee Limb Fitting Centre shown in Appendix 2 (Tayside Rehabilitation Engineering Services Seating Assessment Form).

Although it might not be possible to go into such detail at a level 1 or 2 assessment, the assessor should be able to identify general problems and if necessary refer the user for a higher level assessment.

Background medical factors

The basic user information requested on the referral form (listed in the section on 'Referral' in this chapter), like the primary diagnosis / cause of disability and any relevant secondary conditions, should be checked. In addition the following information about the user's medical history and current status should be considered.

Surgery

For example:

● Having previously undergone an adductor

tenotomy to correct a hip problem, there may be a danger that the problem will re-occur.

- Surgery may be planned for the near future which might significantly change the user's posture.

Neurological summary

For example:

- The extent of motor deficit which may be related to the user's ability to propel, transfer, adjust posture, or lift to relieve pressure.
- The level and degree of sensory deficit might be linked to pressure sore susceptibility.
- If there is a need to take the user out of the seating in a hurry during an epileptic seizure the use of some types of intimate support may be ruled out.

Pressure sores

For example:

- Pressure sore history as sites of scarring will be more susceptible to new pressure problems.
- Current status of existing sores as an open sore will require careful consideration.
- General susceptibility to pressure problems including intrinsic and extrinsic risk factors and ability to adjust posture or lift to relieve pressure. Pressure management is covered in Chapter 12.

Continence

For example:

- Whether the user is incontinent of urine, faeces or both.
- The preferred method of management and incontinence aids used, both of which may influence the choice of cushion/seating materials or the intimacy of support.

Cardiovascular problems

For example:

- It may be dangerous for a user to self-propel due to a heart or respiratory condition.

- An individual might have a respiratory problem which is exacerbated when he/she is reclined or tilted or which requires an oxygen cylinder/nebulizer/suction unit to be carried on the wheelchair.
- A person with certain types of cardiovascular problem is more likely to be at risk of developing a pressure sore.

Pain or discomfort when seated

For example:

- A muscular or joint pain due to posture in the seat.
- A pain due to a pressure concentration caused by a part of the seating.

Behavioural patterns

For example, some users might involuntarily rock backwards and forwards creating concerns about stability.

Orthotic/prosthetic provision

For example, a user may be seen at the assessment without an orthosis although it is intended that they will wear the orthosis when using the wheelchair/seating.

Trends or changes in condition

For example, it is important to know if the condition is stable, deteriorating (and if so what the prognosis is), improving or if it varies (perhaps during the course of the day, month or with temperature, etc.). This should help to determine if the user is being seen at the assessment in a fairly typical state or not.

Other trends

For example, trends in weight or growth may also be significant as a seat or wheelchair based on measurements taken at the assessment may be the wrong size if the user has grown, gained or lost weight rapidly.

Other relevant factors

Other conditions that whilst not directly affecting mobility may affect the prescription, such as the presence of a heart condition placing a limit on the user's allowed level of exertion. Other factors might include:

- presence of oedema
- use of diuretics
- use of TNS
- presence of nerve blocks
- mental or psychological state (refer to Ch. 5).

Physical examination

For a full physical assessment in the specialist clinic it is helpful to have a plinth, which is preferably height adjustable and sufficiently wide for the assessor to sit or kneel behind the individual being assessed. If the plinth is not height adjustable then it will be necessary to place something of an appropriate height under the sitting subject's feet to provide support. Alternatively, a set of interlocking boxes of different heights can be a compact and portable way to achieve a firm surface for sitting of variable height.

The importance of the variables listed below are discussed in more detail in Chapters 3 and 4 and equipment for measuring some of these variables is covered later in this chapter.

Joint ranges

In a specialist clinic situation an investigation of active and passive ranges of joint movement should be carried out in both lying (supine) and sitting positions in order to determine abilities and joint range limitations in these positions. The integrity of the joint (if subluxed or dislocated) and any limitation in joint range, due to a muscle tightness or shortening, may affect the choice of seating and wheelchair. For example, a unilateral hip extension contracture may need to be accommodated by a negative ramp on the same side in order to avoid exacerbating a pelvic obliquity and hence contributing to a scoliosis (Carlson et al 1986).

Skeletal anomalies

For example:

- rib cage deformity
- femur length discrepancy
- bone weakness

will need to be taken into account or accommodated when providing seating.

Shape of spine

If possible the shape of the back and spine should be recorded in both:

- lying (prone), when the spine is not being compressed due to gravity acting on the upper body, and
- sitting when the upper body is subjected to gravity.

It may be necessary to use different references, for example the pelvis when prone and the vertical when sitting. By supporting the user when sitting on the plinth it should be possible to note whether the spinal deformity is structural and fixed or postural and flexible.

Position of pelvis

It is helpful to record the orientation of the pelvis when the user is supported in an acceptable sitting position with the head over the pelvic base. An understanding of whether the pelvis is oblique, rotated or tilted in relation to major axes is essential when formulating any biomechanical seating strategy. For example:

- A fixed pelvic obliquity may need to be accommodated to prevent excessive pressure under the ischial tuberosity on the lower side.
- It may be advisable to attempt to oppose the deterioration of a pelvic rotation or posterior pelvic tilt using a kneeblock and sacral support or an alternative approach.

Trunk stability

The degree of trunk stability, direction of instability and cause of instability should be investigated. For example, a user who leans heavily to one side might need to use one arm to prop him or herself up constantly, preventing that arm from being used effectively. Supporting the trunk directly may allow the arm to be freed and used for other activities.

Head control

The degree of head control, direction of instability and cause of instability are relevant. For example, a head that tends to fall to either side can be supported using a headrest shaped to provide some lateral support.

Muscle tone and pattern

It is important to note whether the user is hyper- or hypotonic, or dystonic and also if there are any influences on muscle tone such as the user's posture or orientation in space which would need to be taken into account when providing seating. The general muscle pattern (extensor or flexor) that is evident should also be noted.

Primitive reflexes

The retention of any primitive reflexes such as an ATNR, STNR, Galant, Moro, startle, etc. should be taken into account, along with any specific factors which are likely to trigger certain reflexes. Reflexes are discussed in Chapter 2.

Ability

General sitting ability can be measured using an established scale such as the Chailey score (Fearn et al 1992, Green & Nelham 1991, Mulcahy 1988) (see Appendix 1). Other scales exist that look at ability to perform everyday activities (Hallett, Hare & Milner 1987). These can be used in relation to an overall programme of postural management aimed at encouraging the development of ability to the next level.

Functional considerations

Activities of daily living

For example:

- A means of achieving a preferred posture and head position for eating may need to be included in the seating.
- The need to use a bottle for toileting may rule out the use of a ramped or intimately contoured seat base, or alternatively influence the type of cushion cover required.

Interests, hobbies, work/school activities

All the activities undertaken by the user when sitting in the wheelchair, and which may potentially be influenced by the choice of wheelchair and seating, should be taken into account. It would be a shame if only after the provision of a new wheelchair it was discovered that the new wheelchair prevented the user from doing something that he or she needed or wanted to do.

Transfer technique

For example, consideration should be given to:

- The height of the cushion, the cushion cover material, and the presence of obstacles like lateral supports when carrying out a sliding side transfer.
- The need for removable/swing-away footrests for transfers in and out of the wheelchair from the front.
- The intimacy of fit of supportive seating if there is a need to apply and remove a hoist sling.

Transportation

For example:

- If the wheelchair and seating is to be transported in the back of a car it will need to fold or dismantle to an extent depending on the space available in the car.
- If the user is to be transported sitting in the

wheelchair and seating this will usually limit the choice of equipment to that which has been tested and approved for such a purpose.

Communication

For example, consideration should be given to the suitability of the wheelchair and seating if a communication device, a computer or switching is going to be fitted and used.

Clothing

The user's normal choice of clothing and shoes may also need to be taken into account when providing equipment. For example, a user may be assessed when wearing a different height of shoe to that which they would normally wear or a child might imminently be expecting a larger size of boot to be supplied. This would influence the height at which the footrests should be set or the size of footcup required. The thickness of clothing normally worn and the type of material should also be taken into account.

An attempt should be made to find out if there are any other practical considerations for user or carer that might be relevant to the choice of wheelchair or seating.

Environmental considerations

As well as discussing how the wheelchair and seating will be used, it is also important to find out about the main environments in which they will be used. Such environments might include the user's home, school, workplace, community, respite care, foster home or day centre.

Access and manoeuvrability

Consideration should be given to the limitations imposed by:

- narrow doors
- narrow hallways
- an awkward layout of doors

- steps
- limited space of turning
- the size of a through the floor lift
- even the type of flooring.

It will be necessary to compromise on other objectives if the alternative is that the wheelchair could not be used in a primary or secondary environment. Good communication between the wheelchair service and community occupational therapists can be helpful where adaptations to the home are needed.

Furniture

For example, if access to a particular table or desk is required the height of the wheelchair or style of armrests will be significant.

A checklist of points to consider when prescribing a wheelchair for use at home, taken from the Wheelchair Training Resource Pack (Department of Health 1996), is shown in Box 6.2.

PRESCRIPTION

The prescription process is summarized in Figure 6.4.

It is good practice to discuss and summarize all the problems that have been reported or identified during the course of the assessment. The specific objectives can then be agreed.

Discussion about the clinical and practical objectives should include:

- An explanation and understanding of any compromises between specific objectives as one objective may not be achievable without compromising on another. Often the postural objectives conflict with practical objectives. For example: (a) the more support provided within a seat the more difficult it can be for the user to transfer; or (b) aiming for a variable tilt in space facility often means providing a wheelchair with a longer wheel base, increased size and hence reduced manoeuvrability.
- A common understanding of priorities. The priority according to the user is most impor-

Box 6.2   Checklist for the wheelchair user at home
A few essential points to consider when prescribing a wheelchair for use in the home. (From Department of Health 1996, with permission)

INDOORS
- Access
  — Steps both to front/back door and inside
  — Space for ramp (gradient 1 : 12)
  — Door widths 30 inches/770 mm is minimum
- Stairs
  — Can the user live on one floor?
  — Is wheelchair lift needed?
- Toilet
  — Position of WC for transfers
  — Height of WC
- Bathroom
  — How will patient transfer?
  — Is shower required – if so can the floor be graded?
  — Access to washbasin
- Bedroom
  — Position of bed for transfers
  — Floor covering
- Kitchen
  — Who is main user?
  — Do work surfaces need to be altered?
- Living room
  — Turning space
  — Height of furniture
  — Floor covering.

GENERAL
- Turning space
  — 3 inch (75 mm) radius for 17 × 17 inch (43 cm × 43 cm) seat size standard self-propelling wheelchair
- Heights for
  — Light switches
  — Door handles
  — Working surfaces
  — Transfers
- Floor surfaces
  — Loose rugs; broken lino; pile carpet
- Windows
  — Height and type of fastening.

These are just a few brief points to remember. There are many more to consider if any adaptation to the home is needed and the plans may take several months to put into operation. Can the patient cope until the alterations are carried out?

OUTDOORS
- Home environment
  — Width of gate and path
  — Gradient of slopes and ramps
  — Width of front door and direction of opening
  — Surface of ground, e.g. gravel path

  — Height of key hole and door handle
  — Steps to the front and back of property
  — Special clothing requirements
- Transport considerations
  — Are parking facilities near the house?
  — Can wheelchair be lifted into car?
  — Will a car hoist be necessary?
  — Is there close access to the car seat for transfers?
  — Should the user be referred for advice for a driving assessment?
  — Is there an alternative means of transport, i.e. Dial-a-Ride/Taxi card?
- Local support groups
- Access guides
  — Availability varies from area to area. Usually free from town halls or council offices. Provide information on the following:

Adult education	Parks
Banks – reach counter/ cash point	Public buildings
	Pubs
Churches	Shopping facilities
Clubs	Sports facilities
Dropped kerbs/ pelican crossings	Theatres/cinemas
	Toilets – National
GP surgeries	Key Scheme
Parking facilities – contact your Social Services for Orange Badge details	

OTHER CONSIDERATIONS
- If returning to work. Should an application be made to PACT through the Access to Work Scheme? (Details in pack.)
- If user has a child at school. Has access to the school building been considered?
- Local environment. Is there availability of dropped kerbs in area, particularly for indoor/outdoor wheelchair users?
- Road/pavement. Are there broken slabs or road works? Contact the local council for any queries concerning access problems.
- Transport
  — Is a conversion or wheelchair car hoist required? Consult the local DLC or Mobility centre. (Details in pack.)
  — Public transport details from transport information centres or see 'Choosing a Wheelchair' (RADAR) or DLF information centre. (See Further reading section.)
  — Dial-a-Ride. Details from local authority/social services.

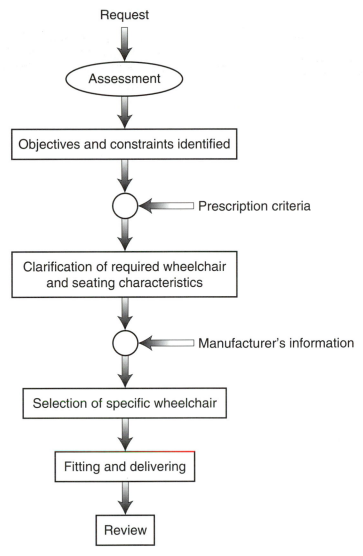

Request

Assessment

Objectives and constraints identified

Prescription criteria

Clarification of required wheelchair and seating characteristics

Manufacturer's information

Selection of specific wheelchair

Fitting and delivering

Review

Figure 6.4 The prescription process.

tant. For example, no matter how strongly clinic staff feel that postural management should be the priority, the decision can only really be made by the user, parent, etc. Clinic staff, however, should aim to clearly explain the risks associated with not tackling potential postural problems and record this in their report.

• Consideration of the wheelchair service guidelines on provision, specific eligibility criteria and budgetary constraints. Where equipment is to be provided by the Health Service consideration should be given to the individual's eligibility for specific equipment based on the service specification agreed with the funding organization.

The next stage is to identify and discuss the options that are to be offered. This should include:

• An explanation about the potential advantages and disadvantages of each of the options identified in terms of the original objectives. The limitations of equipment should be made clear at an early stage to avoid disappointment later.

- If possible a demonstration of the suggested equipment. If the equipment is not available to try it is often helpful to have brochures or pictures.
- Where appropriate, a trial of the equipment which might involve a chance to either: sit in and propel a wheelchair; sit on a pressure-relieving cushion; or alternatively have a trial fitting of an adjustable modular seat.

Initially at least, consideration should be given to standard equipment held in local stock. If the needs cannot be met from a standard range of basic models, then it will usually be necessary to consider equipment outside the standard range. This will require good knowledge of the increasing range of equipment available.

Additional assessment or training may be necessary before a final prescription is reached in the situation where specialized equipment is being provided, such as an indoor/outdoor powered wheelchair.

If at the end of the assessment process there is a choice to be made, the final choice from the range offered should be left to the user or parent. Where possible a choice of colour, upholstery, etc. might also be offered. This is sometimes not possible with standard stocks of equipment but is more manageable with the more specialized types of wheelchairs and certain types of seating.

A range of accessories and modifications are available but it is important to confirm: why they are required; that they will be used; and that they will improve the mobility, comfort, function, independence or posture of the user. As a general rule the simpler the package of equipment provided the better. For example, an extended footrest whilst providing better support for the foot can make folding the wheelchair more difficult, will increase the length and make the overall turning circle of the wheelchair larger, and can restrict access to work tops. Another example would be an extended brake lever which may make it easier to apply the brake but may also get in the way of a sideways transfer.

TRIAL AND FINAL FITTING

Often standard equipment can be delivered directly to the user. With more specialized equipment, however, a fitting appointment is advisable so that the wheelchair, cushion or seating equipment can be adjusted, tried, and its success judged in terms of the original objectives and expectations. Time can also be spent explaining and demonstrating important features of the equipment to the user and carer, such as how a seating system can be dismantled or folded. It may also be necessary to carry out a stability test at the final fitting appointment if a seating system is used which is likely to shift the user's centre of gravity within the wheelchair.

A trial fitting before the final fitting is often advisable where customized seating is required or where the success or otherwise of one element of the seating will determine the choice of other elements.

In the case of a custom contoured seat insert, a trial fitting can allow:

- the shape achieved at the previous positioning and casting session to be checked
- the edges of the seat to be trimmed appropriately
- the location of anchor points for any straps to be marked
- the desired orientation of the seat insert within the wheelchair chassis to be recorded.

At this stage the seating need not be finished or upholstered to allow for further modifications.

It should also be possible at the trial fitting to picture how the user, seating and wheelchair chassis will come together so that other variables, which may have been difficult to predict at the initial assessment, can be clarified. A typical example of this is the optimum positioning of support for the feet, upper limbs and head.

More than one trial fitting might be needed before a final fitting can be arranged when the completed system can be tried and hopefully handed over. With more experience and confidence, however, it may be possible to miss out the trial fitting stage with certain types of seating, hence reducing the time from assessment to provision.

Whichever route is used to hand over the equipment, it is essential that certain basic information about the equipment and service is also provided to the user. This should include:

1. The conditions of loan explaining the basis on which the equipment is made available to the user.
2. The user's obligation of care for the equipment.
3. Information on maintenance such as the importance of keeping the tyres inflated (and what problems may arise if they are under or unevenly inflated), or the battery charged, etc.
4. Advice on what to do and who to contact in case of a technical problem or in case the user's needs change.

It may also be helpful to give the user further information about where to go for advice on related matters or equipment such as a hoist to lift the wheelchair into the car, waterproof clothing and accessories for hobbies.

REVIEW

Suggested review procedures are summarized in Box 6.3.

If possible a review date should be set following provision rather than waiting for a problem to occur. The period agreed between provision and review will depend on factors such as prognosis, age and condition of the user. Ideally all users with needs that are changing, whether due to growth and development or as a result of an improving or deteriorating condition, should be reviewed on a regular basis every 6 or 12 months. Users with degenerative neurological conditions (see Ch. 7) in particular will require an ongoing review of their changing needs.

An active review procedure for all users can be difficult to achieve, however, due to the low staffing levels, high numbers of new referrals and pressure of waiting lists currently experienced by most services. Where a user is being seen by a therapist on a regular basis, ongoing review can sometimes be undertaken during regular treatment and rehabilitation, providing the therapist involved is well informed and understands the purpose of the review.

In many cases the user is the best person to advise when their needs have changed and are no longer being met by the equipment provided. It is important, therefore, that clear information is given stating who the user or carer should contact if a clinical or technical problem arises. Close liaison between wheelchair service staff and therapists, or other professionals, in the community is also essential. If responsibility for notifying the wheelchair service of any problems is passed to other professionals, this should be clearly communicated with both the professional and the user or carer, and also documented.

Where an individual has postural problems and has been supplied with a specialized seating system, it is important to review regularly to ensure the seating is still fulfilling the original objectives and to monitor changing needs.

Box 6.3 Suggested review procedures. (From Newham Wheelchair Service, with permission)

Initial review
- Check that the specifications of the wheelchair delivered are the same as those ordered
- Fit the wheelchair to the user
- Instruct on the use of the cushion
- Check that the wheelchair meets the user's and attendant's expectations
- Check the home environment
- Check on the maintenance and safety aspects of the wheelchair
- Monitor supply factors

Regular review
- Check that the wheelchair meets the user's and attendant's requirements, especially noting developmental and deterioration factors
- Review the prescribed model and accessories in view of new developments (physical and hardware)
- Check on maintenance and safety factors

OBJECTIVE MEASUREMENT IN ASSESSMENT

A thorough physical assessment on a user with severe disability relies on a significant amount of subjective judgement to estimate variables such as joint angle, spinal shape, interface pressure and muscle tone. Although the judgement of some experienced clinicians may be reliable, there is a growing need for a more scientific approach to measurement in the assessment process. This requires measuring tools that are sufficiently accurate, affordable and practical for use in the wheelchair and seating clinic environment.

Measurements can improve understanding of the problem, objectives and limitations, particularly for people with changing conditions who require greater attention paid to the influence of posture on optimum function such as the ability to propel and carry out daily activities. Objective measurement is also useful for comparison when monitoring change.

Joint angles

Joint ranges, tested passively by a clinician, are one example of a variable that is usually estimated by eye with uncertain accuracy.

Some simple hinged goniometers can give a more accurate estimation of the joint angle attained. A simple example of this type of goniometer is where two clear plastic segments articulate and show a reference pointer on a graduated scale (Fig. 6.5A).

Electro-goniometers are also available which incorporate a potentiometer at the hinge which generates a voltage signal proportional to the angular displacement. The signal representing the angle can then be processed and displayed or recorded automatically. These types of goniometer measure angular displacement in only one plane and the hinge must be directly over the centre of rotation of the joint. Most anatomical joints, however, do not behave like a hinge and the instantaneous centre of rotation moves as the joint angle varies. Furthermore, the clinician may be interested in measuring the angle on more than one axis; for example, flexion/extension, abduction/adduction and internal/external rotation of the hip.

Other more sophisticated types of flexible electro-goniometer have been developed, one of which consists of two end pieces, which are aligned with the joint segments, and connected by a flexible strain-gauged beam (Fig. 6.5B). This

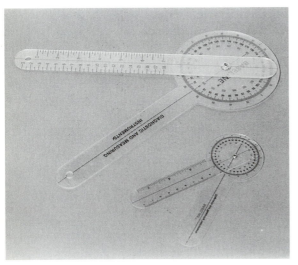

A

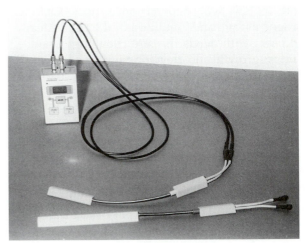

B

Figure 6.5 Examples of goniometers for joint angle measurement. (A) Simple mechanical goniometer. (B) Flexible electro-goniometer (Penny & Giles Biometric Ltd).

type of goniometer theoretically measures the angle between the end pieces in more than one plane and does not rely on a fixed centre of rotation. Tests on early designs, however, showed inaccuracies associated with cross talk between axes (i.e. under certain circumstances such as one end being twisted in relation to the other there were errors in the angular readings).

Although all the above goniometers can give a reasonably accurate measurement of joint angle, they rely heavily on accurate alignment of the arms of the goniometer with the adjacent limb segments. Considerable variability can occur between different operators or even between different applications by the same operator (Goodwin et al 1992, Mayerson & Milano 1984), although this is perhaps still better than the variability achieved when the joint angle is estimated visually (Watkins et al 1991).

It is important to stabilize the pelvis when measuring hip flexion, otherwise a posteriorly tilted pelvis may be compensated by the spine giving a misleading impression that 90 degrees of hip flexion can be achieved. It should also be remembered that the surface tissue is likely to move in relation to the underlying skeletal structure which might obscure the true joint angle.

Back/spinal shape

In the wheelchair and seating clinic, back shape and estimates of spinal shape are usually described in words or using a sketch. It is difficult, however, to quantify spinal deformity from such information.

If time is available more information can be recorded by taking a photograph with markers placed on the posterior superior iliac spine of the pelvis and the posterior processes of the vertebrae. In order to allow comparison over time it is important that all subsequent photographs are taken from an identical position.

Imaging techniques such as X-ray and magnetic resonance imaging are commonly used in the orthopaedic clinic to monitor and measure spinal deformity, especially in children. Angles, such as the Cobb angle (Cobb 1948, Morrissy

et al 1990), indicating lateral asymmetry, can be recorded from the image generated. The surface topography of the back can also be monitored less intrusively using techniques based on the use of light. Two such techniques are ISIS scanning (Weisz et al 1988) and Moire fringe topography (Sahlstrand 1986). Sagittal, coronal and transverse sections can be generated from the surface topography and, using appropriate algorithms, it is possible to predict the path of the spine and hence quantify displacement, asymmetry and rotation (Fig. 6.6).

The above techniques rely on the subject being unsupported in front of the scanner and if such information is available to the seating team it may help to raise awareness of change and avoid an attempt to achieve the impossible.

Theoretically such equipment could also be used to investigate the influence of postural support on spinal shape. Although direct imaging of the back through the postural support would not be possible, as the light would be obscured, it is possible to scan the positive cast taken from the negative impression of the subject. Such casts are taken routinely in the production of most custom contoured seats. Direct comparison between the scan of the unsupported back and that of the supported back should indicate the effect of the postural support provided.

Interface pressure

Although judgement and commonsense might help the clinician to predict where pressure at the tissue/support interface is likely to be higher, it is helpful to measure or map the interface pressure for a more complete understanding of a particular problem and possible solutions.

Besides influencing the choice of seat cushion or seating materials, pressure measurement can also help to investigate the influence of other extrinsic variables, such as posture or orientation, on interface pressures at sites considered to be at risk. For example, someone may have an oblique pelvis (down on the right) and a significant scoliosis (convex to the right) such that the trunk tends to fall heavily to the left. The trunk can be supported by a lateral and upward force on the

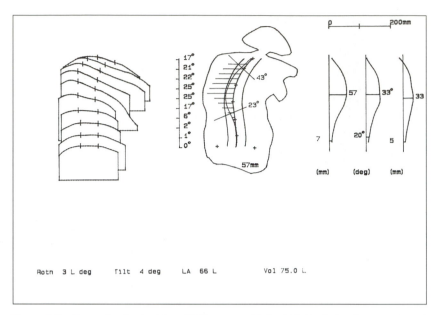

Figure 6.6 Example of output from ISIS scanner (Oxford Metrics) showing: a series of transverse profiles in the coronal plane (left); prediction of path of vertebral bodies with calculation of rotation and lateral curvature (centre); and medial and paramedial profiles in the sagittal plane with estimate of kyphosis and lordosis (right). Indices summarising rotation, lateral asymmetry and volumetric asymmetry are shown at the bottom.

left, however there is concern that too much pressure will be taken under the left axilla. Tilting the whole seating system laterally down on the right might help to reduce the pressure under the left axilla but might also increase the pressure taken under the right ischial tuberosity. In this situation pressure measurement at the right ischial tuberosity and under the left axilla might help to determine an acceptable compromise degree of tilt that does not result in a dangerous level of pressure at either site.

Pressure measurement and pressure measurement devices are described in more detail in Chapter 12 and three types of pressure monitor are shown in Figure 6.7.

Some pressure measurement systems are more practical for use in the clinic setting than others. This depends largely on how easily they can be positioned and measurements taken without disrupting the subject. For accurate placement of individual sensors it is necessary to attach them directly to the skin tissue. A matrix of sensors that can be positioned quickly on or in the seat may be more practical but may be less accurate.

When attempting to measure interface pressure as part of an assessment it is important to recognize the limitations of the equipment being used. For example, if the sensors used are large then the measurement made will represent an average pressure over the full area of the sensor, possibly concealing a significantly higher peak pressure within that area. Alternatively, if the sensors are spaced too far apart then a pressure concentration falling between the sensors may be lost. Characteristics of the sensor such as the thickness, rigidity or inability to stretch may change the pressure at the interface which is being measured. Furthermore, most pressure measurement systems just give a snapshot of static pressure when a specific problem may be due to dynamically changing pressure associated with activity in the wheelchair (Bar 1991).

Care should be taken in drawing conclusions based on absolute pressure readings without taking the potential inaccuracy of the measurement system into account. If used sensibly, however, pressure measurement can be a very useful comparative tool.

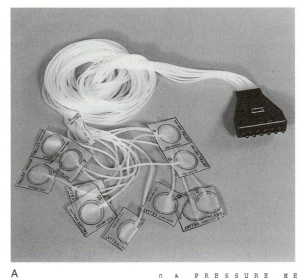

A

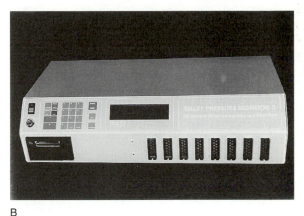

B

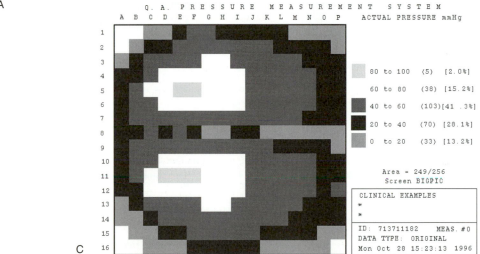

C

Q. A. PRESSURE MEASUREMENT SYSTEM
A B C D E F G H I J K L M N O P   ACTUAL PRESSURE mmHg

80 to 100   (5) [2.0%]

60 to 80   (38) [15.2%]

40 to 60 (103)[41 .3%]

20 to 40   (70) [28.1%]

0 to 20   (33) [13.2%]

Area = 249/256
Screen BIGPIC

CLINICAL EXAMPLES
*
*

ID: 713711182   MEAS. #0
DATA TYPE: ORIGINAL
Mon Oct 28 15:23:13 1996

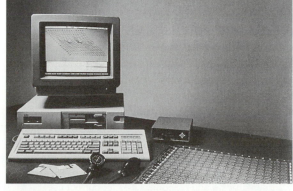

D

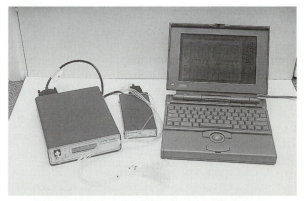

E

Figure 6.7   Examples of pressure monitors. (A,B) A pneumatic system with between 1 and 96 sensors, measuring pressure at each sensor in turn (TPM Mk III, Talley Group Ltd). (C,D) 256 (16 × 16) pneumatic sensors built into a cushion sized matrix which provides a static 'snapshot' of interface pressure distribution (QA System, Helping Hands Company). (E) Dynamic–8–24 individual sensors capable of providing dynamically changing pressure measurements from specific sites (Dynamic Pressure Monitor, Raymar).

Muscle activity, muscle tone, spasticity

Subjective estimates of muscle tone are also often made during the course of an assessment. Spasticity, however, is more easily recognized than it is characterized and quantified (Katz & Rymer 1989).

In the clinic situation muscle tone is characterized as the resistance to passive joint manipulation. As a limb is moved about a joint the stretching of a particular muscle will result in stretch reflex activity, causing the muscle to attempt to contract and oppose the movement.

Attempts to measure muscle tone have been based largely on the use of one of the following:

Box 6.4 Summary checklist for assessment, prescription, provision and review. (From Department of Health 1991, with permission from R. Nelham, C. Nichols and C. Pope and DoH)

1. Establish the reason for referral and the user's/parents'/carer's wishes and life style
2. Observe the current prescription of wheelchair/seating if any and the way that the user is using these
3. Assess, measure and/or record the user's posture and function in current equipment
4. With client out of equipment examine the components and their condition
5. Assess the client in positions of lying, sitting and standing in order to determine his/her abilities in each of these positions. *Do not use prescribed equipment for this process*
6. Measure and note presence of deformity, particularly of the spine and hips, taking care to check for any asymmetrical deformities. Determine whether deformity is fixed or postural and the degree of correction achievable
7. Define pressure distribution needs
8. Determine the treatment/management programmes related to the client's postural support needs
9. Determine environment and social constraints on the prescriptions
10. Use the collected data to determine the posture (upright and/or alternatives) and the support required by the client. Simulate this support with the aim of drafting the prescription, bearing in mind the following:
    a. *For tissue trauma considerations*, determine the appropriate pressure distributing or pressure redistributing cushion either commercially available or purpose made
    b. *For postural considerations*, whenever possible,
        i. Aim for symmetry and distribution of load bearing through both ischial tuberosities and the whole of the thighs and buttocks
        ii. Avoid pelvic tilt, i.e. pelvis to be neutral
        iii. Avoid asymmetry, e.g. windswept hips, scoliosis, etc.
        iv. Provide appropriate support to stabilize the pelvis and lower limbs in all the postures being considered
        v. Once the lower part of the body has been stabilized, determine the postural support required at the trunk level within diminishing functional ability

11. Use support surfaces that provide biomechanically correct application of forces
12. If the foregoing is not readily available, referral to a specialist centre should be considered
13. Choose, or design and manufacture (an iterative process), the most appropriate support system to provide the biomechanically correct postural stability to achieve the above objectives. The equipment should preferably be adjustable to meet the changing needs of the client
14. Determine the type of wheeled mobility into which this postural support system will fit and which will also be compatible with the user's life style, the family's/carer's life styles, physical abilities and mental abilities. Consider the following:
    a. Self-propelled, attendant-propelled or powered mobility
    b. Indoor or outdoor or both
    c. Size – open and folded (for seating system, access to buildings, transportation, space, convenience)
    d. Need for various components to be removable
    e. Weight with or without removable components
    f. Ease of use including manoeuvrability and removable components
    g. Footrest position with reference to sitting posture
    h. Castor position with reference to desired foot position
    i. Stability of chair with occupant
    j. The wheelchair or other wheeled mobility devices should permit the full range of adjustment of the postural support equipment.
15. Determine whether or not provision is through NHS (with or without a voucher option) or by private purchase using published lists of wheelchairs and other vehicles
16. The prescribed wheelchair must be tested for static stability with the user in place. If unstable, determine modifications required or new prescription and retest on completion
17. Instruct the user and/or carers in the particular features and functions of the seating system and wheelchair(s) and other vehicle(s), including maintenance and responsibilities for correct use
18. Identify intervals for review and set dates

- Clinical scales for grading the resistance encountered during passive stretching (Bohannon & Smith 1987)
- Test rigs (Gottlieb et al 1978, Harris & Millar 1990, Lehmann et al 1989, Price et al 1991) or pendulum models (Bajd & Vodovnik 1984, Bohannon 1987, Brown et al 1988, Lin & Rymer 1991) to assess the biomechanical stiffness of a joint.
- Electrophysiological investigation of stretch reflexes and the angular threshold at which they occur (Delwaide 1985, Katz & Rymer 1989, Powers, Marder-Meyer & Rymer 1988). It should be noted, however, that raw EMG information representing resting muscle activity does not necessarily relate directly to muscle tone or spasticity (Basmajian 1976).

Although grading scales like the Ashworth scale (Bohannon & Smith 1987) may allow more objective rating of spasticity, the other methods have been used mainly in the research field and are probably not yet sufficiently reliable and practical for a routine assessment. Besides assessing muscle tone generally, it would be useful to be able to investigate the effects of changes in posture or orientation on muscle tone. There is, therefore, a growing need for a reliable and practical test of muscle tone and spasticity more suited to the wheelchair and seating clinic.

Objective measurement in the wheelchair/seating clinic

Using objective methods of measuring are important for comparison, particularly for users with changing conditions where more radical or alternative solutions need to be sought, for example surgery. In reality many clinicians do not have access to the more sophisticated measuring tools but with experience are able to undertake a thorough assessment and recognize when greater detail or more accurate objective measurements are required.

CONCLUSION

A summary checklist for assessment, prescription, provision and review (Nelham, Nichols & Pope 1996) is shown in Box 6.4.

It is suggested that the reader should refer to the Further Reading section at the end of this chapter for more detailed advice on assessment, wheelchair selection and positioning techniques in addition to the specific references given in the chapter.

REFERENCES

Bajd T, Vodovnik L 1984 Pendulum testing of spasticity. Journal of Biomedical Engineering 6: 9–16
Bar C A 1991 Evaluation of cushions using dynamic pressure measurement. Prosthetics and Orthotics International 15: 232–240
Basmajian J V 1976 Electromyographic investigation of spasticity and muscle spasm. Physiotherapy 62(10): 319–323
Bohannon R W 1987 Variability and reliability of the pendulum test for spasticity using a Cybex II isokinetic dynamometer. Physical Therapy 67(5): 659–661
Bohannon R W, Smith M B 1987 Interrater reliability of a modified Ashworth scale of muscle spasticity. Physical Therapy 67(2): 206–207
Brown R A, Lawson D A, Leslie G C et al 1988 Does the Wartenberg pendulum test differentiate quantitatively between spasticity and rigidity? A study in elderly stroke and Parkinsonian patients. Journal of Neurology, Neurosurgery and Psychiatry 51: 1178–1186
Carlson J M, Lonstein J, Beck K O, Wilkie D C 1986 Seating for children and young adults with cerebral palsy. Clinical Prosthetics and Orthotics 10(4): 137–158

Cobb J R 1948 Outline for the study of scoliosis. American Academy of Orthopaedic Surgeons 5: 261–275
Delwaide P J 1985 Electrophysiological testing of spastic patients: its potential usefulness and limitations. In: Delwaide P J, Young R R (eds) Clinical neurophysiology in spasticity. Elsevier Science, Oxford, ch 16, pp 185–203
Department of Health 1991 Wheelchair training resource pack. Centre of Information for Department of Health, London
Department of Health 1996 Wheelchair training resource pack. Revised DoH 1991 publication. College of Occupational Therapists, London
Fearn T A, Green E M, Jones M, Mulcahy C M, Nelham R L, Pountney T E 1992 Postural management. In: McCarthy G T (ed) Physical disability in childhood. Churchill Livingstone, Edinburgh, pp 401–450
Green E M, Nelham R L 1991 Development of sitting ability, assessment of children with a motor handicap and prescription of appropriate seating systems. Prosthetics and Orthotics International 15: 203–216
Goodwin J, Clark C, Deakes J, Burdon D, Lawrence C 1992

Clinical methods of goniometry: a comparative study. Disability and Rehabilitation 14(1): 10–15

Gottlieb G L, Agarwal G C, Penn R 1978 Sinusoidal oscillation of the ankle as a means of evaluating the spastic patient. Journal of Neurology, Neurosurgery and Psychiatry 41: 32–39

Hallett R, Hare N, Milner A D 1987 Description and evaluation of an assessment form. Physiotherapy 73(5): 220–225

Harris G F, Millar E A 1990 Lower extremity hypertonicity assessment: a computer based system. Journal of Clinical Engineering 15(6): 453–458

Katz R T, Rymer W Z 1989 Spastic hypertonia: mechanisms and measurement. Archives of Physical Medicine and Rehabilitation 70: 144–155

Lehmann J F, Price R, de Lateur B J, Hinderer S, Traynor C 1989 Spasticity: quantitative measurements a basis for assessing effectiveness of therapeutic intervention. Archives of Physical Medicine and Rehabilitation 70: 6–15

Lin D C, Rymer W Z 1991 A quantitative analysis of pendular motion of the lower leg in spastic human subjects. IEEE Transactions on Biomedical Engineering 38(9): 906–918

Mayerson N H, Milano R A 1984 Goniometric measurement reliability in physical medicine. Archives of Physical Medicine and Rehabilitation 65: 92–94

McColl I 1986 Review of artificial limb and appliance centre services, vols I & II. HMSO, London

Morrissy R T, Goldsmith G S, Hall E C, Kehl D, Cowie H 1990 Measurement of the Cobb angle on radiographs of patients who have scoliosis. Journal of Bone and Joint Surgery 72A(3): 320–327

Mulcahy C M 1988 Adaptive seating for motor handicap: problems, a solution, assessment and prescription. British Journal of Occupational Therapy 51(10): 347–352

National Prosthetic and Wheelchair Services Report 1993–1996 DoH funded project. College of Occupational Therapists, London

Nuffield Institute of Health 1995 An investigation into face to face assessment of all non permanent users of wheelchairs. Priority & Community Service Group, Nuffield Institute of Health, University of Leeds

Powers R K, Marder-Meyer J, Rymer W Z 1988 Quantitative relations between hypertonia and stretch reflex threshold in spastic hemiparesis. Annals of Neurology 23(2): 116–124

Price R, Bjornson K F, Lehmann J F, McLauhlin J F, Hays R M 1991 Quantitative measurement of spasticity in children with cerebral palsy. Developmental Medicine and Child Neurology 33: 585–595

Sahlstrand T 1986 The clinical value of Moire topography in the management of scoliosis. Spine 11(5): 409–417

Watkins M A, Riddle D L, Lamb R L, Personius W J 1991 Reliability of goniometric measurements and visual estimates of knee range of motion obtained in a clinical setting. Physical Therapy 71(2): 90–97

Weisz I, Jefferson R J, Turner-Smith A R, Houghton G R, Harris J D 1988 ISIS scanning: a useful assessment technique in the management of scoliosis. Spine 13(4): 405–408

FURTHER READING

Axelson P, Minkel J, Chesney D 1995 A guide to wheelchair selection: how to use the ANSI/RESNA wheelchair standards to buy a wheelchair. Paralyzed Veterans of America ISO/TC173/SCN226

Bardsley G I, Taylor P M 1982 The development of an assessment chair. Prosthetics and Orthotics International 6: 75–78

Behrman A L 1990 Factors in functional assessment. Journal of Rehabilitation Research and Development (Clinical Supplement 2): 17–30

Brubaker C E 1990 Ergonometric considerations. Journal of Rehabilitation Research and Development (Clinical Supplement 2): 37–48

Ferguson-Pell M W 1990 Seat cushion selection. Journal of Rehabilitation Research and Development (Clinical Supplement 2): 49–73

Fife S E, Roxburgh L A, Armstrong R W, Harris S R, Gregson J L, Field D 1991 Development of a clinical measure of postural control for assessment of adaptive seating in children with neuromotor disabilities. Physical Therapy 71(12): 981–993

Goodwill J C, Chamberlain A (eds) 1988 Rehabilitation of the physically disabled adult. Croom Helm, London

Ozner M N 1990 A participatory planning process for wheelchair selection. Journal of Rehabilitation Research and Development (Clinical Supplement 2): 31–36

Pope P M 1985 A study of instability in relation to posture in the wheelchair. Physiotherapy 71: 129–131

Rangnarsson K T 1990 Prescription considerations and a comparison of conventional and lightweight wheelchairs. Journal of Rehabilitation Research and Development (Clinical Supplement 2): 8–16

Taylor S J 1987 Evaluating the client with physical disabilities for wheelchair seating. American Journal of Occupational Therapy 41(11): 711–716

Trefler E, Taylor S J 1991 Prescription and positioning: evaluating the physically disabled individual for wheelchair seating. Prosthetics and Orthotics International 15: 217–224

Warren C G 1990 Powered mobility and its implications. Journal of Rehabilitation Research and Development (Clinical Supplement 2): 37–48

Wells J 1995 Choosing a wheelchair. A Royal Association for Disability and Rehabilitation Publication, London

Zeraeng C, Cattermole J, Cartwright R, Jones M, McCarthy G T, Moffat V 1992 Assessment of child with multiple disability. In: McCarthy G T (ed) Physical disability in childhood. Churchill Livingstone, Edinburgh, pp 65–81

User groups

SECTION CONTENTS

7

Neurological users

INTRODUCTION

Diseases of the nervous system are commonly complex and frequently associated with severe disability with the involvement of several areas of function including posture and mobility. Whilst many similar features are shared by the different conditions, such as muscle weakness, spasm, scoliosis or poor sensation, all of which can affect posture and mobility, it is equally true to say that each condition demonstrates features unique to its particular diagnosis, primarily relating to the site and severity of the neurological lesion. Significant differences also relate to non-clinical features and factors such as the age of onset; whether the condition is congenital or acquired; individual social and economic status, preferences and expectations. These factors, and many others, will elicit different responses and attitudes from each individual as well as their family and other associates and will ultimately affect their quality of life (see Ch. 5). The majority of all wheelchair users are over the age of 60, tend to be occasional users and have limited mobility associated with the ageing process, osteoarthritis and cardiorespiratory diseases. They often depend upon another person to push their wheelchair when out of doors. However, most of those with neurological conditions, whether acquired or congenital, are under 60 years of age and frequently become full-time users.

Wheelchair assessment should be an integral part of a comprehensive assessment of each individual, addressing their varying though specific needs and providing opportunity for regular review and reassessment as a condition changes (see Ch. 6). The information in this chapter will focus on posture and mobility in relation to function in neurological disorders. However, whilst concentrating on correct positioning and improved mobility, it must be remembered that everyone is first and foremost a person striving to get the best from life. Frequently there will be a conflict between postural, environmental and individual requirements. Difficult decisions will have to be made and a compromise reached. The task of the clinician is not to impose their views and attempt to 'normalize' disabled people but to provide relevant information, based on knowledge and experience, thereby enabling each individual to make the best use of their abilities and to minimize the impact of disability on their life style. An understanding of the underlying features of each condition, with the physical and psychological impact these will have on the user, will assist the clinician when assessing and prescribing for posture and mobility needs.

This chapter provides a summary of neurological conditions commonly encountered with wheelchair users, together with an outline of the clinical features that can influence the wheelchair prescription. These are placed in alphabetical order of condition rather than order of importance or number of individuals affected.

ACQUIRED IMMUNE DEFICIENCY SYNDROME (AIDS)

Infection by the human immune deficiency retrovirus (HIV) will result in a severe and frequently fatal illness known as AIDS. There are a number of forms of AIDS and the effects of the illness range from a low grade infection to a severe systemic disorder (Aylward, Dewis & Scott 1992). Transmission is by body fluids and the groups most at risk include sexually active homosexuals, bisexual men, intravenous drug users and haemophiliacs requiring blood transfusions.

Clinical features

The effects of the illness range from severe systemic illness, characterized by weight loss, tiredness, weakness and lethargy with intense night sweats, to secondary disorders such as pneumonia, polyneuropathy, malignant skin disease (Kaposi's sarcoma) and possibly dementia.

Treatment

There is no known cure and each sympton is treated as it appears. Action should also be taken to reduce the development of secondary problems such as pressure sores which occur due to poor general health, loss of weight and low body resistance.

Posture and mobility

As the illness advances, the individual becomes progressively weaker and less mobile, necessitating the use of a wheelchair. The model of chair selected will depend on individual need, environment and life style. In general, a basic self-propelling model is required, with a comfortable, pressure-relieving cushion and adequate protection against pressure sores in all the vulnerable areas including shoulder blades, elbows, heels, buttocks and the sacral area. Maintaining independent mobility should be encouraged as long as is realistic. In many cases the individual becomes bed-ridden due to increasing generalized weakness.

BATTEN'S DISEASE

This is a rare inherited progressive disorder of the central nervous system in which there is an accumulation of storage bodies in the brain cells due to defective lysosomes which restrict the removal of waste products. The condition was first recognized at the turn of the century by a London neurologist, Dr Batten, after whom it is named. There is a 1 : 4 chance of children having the disease only when both parents are carriers. The four types of Batten's are identified by the age of onset. These are: infantile; late infantile (2–4 years of age); juvenile (6–8 years of age); adult.

Clinical features

Visual impairment is the first sign of onset eventually leading to blindness. Epilepsy, loss of acquired skills, rigidity and muscle wasting with decreasing mobility, loss of short-term memory, slurred speech, eating difficulties, hallucinations, incontinence and dementia are the distressing ongoing clinical picture.

Treatment

No known treatment has been found to delay or reverse the disease. Appropriate and sensitive support for the family to enable the child to remain in a loving environment as long as possible is a top priority. Provision of suitable equipment is an important part of this support.

Posture and mobility needs

Weakness of movements and decrease in tone result in characteristic changes in gait. The knees tend to be flexed and the arms hang loosely. As walking deteriorates, the individual takes short shuffling steps. Initiating walking or changing direction becomes a problem as rotation of the trunk is lost. Keeping children on their feet is a priority, though should be sensibly balanced with the opportunity to join in social activities. Regular physiotherapy is important to prevent or reduce contractures and deformities. As with other changing and deteriorating conditions, assessment of posture and mobility should be ongoing, with changes in prescription to suit individual requirements. Close liaison with other professionals is needed to address all aspects of the child's life, including school and social activities. Involvement of a specialist dealing with sight problems or advice from the RNIB will help in providing appropriate activities as sight fails. Timely provision of adjustable wheelchair equipment with correct positioning at all times should be part of the care programme, taking

into account the prognosis and increasing needs of both the individual and their carer.

CEREBRAL PALSY

Cerebral palsy is a term used to describe a group of disorders that affect posture, movement and muscle tone, with possible impairment of intellect, vision, language and perception. These are the result of abnormal structural development or non-progressive lesions in the brain, either prenatal, during delivery or in the first two years of life.

Incidence rate

The rate is 2 : 1000 live births (Lipkin 1991). The risk of cerebral palsy is increased in low weight or premature babies. It is commoner in males and a high proportion are first-born. Life expectancy is normal and 95% live into adulthood (Aylward, Dewis & Scott 1992).

Clinical features

Due to the variety of disorders seen in people with cerebral palsy, the disability can be classified either according to the type of neuromotor disorder displayed, such as spastic, dystonic, ataxic, or dependent on the area of the body affected by the disability, such as hemiplegic, diplegic, quadraplegic, monoplegic or paraplegic (see Ch. 4).

Clinical features will depend on the degree and distribution of the brain damage. The commonest complications relate to involuntary movements, joint contractures, postural deformities, language and communication disorders, which can seriously handicap the individual and create barriers to progress in both social life and employment. In addition, many children and adults have a range of sensory defects, learning difficulties, chewing and swallowing problems, behavioural disturbances and seizures. On the other hand, many people with speech and movement disorders are of average intelligence and independent, with opportunities to do well in employment if public prejudice can be overcome and providing they have access to suitable equipment including communication aids.

Treatment

Appropriate treatment should be used to address individual problems. This should be centrally coordinated to prevent isolated action that improves one aspect of care or function at the expense of another. All treatment should be targeted at improving quality of life by optimizing development of ability and personality whilst easing care. Surgical intervention may be required to prevent or correct deformity which, if left unattended, will further reduce function and cause problems with general care and hygiene. Botulinum toxin injections have recently been successfully introduced to reduce spasm in selected muscles. The injections are accompanied by intensive physiotherapy or the use of orthoses for maximum benefit. Whilst often children with mild cerebral palsy attend mainstream schools, there are also specialist schools, clubs and centres dealing with all age groups. Information can be obtained from Scope (previously the Spastic Society).

Posture and mobility needs

Standing daily, with or without a standing frame, should be encouraged to reduce or delay development of scoliosis. Children with mild cerebral palsy will learn to walk, possibly with an unusual gait, though have a chance of developing postural problems and may require a wheelchair later in life. At the other end of the disability scale, children and adults with cerebral palsy form the largest number of those seen in seating clinics and present some of the most challenging and complex disabilities. The principal aim of any treatment is to aid development and improve quality of life whilst reducing deformity and maximizing function. Physical treatment and equipment should endeavour to control abnormal movement and reduce the influence of primitive reflexes without restricting purposeful function. Pelvic stability with an upright sitting position is generally recommended to control

spasm and encourage development of correct postural tone and normal pattern movements but consideration must be given to change of position and support to control the head, particularly for feeding, social interaction, transportation and outdoor activities. Early advice should be provided on 24-hour postural management to include positioning in lying, sitting, standing and also walking as relevant (see Ch. 9). An holistic approach with good ongoing communication between family members and all agencies involved with cooperation and agreement concerning the provision of treatment and equipment will provide opportunity for maximum development of the child and good quality of life. Although this ideal can be achieved to a degree up to 16 years of age, reduction in opportunities for physical treatment and access to many rehabilitation services after this age can result in rapid deterioration in range of movement and level of ability with a noticeable increase in scoliosis, joint contractures and general function. Every effort should be made to provide life-time support to the individual and their family. Emphasis must be on ability rather than disability and there are many adults with severe disabilities resulting from cerebral palsy who, through a combination of persistence and determination and often without professional support, have managed to overcome their many difficulties, enabling them to lead a full and active life (Vernon 1990).

CEREBROVASCULAR ACCIDENT

Stroke is the popular name for a cerebrovascular accident (CVA), which is an interruption of the blood supply or a haemorrhage into part of the brain resulting in development of impaired function of the brain and nervous system.

Incidence

The incidence rate is 150–200 : 100 000. Although there are an increasing number of people in the high-risk group there is a reduction in incidence, probably due to better health education and prevention as a result of improved treatment of hypertension.

Clinical features

The clinical features are loss of function or weakness of the muscles of one side of the body, dysphasia, sensory inattention, difficulty with swallowing, ataxia, disorders of gait and possible loss of coordination. The degree of disability and level of recovery depends on the site and severity of the incident, the attitude, expectations and age of the individual. The sudden onset will have psychological implications for both patient and family, who may have difficulty in adjusting to their sudden change in life, especially when the 'bread winner' of the family has the stroke.

Treatment

Medication reduces the risk of a recurrence. There is generally a degree of recovery which continues for up to 6 months. Continued improvement in functional performance occurs for many people as they continue to adapt to their disability. Physiotherapy and occupational therapy are aimed at improving function by strengthening the unaffected muscles, increasing confidence and gaining independence, possibly with the use of aids and equipment.

Postural and mobility needs

Many will recover sufficiently to walk independently. Others may require a stick or walking frame with a wheelchair for outdoor use. A few will become permanent wheelchair users. Weakness of muscles on one side of the body can result in the development of an asymmetrical sitting position with general poor posture. Those with sufficient balance to walk tend to weight bear heavily on the non-paralysed side resulting in osteoarthritis of the knee in many cases. Advice on correct positioning from day one is essential. As with other neurological conditions, there is frequent debate as to at what stage a wheelchair should be prescribed (Blower 1988). Temporary provision of a wheelchair is not always possible through the wheelchair service (see Ch. 1), but should be considered for the psychological and social benefits and also to encourage inde-

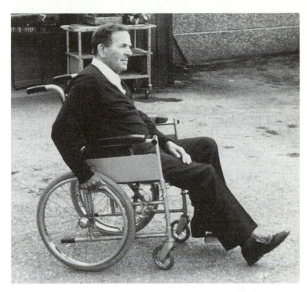

Figure 7.1 A wheelchair user with hemiplegia using the unaffected arm and leg to propel and steer his wheelchair. (Reproduced from Department of Health 1991 Wheelchair training resource pack, Centre of Information for Department of Health, London, with permission.)

pendence. Although difficult to achieve, some people with a permanent hemiplegia learn to propel a wheelchair with the unaffected hand and steer with one foot (Fig. 7.1). In these cases, apart from taking mental and physical ability into account, assessment must consider the most appropriate seat height for the individual as a low seat can create problems when working at a table or standing from the seat, whereas a high seat encourages sacral sitting in order to reach the floor with the propelling foot. This can result in discomfort and pressure under the thigh and sacrum. A one-arm-drive wheelchair is appropriate for some though confusing for those with cognitive and proprioceptive difficulties. It also presents problems relating to turning space, door widths and additional weight for lifting into a car. For others a powered wheelchair may be more suitable (see Ch. 13). A stable base cushion is required and possibly thoracic supports to aid balance and encourage symmetrical posture. Support for the affected arm and hand with either a Bexhill armrest or wider armrest, will reduce shoulder pain on the affected side but should not restrict function (Fig. 7.2). Comprehen-

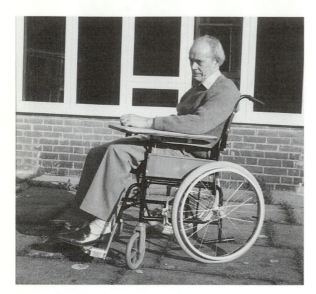

Figure 7.2 A Bexhill armrest is designed to provide support to the paralysed arm and shoulder joint with less restriction than the standard tray.

sive assessment and regular review should identify the most appropriate accessories required at different stages of recovery. Some equipment will be required only on a temporary basis and therefore supplied by the rehabilitation unit rather than the wheelchair service or social services.

FRIEDREICH'S ATAXIA

This is an inherited disorder with onset in childhood or early adult life. The cerebellum is affected but there is also atrophy of the dorsal columns of the spinal cord and possibly the corticospinal tracts.

Prevalence is in the order of 250 : 100 000 (Goodwill & Chamberlain 1988).

Clinical features

The first sign is ataxia which results in walking with a wide-based gait. In time, balance deteriorates and weakness in the dorsiflexors causes foot drop. Other signs are dysarthria and tremor which affect hand function. There is a degree of mental impairment over a period of time and an understandable tendency to depression due to the awareness of the progressive nature of the disease and the possibility of having observed deterioration in other members of a family.

Posture and mobility needs

As balance deteriorates and ataxia increases, assessment will be required for a wheelchair. In time, hand involvement will inevitably limit the ability to self-propel and it will not be long before a powered wheelchair is required with a facility for both user and attendant control; the latter is for safety out of doors or in tight spaces. Environmental controls may also help to increase independence and delay the need for a full-time carer. Spinal deformity is common and early support in the wheelchair together with good positioning in the lying posture will reduce and delay deformity. A reclining backrest or tilted position, whilst reducing the force of gravity on the spine, can restrict any remaining purposeful function. Any compromise should reflect the preferences of the user.

GUILLAIN–BARRÉ SYNDROME

This is a type of peripheral neuropathy which has an acute onset and affects many peripheral nerves simultaneously. The majority of cases have spontaneous recovery over a period of time but in others there is permanent paralysis of a varying degree.

Clinical features

Involvement of the respiratory muscles and failure to improve within 3 weeks are poor prognostic signs. The severity and distribution of muscle weakness is variable. The acute onset in a previously active person will result in shock, fear and possibly a period of depression.

Treatment

Once the acute phase is over, the patient is mobilized with treatment directed at preventing joint contractures and pressure sores whilst building up muscle strength and morale. This is one of the neurological conditions in which there is a good chance of recovery, though some are left with a permanent weakness.

Posture and mobility needs

Involvement of the trunk muscles and lower limbs may necessitate the use of a wheelchair. An attendant-pushed wheelchair with a high supportive back and a degree of tilt or recline is generally required in the early acute phase. In some cases the individual is reluctant to accept a wheelchair due to its association with permanent disability. As muscle strength returns, the prescription will require reviewing on a regular basis with a reduction in support and consideration for independence by self-propelling or using a powered wheelchair. Weight loss and muscle atrophy, particularly of the gluteal muscles, necessitates the need for a pressure-relieving cushion (see Ch. 12). Uncertainty of prognosis makes it difficult to prescribe appropriately. It can also influence and may delay agreement for home adaptations. Provision of a modular wheelchair will help to accommodate changing needs. Prolonged physiotherapy with the use of orthoses and walking aids will, in time, replace the need for the wheelchair, though there may be a continuing need when covering longer distances until full recovery is reached. Some people may require a wheelchair on a permanent basis and, even without a relapse, fatigue may persist for up to 2 years. Correct positioning at all times and postural support will be needed to encourage a symmetrical position and prevent deformities of the pelvis and spine, particularly in the early stages. Consideration should be given to outdoor mobility needs as well as environmental controls for those with a long-term or permanent upper and lower limb weakness.

HEAD INJURY

A head injury can result in a complex and varied pattern of disability. The major cause of brain damage is as a result of an accident. There are three main types of head injury:

1. Concussion, which is a transient loss of consciousness following a blow to the head, generally with full recovery.
2. Contusion, which is damage to the cerebral tissue from local bleeding or oedema.
3. Compression, which involves bleeding into the skull, leading to compression of the brain and a steady deterioration in the patient's condition (Dandy 1994).

The Glasgow Coma Scale is the usual method of assessment and includes monitoring of the eyes, verbal responses and motor responses.

The incidence of head injuries of all degrees is in the region of 1500 : 100 000. Of these, about 17 are severe or very severe and result in some degree of permanent physical and cognitive disability (Eames 1988). The majority of people with head injuries affecting mobility are in the 15–24 age group with a 3 : 2 male to female distribution.

Clinical features

The degree and features of any disability will depend on the site and extent of the injury (see Ch. 4). Disruption to mobility can be very complex with a variety of postural patterns and frequently secondary complications which may be of a neurological nature or due to fractures of the spine or lower limb. Patients are often aggressive in the early stages due to general irritability, resulting in restlessness and unreliable behaviour which can be a greater barrier to rehabilitation than loss of physical function.

Treatment

Priority in the early stages is to prevent contractures by carrying out regular passive exercise. Splinting may also be used to prevent or correct deformities. The length of time for recovery and the degree of independence finally achieved is difficult to predict in the early stages. Psychological and social aspects of treatment are equally important, with appropriate family support. Headway is a voluntary organization which can provide advice and active support in this field.

Postural and mobility needs

When there is damage to the brain stem it can be difficult to obtain a good sitting position and contractures may develop due to rigidity and a range of involuntary movements with lack of cooperation by the individual. Sitting tolerance may be low but should be encouraged to increase respiratory function and prevent static secretion. Variations in postural tone with a range of patterns make it difficult to achieve a stable sitting position. More often than not the head will flop and the body fall forward. Using a chair with adjustable positions of tilt and recline will help in positioning the individual together with maximum support to maintain a symmetrical position (Fig. 7.3). It may be necessary to use a head band or a form of collar to prevent the head hanging forward (Fig. 7.4). Care must be taken to protect against pressure sores as there is likely to be loss of sensation or inability to change position. Due to uncertainty in the degree of recovery and final level of independence, it is necessary to carry out regular reassessment and to review all equipment provided. Positioning in the wheelchair should follow the general principles to encourage symmetry, balance, eye contact and communication as well as providing comfort, preventing pressure sores and assisting with general care and retraining. Families need long-term support to cope with antisocial and behavioural problems as well as physical problems resulting from the injury. Headway, the National

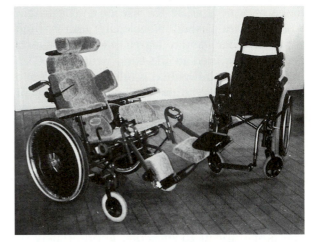

Figure 7.3 The tilt-in-space chair (left) and the recliner (right) provide comfort and increased support for the head, spine and upper trunk for full-time users with deteriorating muscle weakness. However, these chairs are large and difficult to manoeuvre in the average home.

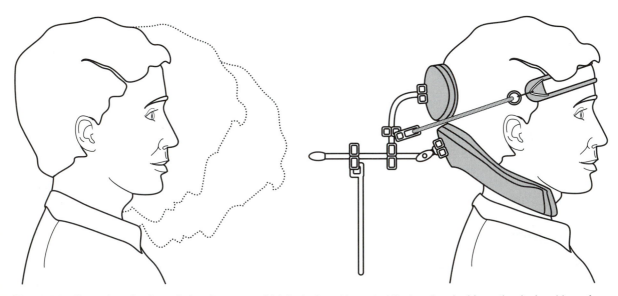

Figure 7.4 Illustration of a dynamic head support, which is designed to control the head and address the dual problem of forward and sideways flopping, whilst allowing limited movement. (Illustration provided by James Leckey.)

Head Injuries Association, can provide advice and practical support in many cases.

HUNTINGTON'S CHOREA

This is an inherited condition with an incidence of 1 : 20 000 in the UK (Aylward, Dewis & Scott 1992). Children of an affected parent have a 50% chance of developing the disease. The disease is progressive with onset between the ages of 30 and 50, leading to severe disability and death within about 14 years from onset (see also Ch. 10).

Clinical features

The deterioration is due to the destruction of the cells of the brain and is characterized by the gradual onset of uncontrollable chorea like movements. These are either in the form of abrupt jerking or a slow writhing nature and are accompanied by gradual mental deterioration with a change of personality and behaviour. The symptoms worsen as the disease progresses. The normal walking gait is interrupted by uncontrolled lurches and it becomes impossible to hold or pick up any object. The affected individual has a general lack of insight into their condition.

As there is no known treatment for the disorder, symptoms should be treated as they occur. In the final stages the individual becomes emaciated and bed-ridden, generally requiring 24-hour care.

Postural and mobility needs

Assessment for a wheelchair with postural support will be required as soon as balance is lost. In time, postural support becomes ineffective due to the increase in jerky and writhing movements of the individual. Comfort and padding to prevent the individual injuring themselves are the main priority, together with easing life for the carer. In general, a wheelchair is only required for a limited period of time, for as the disease progresses the chorea-like movements make it impossible to keep the individual in a sitting position or to push them about safely. A more practical solution is to seat them in a deep comfortable armchair on wheels (see Ch. 4) but whenever possible with a tilt position and recline option as the muscles later become rigid and the limbs stiffen. Weight loss is a problem and protection against pressure sores should be provided.

MOTOR NEURONE DISEASE (MND)

This progressive degenerative disease affects:

- Lower motor anterior horn cells of the spinal cord.
- Upper motor neurones in the motor areas of the cerebral cortex.
- Lower motor neurones in the nuclei of the motor cranial nerves.

Onset is insidious but as the nerve cells degenerate, the muscles atrophy, resulting in progressive weakness of limbs with bulbar involvement.

Incidence rate

This is 1–2 : 100 000 annually. The prevalence is in the region of 6 : 100 000 (Langton & Hewer 1988), with a male to female ratio of 2 : 1. The cause remains unknown, though there is a familial tendency in 5% of all cases. The onset generally occurs between 50 and 60 years of age. MND cannot be transmitted or artificially induced and, within the animal kingdom, it has only been identified in man.

Clinical features

Early symptoms are weakness of the hands and arms with the loss of finer movements, resulting in practical difficulties such as fastening buttons. Loss of strength of the lower limbs follows with impairment to walking, due to weakness of dorsiflexion of the foot. Other problems include slurred speech and difficulty with swallowing and breathing as the respiratory muscles become involved. Dysphagia results in social isolation as well as loss of choice and increased dependence on others. The rate of progression varies depending on the prominence and distribution of upper and lower motor neurone lesions. Although there is no remission, the disease may plateau.

Treatment

No medical treatment will influence the course of the disease. Individual symptoms should be addressed as they occur. General care and support for the family is important, with quick response to changing need. Environmental controls can reduce and delay dependency on others whilst communication aids can help to maintain social contact at a later stage.

Postural and mobility needs

The provision of appropriate equipment at the relevant time can ease the burden for both the individual and their carer. Pressure management should be addressed at an early stage as loss of weight together with muscle atrophy place the user at high risk (see Ch. 12). Once there are signs of poor balance and falling, a wheelchair should be considered to enable normal life and independence outside the home to continue for as long as possible. Mobile arm supports and environmental controls may be an option if appropriately prescribed. The assessor should bear in mind the need for postural support and change of position in a wheelchair in order to maintain function, including respiratory function and swallowing. Prescription should reflect the changing condition without overprescribing at an early stage. Funding for additional equipment or wheelchair accessories for hobbies can be discussed with local or national charities, including the MND Society who provide good family support and appropriate equipment. Many people will require a wheelchair for only short periods of time, preferring to use an armchair for comfort. Initially a lightweight self-propelling wheelchair will provide greater independence and improved quality of life. When weakness increases, a powered outdoor wheelchair will help to maintain independent mobility for a longer period of time. As dependence increases, attention should be paid to the need for a good head support (Fig. 7.4) and a tilt facility with leg

supports. There may also be a need to attach an oxygen cylinder to the chair. A far wider range of multi-adjustable chairs is now available for people with deteriorating conditions, though the size of chair may be a restricting factor in the home situation. Funding problems should not delay provision of a special chair or necessary modifications, as failure to respond quickly can make provision unsatisfactory and affect the quality of life. A means of quick access to special wheelchairs should be considered for all deteriorating conditions.

MULTIPLE SCLEROSIS (MS)

This is a chronic progressive degenerative disease affecting primarily young adults. It is characterized by remissions and relapses as a result of patchy inflammation and destruction of myelin throughout the brain and spinal cord. Degeneration of the nerve fibres results in failure of transmission of the nerve impulses. The severity and site of degeneration is variable. Within a few weeks of an acute attack inflammation will diminish, allowing a degree of recovery to take place.

Prevalence rate

This is 40–60 : 100 000 of the population (Badley, Thompson & Wood 1978). The onset is highest in the 17–30-year age group, with a slightly higher incidence among women. The average time from onset to severe disability is 9.5 years (Confavreux, Aimard & Devic 1980). The global incidence of MS has remained fairly constant, though it is rare in countries close to the equator (tropical climate).

Clinical features

The course and effect of MS is variable and unpredictable. Spontaneous remissions of varying length are common, particularly in the younger age group. The degree of disability varies. Providing appropriate support is available, many sufferers will remain independent for long periods.

Complications include spasticity, ataxia, incontinence, loss of vision, vertigo, anxiety and depression, together with psychological and personality changes depending on the severity of the condition. Disability in the majority of cases will increase at a greater or lesser speed over a 20-year period, resulting in chronic incapacity and dependency.

Treatment

A range of drug therapy is available. These have varying degrees of success but can have side effects and should be carefully monitored. Excessive spasticity can cause pain and although extensor spasm can be useful for function, flexor spasm if not controlled can result in contractures forming. Botulinium toxin injections into selected muscles provide short-term relief and are most effective when accompanied by intensive physiotherapy or other antispasmodic measures such as the use of orthoses or oral medication. The implant of a baclofen pump can be used to control spasm and pain, though it is not appropriate for everyone. Although baclofen is commonly used, careful monitoring is required as it can have an adverse effect by reducing tone in the lower limbs, so limiting the ability to stand, walk or transfer independently, as well as increasing problems in general care and management. Regular physical treatment should be directed at reducing spasticity and maintaining a full range of movement to prevent contractures. Surgical intervention and the use of orthoses to prevent deformity may be useful in a few well-selected cases. Support for all family members should not be overlooked.

Postural and mobility needs

An average wheelchair service will have between 5% and 8% of people with multiple sclerosis on their books at any one time (Bar 1993). The degree of support and the need for a wheelchair will vary for each individual and at different stages in the course of the disease. The presence of spasticity, contractures and pressure sores will complicate the picture in many well-established cases when endeavouring to provide the correct level of postural support and mobility. Initially, a lightweight or powered wheelchair may be required for intermittent use to maintain function and independence during a relapse when balance and walking are affected or to conserve energy. Consideration should be given to total mobility needs for work, home, social and outdoor requirements and contact should be made with the relevant bodies. Factors affecting mobility and contributing to poor postural habits include:

- asymmetry of position due to muscle weakness and imbalance in trunk and upper limbs
- sacral sitting
- severe and sudden spasticity
- muscle rigidity
- pain
- general fatigue
- contractures
- impairment of sensation
- impaired vision and vertigo
- poor bladder control
- tremor
- unsteady gait with increased walking difficulties as the disease progresses.

Poor positioning in all positions, including lying, can result in scoliosis and pelvic obliquity with windsweeping of the hips. Failure to address the need for good positioning at an early stage can create later difficulties with sitting and consequently all function, as well as general hygiene and care. Achieving 90% hip flexion may help to reduce spasm in the lower limbs. A degree of tilt is helpful for those with weak trunk muscles but can restrict hand function and also independent standing transfers, as well as causing backflow of urine in a catheter or when using a urine bottle.

People with MS have a high incidence of pressure sores (McGregor 1984) in the later stages of the disease due to a combination of the above factors, together with a tendency to depression and deterioration in general health. The use of a hoist and slings for transfers can aggravate the situation if the sling is not removed during the day, or carelessly removed causing shear over bony prominences.

Comprehensive assessment and advice should be offered at an early stage with multidisciplinary involvement and appropriate physical treatment. The provision of postural and mobility equipment should take into consideration communication and social needs, whilst encouraging maximum function and independence and minimizing disability and further complications.

Ongoing maintenance of range of all joint movements, regular review and a quick response to changing needs will prevent or delay dependency.

MUSCULAR DYSTROPHY (MD)

There are more than 20 types of muscular dystrophy. The Duchenne type, named after Dr Duchenne de Boulogne who worked in Paris in the mid nineteenth century (Muscular Dystrophy Group 1995), is the type most commonly seen in wheelchair clinics. This is a genetic disorder characterized by progressive weakness due to atrophy of the muscles. It affects boys only and results from defect of a single important protein in the muscle called dystrophin. The rate of progressive muscular weakness is variable with noticeable weakness of the lower limbs in the first instance and gradual limitation in general mobility, with growing weakness and fatigue and development of contractures and scoliosis.

Incidence rate

This is 1 : 3500, resulting in about 100 new cases each year in the UK and a known 1500 living in the UK at any one time (Muscular Dystrophy Group 1995). Lower numbers have been recorded in Australia and Alberta (Monckton, Hoskin & Warren 1982). It is said that genetic counselling could reduce these figures by 15%.

Clinical features

The first signs are seen between the ages of 1 and 3 as a wide-based gait develops. Between the ages of 8 and 11 walking becomes increasingly difficult. Further difficulty is experienced when getting up from the floor and the child tends to go into the prone position using his hands to 'walk-up' in order to compensate for weakness in the hip extensors (Gower's sign). Weakness progresses from proximal to distal muscle groups with a generally symmetrical distribution. Hyperextension of the lumbar spine is common in order to keep upright and maintain a balanced head position.

Treatment

There is no known cure and few of those with this disorder survive beyond 20–22 years of age. Once the weakness develops in the quadriceps, fitting a lightweight above-knee orthosis may help to maintain walking for a further 6–30 months, but provision of a suitable wheelchair will reduce fatigue and frustration and give greater quality of life. In a family where more than one sibling is affected greater attention must be paid to practical issues of coping with equipment as well as the psychological and social impact this has on the family.

Posture and mobility needs

When assessing for provision of a wheelchair, high priority must be given to function, life style and appearance, enabling the individual to continue to take part in schooling and social activities with his peer group. A lightweight self-propelling wheelchair will help in the early stages and for a limited period of time, though the need for increasing postural support can reduce the efficiency of self-propelling. A powered indoor/outdoor chair, with the option of attendant control for the carer, will prolong independence providing the home environment is suitable. Once the wheelchair is used all day, the downward force of gravity will increase the speed of spinal deformity and collapse, increasing pain and discomfort (Hsu 1990). Progressive scoliosis (see Ch. 8) can restrict lung capacity, causing breathlessness and possible cardiac abnormalities, also reducing the time tolerated in an upright position. Spinal surgery with fixation by fusion or the insertion of a rod at an earlier stage may delay scoliosis. Alternatively, a spinal jacket can provide stability, though in many cases this cannot be tolerated as the spine continues to collapse. The success of a seating system is variable as it cannot prevent spinal deterioration but should aim to provide comfort and prolong function. Reclining or tilting the chair during the day will reduce loading on the spine, pain and discomfort, but it is not always acceptable as many of the boys adopt a position with an exaggerated lumbar lordosis to maintain an upright position and balance the head to maintain eye contact and function. There is a tendency to prop on one elbow for support. A pad fixed in front of the chest can provide additional support and can reduce loading on the spine to a degree, though this may interfere with function. Environmental controls should always be considered. Maintaining independence in a powered wheelchair is the top priority for this group who are difficult to support in the sitting position.

MYALGIC ENCEPHALOMYELITIS (ME)

ME is generally classified as a chronic fatigue syndrome which can follow a feverish illness.

Clinical features

Common complaints include weakness, lethargy, the inability to tolerate light and noise and fatigue even after minimal exertion. Depression may also be present and in some cases there are signs of minor muscle damage.

Treatment

This can vary from complete rest, which can cause muscle wasting, to a course of graduated exercise to assist the return of normal muscle function and power.

Posture and mobility needs

These will vary depending on the degree of fatigue and weakness which can be variable from day to day. Some sufferers are full-time wheelchair users, though most walk for a limited distance and time. The prescription should reflect the symptoms presented and the overall needs and environment of the user.

PARKINSON'S DISEASE (PARKINSONISM)

This is a complex though relatively common clinical syndrome, associated with a decreased concentration of a naturally occurring chemical (dopamine) in certain areas of the brain. It is characterized by rigidity of muscles, reduction or inhibition of movement and a noticeable tremor that increases with effort.

Prevalence rate

The rate is 65–187 : 100 000 in the UK with a male to female ratio of 3 : 2 (Goodwill & Chamberlain 1988). It is commoner in older age groups with onset occurring in the fifth to sixth decade.

Clinical features

In the early stages there is a barely perceptible impairment of movement. Common characteristics include: loss of facial expression; slow or shuffling gait; gradual increase in time taken to perform basic tasks; 'pill rolling' movement with the fingers; slurred speech; pain and stiffness in limbs with dementia in later stages. Tremor is not always present but is sometimes associated with muscular rigidity. The symptoms become more apparent as the disease progresses. Sudden progressive acceleration and a sequence of rapid short steps (festinating gait) caused by an involuntary response to external stimuli alternates with a total inability to move. Fine movements become affected, the speech becomes monotonous and weak, there is a loss of facial expression, impairment of memory and signs of dementia in the older age group with changes in behaviour which affect family and social life. Pain increases due to muscle tightness.

Treatment

The drug L-dopa increases the level of dopamine in the brain and reduces symptoms in 80% of sufferers. Treatment can lose its effect over a period of time, resulting in an increase of symptoms and loss of independence. There have been recent reports of successful advances in brain surgery in carefully selected cases.

Postural and mobility needs

The slowing of voluntary movement and difficulty initiating movement affects getting out of a chair, using a walking frame or a wheelchair. During the early stages, use of a powered wheelchair may prove helpful. Self-propelling is not usually a realistic option. Few become chair-bound though increasing dependency on others can prove a burden to the carer, whose needs should be given a high priority in the assessment procedure. Those in the younger age group may still be employed and require assistance with all mobility in order to continue normal life.

The risk of pressure sores is associated with weight loss possibly due to problems with eating, general debility and an inability to change position, particularly in bed. Effective equipment should be provided for all support surfaces.

POLIOMYELITIS

This disease is the result of a virus infection of the nerve cells in the anterior grey matter of the spinal cord, contracted through the nasopharynx or gastrointestinal tract (Crawford Adams & Hamblen 1995). It is characterized by inflammatory and degenerative changes in the muscles which lead to weakness and possibly muscle atrophy. Few new cases of poliomyelitis are now seen in the western world due to the introduction of a vaccination programme during the 1960s, though a number of those affected who have residual paralysis of the lower limbs are wheelchair users. Higher numbers of wheelchair users of all ages are seen in the inner cities where there are increased numbers in the ethnic population, especially those originating from Asia and Africa. A clinical study reported in 1983 provides interesting figures (Rastogi et al 1983).

Clinical features

The disease may appear at any age though it is more common in children or adults between the ages of 40 and 60. There is a variable degree of muscle atrophy and weakness, commonly seen in the limb girdles, and in some cases affecting the muscles of respiration. Poliomyelitis differs from cerebral palsy in two ways:

1. The paralysis is flaccid and not spastic.
2. Any muscle can be involved and the condition does not affect flexor muscles more than extensors as individual nerve roots are involved (Dandy 1994).

There is increasing concern regarding the late effects of poliomyelitis (LEP), sometimes known as post polio syndrome (PPS), which is thought to be associated with the diminishing number of nerve cells at a later age in someone whose number of nerve cells is already limited. This can affect all functions including respiration and general ability, with sudden onset of fatigue factors (Field 1995).

Posture and mobility needs

After many years of independence increasing age, together with deterioration in muscle strength, generally due to continuous strain on unaffected as well as partially affected muscle groups, can result in joint pain, signs of deformity and reduction in ability. This is particularly true of full-time wheelchair users who self-propel, often in an obsolete, though very functional, model of wheelchair (Fig. 7.5) and who place additional strain on their shoulder muscles for sideways transfers. Reassessment will leave the individual with a choice between changing their familiar though elderly wheelchair for a lighter self-propelling model or a powered version. After many years it can be difficult to adapt to change as this may affect life style habits and may not be compatible with environmental factors such as kitchen equipment, storage space,

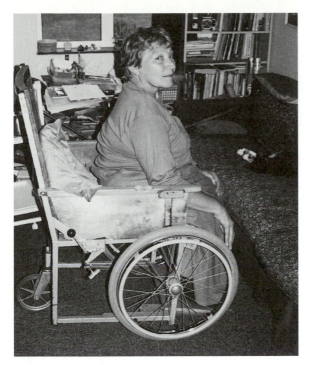

Figure 7.5   Modern wheelchairs are not always the most appropriate prescription. Many long-term full-time users prefer to continue to use an outdated but familiar model which, over the years, has become part of their life style and continues to provide greater independence in their home. This lady with poliomyelitis continues to use her original wheelchair, but is aware of the growing difficulties associated with maintaining this model.

transfer heights or other mobility equipment. Poor postural patterns often used to compensate for muscle weakness result in deformities with increasing problems aggravated by age. Options include surgical correction or the use of orthoses and should be considered depending on the area affected and the severity of the problem.

RETT SYNDROME

This was first recognized as a syndrome as recently as 1966 by Andreas Rett in Vienna, and is a relatively rare disorder of genetic origin which affects only girls. Rett syndrome is, as yet, incurable and results in profound mental and physical disability (see Ch. 10). It is characterized by a slowing of development and a regression of previously acquired skills, together with marked changes in emotional development and behaviour. Onset occurs between 6 and 18 months of age with changes often observed at about 9 months of age. The incidence rate is about 1 : 1000 of female births; the prevalence rate is 1 : 10–15 000 girls (Hagberg 1989).

Clinical features

Apart from the loss of previously acquired skills, wringing of the hands is a common feature and also loss of purposeful hand use. Muscle wasting, cold feet, a decrease in mobility and increased spasticity, together with the development of scoliosis, are additional features. Seizures occur in about half the cases and hyperventilation occurs commonly between the ages of 4 and 12 years.

Treatment

Drugs have little effect and treatment is directed at encouraging movement and activity and supporting the family.

Posture and mobility needs

In the early stages girls with Rett syndrome can walk with varying degrees of help. This should be encouraged to minimize deformity and delay development of scoliosis of the thoracolumbar area which is a characteristic of this disease. Scoliosis can be delayed by provision of a spinal jacket and spinal fusion is carried out in selected cases (see Ch. 8). There is a rapid increase in scoliosis after the age of 8 years, with greater deterioration of the spine in those who are more sedentary or hypotonic. Wheelchair prescription should be regularly reviewed and good postural support provided at an early stage with advice on positioning in all situations. As with all children, it is necessary to consider a range of needs including family, schooling and social requirements. Soft moulded seating which supports the back at rest without interfering with activity is generally recommended. Spinal surgery or the use of an orthosis are other options. The Rett Syndrome Association provides good information and support for all family members.

SPINA BIFIDA

Spina bifida is a developmental abnormality of the neural tube which fails to unite, leaving a gap over which the skin is defective. The defect occurs during early development of the embryo when the posterior part of the neural tube, part of which is formed from the spinal cord and spine, instead of being whole is divided, that is bifid. The defect varies in its degree and size and there are two main types of spina bifida – occulta and cystica. Spina bifida cystica has two forms, known as meningocele and myelomeningocele.

Spina bifida occulta is relatively minor with the defect not being obvious at the skin surface. There is a failure of fusion of the vertebral arch posteriorly and there may be an impairment of nerve function also by the tethering of the dura and through this the spinal cord to the skin surfaces by a fibrous membrane (Crawford Adams & Hamblen 1995). As the spinal cord elongates, there is traction on the spinal cord as the lengthening is not equal. The neurological deficit may therefore be progressive though many people have no symptoms and are unaware that they are affected.

Clinically there is muscle imbalance of the lower limbs, selected muscle wasting and foot deformity either equinovarus or cavus (Crawford Adams & Hamblen 1995).

With spina bifida cystica the visible signs are a sac or a cyst. In the meningocele form the sac contains tissues which cover the meninges. Usually the nerves are not badly damaged and little disability is present. This is the least common form of spina bifida. Myelomeningocele is more severe with grave involvement of nerve function leading to motor, sensory and visceral paralysis. There is a major defect involving the bony vertebral arches, the overlying soft tissue and skin. Often the meningeal membranes enclosing the spinal canal are also involved so the neural tube itself is exposed and open. The defect is commonly found in the thoracolumbar region. In the severest form there is a protruding sac at the base of the spine containing cerebrospinal fluid and possibly some nerve tissue (myelomeningocele).

Incidence rate

This rate is 1 : 1000 (Lorber & Ward 1985). The majority have a normal survival rate. The incidence is expected to fall with the antenatal screening that now takes place.

Clinical features

Children born with spina bifida may be paraplegic with or without spasticity, have impaired or loss of sensation, impaired circulation, double incontinence, mental retardation, perceptual problems and, in some cases, show a degree of apathy and lethargy. Most also have hydrocephalus due to an accumulation of cerebrospinal fluid which arises from an imbalance in the production and drainage of that fluid and caused by excessive pressure and swelling of the cavities in the brain. Hydrocephalus can occur independently either at birth or later in life due to other causes. The degree of paralysis corresponds to the degree of dysplasia or secondary damage in the spinal cord and ranges from the mild or minor weakness of a single group of muscles to severe and total paralysis (Crawford Adams & Hamblen 1995).

Treatment

The aim of treatment is to correct the deformity, maintain correction and work towards maximum function. The introduction of new surgical and medical treatment of spina bifida and improved methods of controlling hydrocephalus have dramatically improved life expectancy since the 1960s. Of those promptly treated three out of five survive (Hunt 1990). Insertion of a shunt will drain any excess cerebrospinal fluid into the abdominal or heart cavities. Surgery is generally started once the child is between 1 and 3 years old and is thriving. Many are ambulant with the help of physiotherapy and encouraging walking and standing will delay development of scoliosis. Bracing may be used to control contractures and deformities and a range of orthotic devices used to give postural support.

Postural and mobility needs

Scoliosis is common and results in poor sitting balance and compromised respiratory function. Flexion deformity, due to muscle imbalance in both the hips and the knees, is likely to develop and although many walk, a wheelchair may be required for going further afield. A spinal jacket will in some cases stabilize the spine and improve balance and function (see Ch. 8). Seating objectives are to provide a stable base, maintain good alignment of the spine, relieve discomfort over sensitive areas and prevent pressure, encourage good respiratory function and improve self-image and independence. ASBAH, an association for spina bifida and hydrocephalus, plays a leading role in providing practical support, advice and information through leaflets, clinics and fieldworkers, as well as initiating research programmes. As with many of the congenital conditions, earlier support comes to an abrupt end at adolescence and ongoing problems relating to incontinence and renal failure are often not addressed until an emergency situation arises.

SPINAL MUSCULAR ATROPHY

There is progressive degeneration of motor nerve cells within the spinal cord, resulting in muscle weakness and wasting. The motor nuclei of the cranial nerves may also be defective. There are various types of spinal muscular atrophy which differ according to age of onset, severity and speed of deterioration and prognosis.

Acute Werdnig–Hoffmann disease appears during the first 6 months of life. It is a degenerative condition and tends to affect the proximal more than the distal muscles and the lower more than the upper limbs. Intelligence is not impaired. There is progressive symmetrical weakness of the muscles and a life expectancy of 2–3 years only.

The main aim of any treatment or postural support is to make the child comfortable and to ease care for the family.

Increasing muscular weakness means additional support is required in the sitting position. The Snug seat, which has a range of evazote shapes and inserts that can be strategically placed for support under an attractive cover, is found to be suitable for this condition. The system has an inbuilt tilt facility and the shell-shaped seat can double up as a car seat with safety fittings available.

Chronic Werdnig–Hoffmann disease appears during the first 12 months of life. The rate of progression varies, though most of those affected require a wheelchair by the age of 8 years old. Life expectancy is variable and many with this condition reach adulthood, though their condition deteriorates in a similar way to boys with Duchenne's muscular dystrophy (MD).

Treatment and provision of equipment for postural and mobility needs should reflect the current situation and be regularly reviewed as required. Every effort must be made to support the family with advice and information, to be realistic and avoid overprescription.

In Kergelberg–Welander disease onset takes place between 5 and 15 years of age. In the early stages the lower limbs are more affected than the upper limbs and distribution tends to affect the proximal before the distal muscles. In general, most of those affected require a wheelchair before they reach 30 years of age. The rate of progression and life expectancy vary, though few, if any, live beyond the mid forties. With spinal atrophy the intelligence is not normally affected, though as the disease progresses, concentration may be reduced.

Treatment

Physiotherapy and occupational therapy are aimed at maintaining range of movement, preventing deformity, encouraging maintenance of functional ability and independence by advising on good positioning whilst providing equipment at the relevant time. Supportive and comfortable seating is a top priority to aid development of skills and social integration in the earlier years, as well as maintaining good respiratory function, feeding, swallowing, digestion and bowel movements.

Postural and mobility needs

Appropriate seating for school is essential

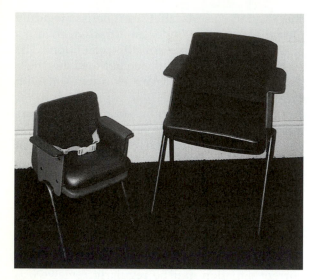

Figure 7.6 For children attending mainstream schools, the lack of support in the standard school chair can be remedied by fitting a lightweight and barely noticeable insert. (Adaptation by Medical Engineering Resource Unit, Carshalton.)

(Fig. 7.6). Constant reassessment and provision of additional support will help to maintain function and quality of life. In the early stages the individual may prefer to self-propel using a lightweight wheelchair. This also presents a more acceptable image for the young teenager. As the disease progresses increased support will be required to prevent scoliosis and a powered wheelchair may be more appropriate with an option for attendant- as well as user-operated controls. Consideration may be given to providing a spinal jacket in the early stages, though as the disease progresses and the spine continues to collapse, a jacket may restrict respiration and cause pressure sores. Mobility for travelling further afield should be considered at an early stage, possibly through provision of an indoor/ outdoor powered wheelchair, in order to provide the best possible life style for each individual.

SPINAL CORD INJURY (SCI)

The majority of injuries to the spinal cord are due to a traumatic incident and can result in paraplegia or quadraplegia (see Ch. 4). Paralysis may be partial or complete, depending upon the level and severity of the lesion.

There is an annual incidence rate between 3.5 and 8 : 100 000, with a male to female ratio of 6 : 2 (Peach & Grundy 1991). The peak age for accidents is 15–19 years. The most frequent causes are sporting or road traffic accidents, many of which could be prevented or reduced by taking precautions such as reducing speed or wearing a helmet.

Clinical features

Paralysis and loss of sensation occur below the level of the lesion (see Ch. 4) with muscle wasting and spasm in the lower limbs in paraplegia. Depression is common and can delay recovery.

Treatment

Medication as required and counselling, together with intensive rehabilitation and provision of an appropriate wheelchair with the necessary technology such as environmental controls for high lesions, will enable the majority of cases to gain a high degree of independence. Once the general medical condition is stabilized, particularly with paraplegia, independence increases with regular exercise, including sport, to build up undamaged muscles. The degree of recovery and future independence depends also on severity of injury, personality, motivation of the individual and family attitude and support.

Postural and mobility needs

Many people with spinal cord injuries regain a high degree of independence. Paraplegics generally have good balance and trunk control and benefit from a lightweight self-propelling wheelchair. Higher lesions have variable balance with upper limb weakness and little trunk control. An asymmetrical posture is often adopted for comfort and stability unless postural support is provided. A 'bucketed' seat position can increase stability and function, though a close watch should be kept for pressure sores in the sacral area. With a high lesion a degree of recline may be required on the backrest with some lateral support to prevent the upper body falling forwards. With new technology chairs there is often a sufficient degree of adjustability of both seat position and angle as well as the degree of backrest tension to accommodate individual requirements and improve posture and function. A high backrest with a head support helps to distribute body weight but may reduce function, cause discomfort over the scapula area or interfere with position adjustment by carers. Pressure sores are common due to loss of sensation, muscle atrophy and depression (see Ch. 12). Prevention may be achieved or incidence reduced by establishing a preventive routine with regular change of position, good diet and avoidance of rough clothing, together with a stable seating base and pressure-relieving cushion. Comprehensive assessment is required at an early stage and an holistic approach required to include future employment opportunities and social life.

SUMMARY

Most neurological conditions are complicated by a variety of changing needs: some clinical, some personal and some environmental. Change may be over a period of time or the situation may vary from day to day depending on the general condition of the individual and their diagnosis. Secondary problems such as urinary infections, pressure sores or depression may necessitate the need for continuing medical intervention and can affect the quality of life for the individual and their immediate family. The opportunity for regular review and reassessment of postural and mobility needs should always be available. Compensatory patterns of movement associated with muscle imbalance and spasm are often adopted to maintain function and independence. Consideration should be given to this fact and the additional stress on ligaments and joints this causes, aggravated in time by the ageing process. Fluctuation in a condition, particularly in the early stages, can make prescribing difficult and delay progress. In cases where an individual is attending a rehabilitation centre, it is reasonable to expect the specialist unit to provide temporary and possibly adjustable equipment until the condition becomes stable or discharge is due. There should be close and regular communication between centre and wheelchair service to ensure that appropriate equipment is available when required. Failure to provide necessary equipment can delay progress and opportunity for improvement, but requests for specialist or custom-made equipment too early in rehabilitation may prove to be inappropriate and therefore not cost effective in the long term. Wheelchair and seating equipment should never be assessed or provided in isolation and all aspects of the individual, their expectations and life style, care needs, communication, employment and family commitments, are an essential part of the total picture to be considered when prescribing equipment and planning a way forward that enables each individual to follow their preferred life style.

REFERENCES

Aylward M, Dewis P, Scott T (eds) for Benefits Agency and Central Office of Information 1992 Disability handbook. HSSS J1543NJ. HMSO, London
Badley E M, Thompson R P, Wood P H N 1978 The prevalence and severity of major disabling conditions: a reappraisal of the Government Social Survey of the handicapped and impaired in Great Britain. International Journal of Epidemiology 7: 145–151
Bar C 1993 Rationalisation and reorganisation of the Welsh Wheelchair Service. Progress report May 1991–June 1993. Welsh Health Common Services Authority, Wales
Blower P 1988 For debate: the advantages of the early use of wheelchairs in the treatment of hemiplegia. Clinical Rehabilitation 2: 323–325
Confavreux C, Aimard G, Devic M 1980 Course and prognosis of multiple sclerosis assessed by computerised data processing of 349 patients. Brain 103: 281–300
Crawford Adams J, Hamblen D L 1995 Neurological disorders In: Outline of orthopaedics, 12th edn. Churchill Livingstone, Edinburgh, pp 133–136
Dandy D J (ed) 1994 Deformities in children In: Essential orthopaedics and trauma. Churchill Livingstone, Edinburgh, pp 141–160
Eames P 1988 Head injury. In: Goodwill C J, Chamberlain M A (eds) Rehabilitation of the physically disabled adult. Croom Helm, New York, ch 24, p 399

Field P 1995 Post polio syndrome. From paper on research undertaken on behalf of British Polio Fellowship, London

Goodwill C J, Chamberlain M A (eds) 1988 Rehabilitation of the physically disabled adult. Croom Helm/Sheridan Medical, New York

Hagberg B A 1989 Rett syndrome: clinical peculiarities, diagnostic approach and possible cause. Paediatric Neurology 5: 75–83

Hunt G M 1990 Open spina bifida: outcome for a complete cohort. Developmental Medicine and Child Neurology 32(2): 108–118

Hsu J D 1990 Spine care of the patient with Duchenne muscular dystrophy. Spine: State of the Arts Review 4(1): 161–172

Langton Hewer R 1988 Motor neurone disease. In: Goodwill J, Chamberlain M A (eds) Rehabilitation of the physically disabled adult. Croom Helm, London, ch 19, pp 308–322

Lipkin P 1991 Epidemiology of the developmental disabilities. In: Caputer A J, Accardo P J (eds)

Developmental disorders in infancy and childhood. Paul N Brookes, Baltimore

Lorber J, Ward A M 1985 Spina bifida: a vanishing nightmare. Archives of Disabled Children 50(11): 1086–1091

McGregor J C 1984 Surgical treatment of ischial pressure sores. Journal of the Royal College of Surgeons of Edinburgh 29: 242–245

Monckton G, Hoskin V, Warren S 1982 Prevalence and incidence of muscular dystrophy in Alberta, Canada. Clinical Genetics 21: 19–24

Muscular Dystrophy Group 1995, Muscular Dystrophy Group Fact Sheet DU1 Apr 1995 1/8

Peach F, Grundy D 1991 How preventable are spinal cord injuries? Health Trends 23: 62–66

Rastogi S, Agarwal A K, Sipani A K, Varma S, Goel M K 1983 A clinical study of post polio infantile paralysis. Prosthetics and Orthotics International 7: 29–32

Vernon G 1989 Stand up the real Glynn Vernon: video for Scope. Pavilion Publishing, Brighton

FURTHER READING

Bleck E E, Nagel D A 1984 Text book of paediatrics. Churchill Livingstone, Edinburgh

Bromley I 1991 Tetraplegia and paraplegia. A guide for physiotherapists, 4th edn. Churchill Livingstone, Edinburgh

Communication 1990 Equipment for Disabled People. The Disability Information Trust, Oxford

De Souza L 1990 Multiple sclerosis. Approaches to management. Series therapy in practice 18. Chapman and Hall, London

Gardiner-Medwin D 1980 Clinical features and classification of the Muscular Dystrophies. British Medical Journal 36(2): 109–115

Hopkins A 1993 Clinical neurology: a modern approach. Oxford University Press, Oxford

Otto Bock 1989 Seating in review. Current trends for the disabled. Otto Bock Orthopaedics, Canada

8

Users with musculoskeletal problems

INTRODUCTION

Individuals suffering with musculoskeletal problems, chiefly arthritic conditions, constituted the largest group of wheelchair users in recent surveys (Fenwick 1977, Dudley & McMahon 1994, Kettle, Rowley & Chamberlain 1992). Each district service will have approximately 18–27% with such problems in their area. The group present with a number of clinical features that should be fully assessed before the correct prescription is arrived at. Such features include: pain, muscle strength and weakness, joint range of movement (ROM), contractures and joint fusion, muscle imbalance, trunk instability, loss of symmetry, local or systemic disease, limb shortening, deformity and abnormal bone formation. Details of the assessment procedure are given in Chapter 6.

Wheelchair locomotion compared to locomotion with or without walking aids has been studied. Some studies have found that the energy expenditure was less than that used in walking at corresponding speeds (Hildebrandt et al 1970), others found it to be the same (Glaser et al 1975) and a further study found it to be 9% more (Traugh, Corcoran & Reyes 1975). It can be concluded that wheelchair locomotion requires approximately the same energy as normal ambulation (Fisher & Gullickson 1978).

ASSESSMENT POINTS

In musculoskeletal assessment the Medical

Research Council (MRC) muscle power scale is generally used. The grades are defined as:

Grade 0   No power
Grade 1   A flicker of movement
Grade 2   Power to move a joint with gravity eliminated
Grade 3   Move limb against gravity
Grade 4   Move limb against gravity with some active resistance
Grade 5   Full and normal muscle power.

Through the examination and assessment of the orthopaedic case the therapist may find the following reminder useful when examining a limb: deformity? shortening? swelling? wasting? scars? (Dandy 1994). Leg shortening is measured in the lying position in two ways: 'true' from the anterior superior iliac crest to the medial malleolus and 'apparent' from any point in the midline, for example the pubis symphysis to the medial malleolus.

A fixed flexion deformity of the hip is assessed with the individual in supine lying. The opposite hip and knee are flexed to the abdomen. If the affected hip also flexes, a fixed deformity is present. In this way the back is not able to arch to accommodate the contracture as it does in the supine lying position. This is known as the Thomas' test.

The assessment of a scoliosis is given later in this chapter.

Good seated posture

A good seated posture is desirable at all times to use the minimum of effort and energy, leaving the maximum of effort and energy for functional activities (Disabled Living Foundation 1993). The size of the seat should ensure that the maximum area of the user's body is in contact with the base of support, which will also ensure that there is pressure relief over the maximum area possible especially if contoured seating is used (Sprigle, Chung & Brubaker 1990). The seating surface should be level, with sagging and asymmetry avoided. The hips and knees should be at 90 degrees with consideration paid to the following: footrest length and angle, footplate angle, back-

rest height, shape and angle, arm support and armrest height. (See Ch. 6.)

TEMPORARY LOANS

Individuals with musculoskeletal problems may require wheelchairs to enhance their quality of life by allowing them to travel greater distances than they would be able to walk on a permanent basis, due, for example, to osteoarthritis. Others may simply require a wheelchair temporarily for the duration of the postoperative recovery, for example.

The majority of NHS wheelchair services provide equipment for individuals who have a disability that will last longer than 6 months. Some services, however, do not loan equipment for the long-term occasional user – use less than three or four times a week. It is advisable that the local service is contacted so that the local criteria can be established.

Wheelchairs required for periods of less than 6 months are acquired from temporary loan stocks. However, many wheelchair services do not provide wheelchairs for such temporary loans, and these loans are administered separately either from the local clinic (with or without a charge or deposit) or from a national charity such as the Red Cross. In London alone, the Red Cross loaned 12 000 wheelchairs during 1995 (Sargent 1996). Loans may also be available from a local charity which works alongside the NHS

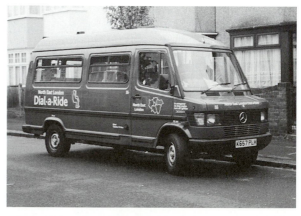

Figure 8.1   Transportation with tail lifts such as Dial-a-Ride has increased users' horizons greatly.

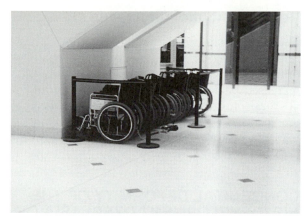

Figure 8.2 Wheelchairs ready for loan in a shopping centre.

service, both financially and through the use of resources, such as Newham Association for Disabled people (NAD) (Ham 1996). Wheelchairs may be loaned for periods ranging from days to 1 month (Southend wheelchair service), to 2 months (North Durham wheelchair service) and 6 months (Ham 1996).

Non-standard items are generally not available from the loan service; for example, stumpboards, elevating legrests, recliners or extended wheel-base models. Departments that will require such equipment on a regular basis should establish a local stock for this temporary period, post surgery for example.

Medical conditions that cause musculoskeletal abnormalities involve bone only, bone and local soft tissues, bone and systemic diseases. This chapter will cover the conditions commonly requiring wheelchairs in alphabetical order and not in the order of numbers of presenting cases.

ACHONDROPLASIA

Background

This is an hereditary disorder of the bone and cartilage (Golding 1989).

Clinical features

There is a failure of normal ossification in the long bones, which may be only half of their normal length (Crawford Adams & Hamblen 1995). Achondroplasia is apparent at birth and the condition leads to marked shortening of the limbs, giving dwarfism. The trunk growth is only slightly impaired and adults seldom reach 130 cm (4 ft 3 in). The hands are short and broad and the three central digits are of almost equal length, producing a 'trident' hand (Crawford Adams & Hamblen 1995). The head is slightly larger than normal and a marked lumbar lordosis is seen, often with a thoracic kyphosis which may lead to complications involving the spinal cord. A waddling gait is often observed. The joints are often stiff but not painful (Golding 1989). There is no mental impairment and life expectancy is normal (Crawford Adams & Hamblen 1995).

Treatment

Surgical leg-lengthening procedures are now being undertaken to increase the individual's height but these are lengthy procedures.

Posture and mobility needs

Although these individuals are able to walk, a wheelchair or buggy may be required in order to keep up with their parents or peers or in daily activities with others. Self-propelling models are generally selected, ensuring that the wheels and the seat height are ergonomically correct for the individual user to ensure efficient propulsion. The diameter of the propelling wheel also needs to be considered, as wheels with a larger diameter help when the arms are short, as do lower armrests. If the arms are too short to make propulsion effective, a powered model may be required for some individuals. If the user is to sit in the wheelchair for a long period of time, an accommodating soft or custom moulded back-rest cushion may be required for both comfort and support, especially where there is a marked lumbar lordosis and thoracic kyphosis. A scoliosis may also develop and other support mechanisms may be used to control the development. While leg lengthening is taking place a temporary wheelchair with extended King's type stump boards (Ham & Richardson 1986) may be required to accommodate the leg-lengthening devices. The stability of the chair must be checked fully to ensure the equipment is safe. This is especially important when such modifications are made to the chair, as even changes in the body position in normal activity can profoundly affect the wheelchair stability (Kirby et al 1995).

ANKYLOSING SPONDYLITIS

Background

This disease, which is not uncommon, affects young male adults generally between 15 and 40 years. The male to female ratio is 5 : 1. The incidence is 2–5/1000 adult males. It occurs in relatives of patients 30 times more commonly than the general population. When fully developed, the disease is characterized by ankylosis of the sacroiliac joints, inflammatory arthritis of the synovial joints of the spine and ossification of the spinal ligaments.

Clinical features

Young male patients present with low back pain and stiffness with progressive immobility and muscle wasting. The joints that are affected are the sacroiliac, the vertebral joints (leading to the 'bamboo' spine) and peripheral joints, especially the large joints, the hip and shoulder (Golding 1989). Chest pain, iritis and pyrexia of an unknown origin may also be features.

Treatment

General education about the progression of the disease is important as are exercise programmes to retain mobility and prevent deformity. These will include breathing exercises as well as exercises for the neck, thoracic spine, hip stretching and general spine mobility. Drugs in the form of NSAIDs (non-steroidal anti-inflammatory drugs), secondary line anti-inflammatory and steroid drugs may also be prescribed (Golding 1989).

Posture and mobility needs

The wheelchair needs will vary from a basic self-propelling or attendant-controlled chair for outings and greater distances, to models with increased backrest angles and modifications for postural support as the condition becomes worse. Models with increased backrest angles may also require special cushions for comfort or positioning.

CONGENITAL DEFORMITY OF THE HIP (DEVELOPMENT DYSPLASIA OF THE HIP) (CDH)

Background

CDH is generally diagnosed a few days after birth or in the first 2 years of life. If the condition is neglected or the treatment is inefficient, disability will result. There are four causes:

- Genetically determined joint laxity.
- Hormonal joint laxity.
- Genetic dysplasia of the hip leading to poor development of the acetabulum and femoral head. This defect is often bilateral and this cause is as common in males as females.
- Breech position during delivery (Crawford Adams & Hamblen 1995). This cause is six times more common in girls than boys and it is bilateral in a third of cases.

Clinical features

The Barlow test is a diagnostic manoeuvre for the detection of dislocation or instability of the hip in the first few days of life. It is a medical examination and well documented elsewhere (Crawford Adams & Hamblen 1995). There is reduced abduction in flexion at the hip joint. If it is not diagnosed early enough there will be a delay in walking and an abnormal gait. The earlier the dislocation is reduced, the better the prognosis. Even in the best conditions, half or a third of children treated after the first year of life can be expected to remain permanently free of trouble. Gradual redislocation or subluxation is frequent and pain from secondary degree changes often develops later in life (Crawford Adams & Hamblen 1995).

Treatment

In the neonatal child of less than 6 months old, bulky nappies help to increase abduction and splinting takes place at approximately 3 months. In children aged between 6 months and 6 years, closed reduction is performed early and operative reduction after 3 years. In children between 7 and 10 years with untreated dislocations, the treatment will depend upon the individual and be either conservative or operative reduction. In adolescents, a total hip replacement in later life may be the treatment of choice or an arthrodesis. If the condition is bilateral then abduction osteotomies at the level of the ischial tuberosity may be appropriate (Crawford Adams & Hamblen 1995).

Posture and mobility needs

It is essential that the wheelchair therapist is aware of the current position/state of the hip joint to ensure further damage does not occur. Working with other team members is therefore vital with these cases. To ensure that a good position and symmetry is maintained, lateral pelvic supports, a pommel and/or kneeblocks may be used depending upon the assessment and the goals of management. Windsweeping may also occur. If these children require surgery, frog plasters or hip spicas are often used for immobilization. In these cases the loan of a temporary non-standard wheelchair may be required. Paediatric orthopaedic units should hold such equipment for loan while the plaster is required (see Ch. 9).

FRACTURES

Background

Fractures cost the NHS approximately £750 million annually and although they are a large group to be noted in this chapter, they do not often necessitate a wheelchair on a permanent basis. The most common fractures that necessitate wheelchairs are those associated with the elderly, notably about the hip, femur, knee and ankle areas. While fixation or plaster of Paris (POP) are being used as a part of the treatment, a wheelchair may be necessary on a temporary basis. However, the therapist should have knowledge of fractures and the healing that has subsequently taken place.

Clinical features

Fractures occur in different degrees of severity depending upon the nature of the injury or impact. Where the skin is intact, the fracture is termed closed (or previously simple). Where there is an open wound with soft tissue damage, the fracture is termed open (or previously compound) (Dandy 1994). Fractures may not all heal as expected. They may be slow to heal (delayed union) or fail to heal (non-union) or there may be malunion, that is, union in the incorrect position.

Treatment

Individuals who have suffered a fracture are usually directed to a wheelchair short-term loan service as they are not permanently disabled. However, it should be remembered that the healing of bone takes a number of weeks. Callus forms in 2–6 weeks and ossification with the solid bone occurs at 6–12 weeks. However, callus does not mature for 12–26 weeks and the gaps between the cortical ends bridge at between 6 and 12 months. During the following 12 months, remodelling occurs (Dandy 1994). Some individuals may therefore require a wheelchair for longer than a 2–6-month period.

Posture and mobility needs

If the fracture is slow to heal in any part of the trunk or lower limb, and it is in an elderly person, a wheelchair may be necessary, especially if weight bearing is to be avoided or is too painful. Elevating legrests, extended stumpboards, cushions and padded extended backrests may be required.

HYPERPARATHYROIDISM

Background

This occurs when there is excessive parathyroid secretion into the body, usually from an adenoma of one of the parathyroid glands, which results in lassitude, dyspepsia and generalized osteoporosis.

Clinical features

Adults present with pathological fractures and bone pain as the bone is absorbed and gradually becomes spongy with thin cortices. Indigestion and weakness also occur (Crawford Adams & Hamblen 1995).

Treatment

This involves the removal of the causative parathyroid tumour.

Posture and mobility needs

Basic wheelchairs may be needed for increasing the individual's quality of life and to reduce the amount of weight bearing occurring.

JUVENILE CHRONIC ARTHRITIS (JCA)

Background

JCA is a persistent arthritis of longer than 3 months' duration in children under 16 years of age. JCA is divided into four groups, which are described below.

Clinical features

Still's (systemic JCA)

This disease affects girls more often than boys and is generally seen in infants or the very young. There is a fever, rash and the joints are involved with growth disturbance. The eyes may also be involved.

Polyarticular JCA (juvenile RA)

This disease is common in girls and joint swelling is often marked. The cervical spine, the temporomandibular and hip joints are commonly affected and it is seropositive.

Pauciarticular JCA

This is a monoarthritis where premature fusion of the epiphysis occurs. It is seronegative.

Monoarthritis (articular JCA)

This is a systematic connective tissue disorder which is usually seronegative.

Treatment

The treatment is similar to RA in adults. Aspirin and NSAIDs drug therapy is used with rest, splinting and gradual exercise. Surgery may be necessary in some cases.

Posture and mobility needs

As rest and graded exercise are part of the treatments for this disease, a wheelchair may be required when walking is not possible or limited. The model required is generally attendant controlled and a comfortable cushion, backrest pad and possibly arm pads may be required.

NEUROFIBROMATOSIS (VON RECKLINGHAUSEN'S DISEASE)

Background

This is a congenital inherited condition.

Clinical features

The disease is characterized by pigmented areas on the skin, cutaneous fibromata of the connective tissue, multiple neurofibromata in the course of the cranial and peripheral nerves which may also involve compression of the spinal cord. A scoliosis often develops which may produce neurological disturbance of the limbs and be so severe that the function of the spinal cord is impaired. Pathological fractures may also occur.

Various manifestations are seen depending upon the area affected (Crawford Adams & Hamblen 1995).

Treatment

The neurofibroma causing the trouble is surgically removed.

Posture and mobility needs

If a scoliosis develops and the spinal cord function is impaired, supportive and corrective seating modifications may be required.

OSTEOARTHRITIS (OA)
Background

This is a common degenerative joint disease with a frequency that increases with age. The estimated incidence in a health district with a population of 250 000 would be 52 250 individuals with OA. It is estimated that 860 of these would have severe or very severe forms of the disease.

Clinical features

Pain, loss of joint range and function and stiffness are the main clinical features (Chamberlain 1988). The pain is worse on weight bearing. The hip is often affected, leading to groin pain which radiates to the knee, and may also produce backache with an increased lumbar lordosis. Activities such as climbing stairs, kneeling, getting out of a chair, out of the bath and off kerbs when walking are typical features of the condition.

Treatment

Treatment aims to relieve the pain and stiffness and to restore function. This is with the use of analgesia, local steroids and to reduce weight bearing to the affected joints. Physiotherapy is used to relieve pain and maintain joint range and muscle strength. Occupational therapy assists with ADL activities. Surgery is the treatment of choice when the pain becomes uncontrollable and the disability has increased and before a permanent wheelchair existence is necessary. However temporary short-term loans may be required when the symptoms are at an acute phase or while awaiting surgery.

Posture and mobility needs

Approximately 25% of wheelchair users suffer with arthritis. The wheelchair and environmental modifications make an enormous difference to these individuals. Chairs that have a high seat to floor distance are often required and this may be achieved with a deeper cushion. These users are often overweight and require larger width models. This produces problems for the carer in assisting or pushing the wheelchair and user, handling the chair into cars and for storage purposes. Also in the environment generally, large chairs are a problem for shop access and doorways. OA wheelchair users range from those requiring a basic chair to increase their outdoor range and therefore quality of life to those requiring many modifications. Deformities need to be accommodated and may include hip and knee deformities, possibly fused knee joints following surgery, ankle and hand deformities. Modifications may include: greater angle of the backrest, shaped cushions, higher seat to floor height, elevating legrests, footboards or extended footplates, alternative angled leg rigging, increased diameter for the handrims, lighter weight wheelchair for the carer's use in transportation. Powered models in the form of add-on devices to manual chairs and powered outdoor or indoor/outdoor models may also be required.

OSTEOGENESIS IMPERFECTA (BRITTLE BONES)
Background

This is a congenital inheritable disorder of the bones and cartilage. The production of the bone tissue is faulty and this stops at the 'woven' bone stage. The bones are therefore soft and brittle due to this and the defective collagen formation

(Apley 1973). Other collagen-containing tissues may also be affected such as the teeth, skin, tendons and ligaments. The severity of the disease varies greatly. In some, fractures occur before birth, in others only a few fractures may occur but in others more than 100 fractures may be experienced in childhood. Most children survive into adulthood and there is a good life expectancy if the risks of fractures from minor trauma is lifted (Wisbeach et al 1992).

Incidence

The incidence is between 1 : 20 000 and 1 : 50 000.

Clinical features

Fractures occur frequently especially with the more severe cases, which makes the instructions in correct caring, handling and management vital. Deep blue coloration of the sclerotic tissue of the eye may occur, deafness from the otosclerosis, which becomes worse in later life, and leg laxity are also found (Crawford Adams & Hamblen 1995).

Treatment

Fractures unite readily but in the more severe cases marked deformity may develop with malunion or bending of the soft bones.

Posture and mobility needs

Such children will require wheelchairs that are well padded to ensure that innocent knocks do not develop into fractures unnecessarily. These may include padding of the side panels, the back and headrest and a harness or pelvic belt to ensure security for outings, as these children are often deaf and have sight problems. Those children at higher risk of fracture may need to use a powered wheelchair and others, lighter models.

OSTEOMALACIA
Background

This is caused by a dietary deficiency of calcium and vitamin D or malabsorption, chronic renal failure or chronic liver disease.

Clinical features

Patients present with bone pain with possibly limb weakness, deformity, marked bone tenderness, hypocalcaemia and pseudomyopathy of the pelvic girdle and thigh muscles (Golding 1989).

Treatment

The treatment involves treating the cause and through dietary supplements.

Posture and mobility needs

These are similar to those of OA.

OSTEOMYELITIS – ACUTE AND CHRONIC
Background

This is an inflammatory bone disorder that may occur in infants, adolescents or adults. In infants the infection may be due to staphylococcus or streptococcus organisms, which leads to oedema in the area and to the separation of the sequestrum of the bone. In the adolescent, acute and subacute forms are seen and in the adult, a thoracic back pain often develops (Golding 1989).

Clinical features

The acute disease is confined to children especially boys. The bones most commonly affected are the tibia, femur and humerus. The onset is rapid. The child feels ill with severe pain over the affected bone. There is generally a history of boils or minor illnesses. In the chronic disease there is a purulent discharge from a sinus over the affected bone. Pain occurs with abscesses and flare ups.

Treatment

Bed rest and antibiotics are the main treatments. In the chronic abscess cases, operations to release the pus, drain the abscess and remove dead bone may be necessary. This will reduce the pain and splinting may be necessary until the infection is over.

Posture and mobility needs

This will depend upon the severity of the disease. The model of wheelchair needed will range from an attendant-controlled model to reduce weight bearing and relieve pain to a self-propelling model with a cushion for the more chronic cases.

(SENILE) OSTEOPOROSIS

Background

This condition affects the elderly, especially post-menopausal women over the age of 60 years. Bone is lost at an average rate of 2% per year for up to 10 years with the greatest loss in the early menopausal years (Ballard & Purdie 1996). The whole skeleton is affected but the changes in the spine are more obvious than elsewhere. There is a reduction in the total bone tissue with a lack of the bone osteoid matrix, thin trabeculae and secondary loss of the mineral calcium phosphate (Golding 1989).

Clinical features

Microfractures and compound fractures are common. The thoracic vertebrae gradually become wedge shaped so the spine begins to flex forwards producing a rounded kyphosis (Crawford Adams & Hamblen 1995).

Treatment

Treatment is by calcium supplements and hormonal oestrogen supplements for post-menopausal women (Golding 1989) in the form of tablets or patches.

Posture and mobility needs

Generally such individuals would require a wheelchair for outside purposes to increase their range of mobility with friends and relatives as they become older and less able bodied. They may require accessories for comfort but seldom require modifications.

PAGET'S DISEASE

Background

This is a common condition that affects the skeleton, arising in those over 40 years of age. It is a slow progressive disorder of one or several bones. The bones become thickened, spongy, and show a tendency to bend.

Clinical features

Pathological fractures may develop and the individual may also complain of bone pain (Crawford Adams & Hamblen 1995). Osteoarthritis of the hip, collapsed vertebrae in the lumbar spine leading to a kyphosis, which may become fixed, and possible paraparesis may also develop (Golding 1989). This may make it difficult for the user to tolerate an upright position for long. Also, a kyphosis of the cervical spine results in a poor head position and subsequently affects both eye contact and feeding. This cannot be solved with a head support although it sometimes helps to put a wider canvas in the wheelchair with a padded back support for comfort and to accommodate the kyphosis.

Treatment

Drug therapy and radiotherapy are used to reduce the bone pain. Calcitonin is used to relieve the pain in active Paget's disease.

Posture and mobility needs

These are similar to those of OA.

BACK PAIN AND PROLAPSED INTERVERTEBRAL DISC (PID)

Background

Back pain accounts for one million people in the

UK seeking advice from their general practitioner each year. Of these, 500 000 require a hospital appointment and 50 000 are admitted. Surgery is required in 7000 and sciatica is associated with the back pain in a sixth of individuals (Chamberlain 1988). More working days are lost now than 20 years ago from back pain, and this reflects the increased disability associated with episodes of back pain (Jayson 1996). The causes of back pain are: mechanical or soft tissue, arthritis, bone disease or visceral.

The major causes of back pain are mechanical strains and sprains, lumbar spondylosis, herniated intervertebral disc (PID) and spinal stenosis. PID is the herniation of the intervertebral disc and it is a common cause of low back pain and sciatica. The prolapse is commonest at the L5/S1 and L4/5 levels. Part of the gelatinous nucleus pulposus protrudes through the annulus fibrosis at the weakest part – the posterolateral point. The size of the protrusion affects the symptoms. If it is small, it will affect the pain-sensitive posterior longitudinal ligaments and give back pain. If it is larger and it protrudes through the posterior ligament and touches the nerve, sciatic pain occurs. Natural healing is by shrinkage and fibrosis of the extending disc material. It usually starts between the late teens and the forties, with the peak prevalence in 45–60 year olds with little difference between the sexes (Jayson 1996).

Clinical features

Back pain has many manifestations and localized problems should not be confused with other pathology. Pain is generally in the lumbosacral region, buttocks and thighs. The pain is mechanical in nature and varies with physical activity and with time (90% of patients recover from acute attacks in 6 weeks; Jayson 1996). Pain in the calf on walking is generally due to arterial insufficiency. Pain at night and persistent pain in the day may have a neoplastic cause and early morning stiffness is characteristic of inflammatory joint disease. Disturbance of the bowels and bladder suggests a serious pathology as does weight loss, anaemia and ill health (Chamberlain 1988).

Treatment

Conservative treatment includes a minimum period of rest (1–3 days), early physical activity, physiotherapy, traction or a corset. Drug therapy to reduce the pain and local injections may be used. By 6 weeks most people are back at work. If there is no improvement conservatively, a biopsychosocial assessment is required and operative treatment may be needed to remove the extended material and relieve pressure on the nerve.

Posture and mobility needs

Individuals suffering with PID may require the temporary loan of a wheelchair through services previously described. If the condition persists and becomes chronic, a wheelchair may be needed on a permanent basis. Such models may be attendant controlled for outdoor use only or may be self-propelling for greater need. As pain is a constant feature, a soft, comfortable cushion may be required (such as foams or pudgee types which will improve the comfort and absorb jolts), an extended backrest and holomatic castors to improve the comfort of the ride. As sitting generally increases the loading pressure on the disc and increases the pain, it is not a position that many sufferers choose. However following surgery and the wearing of spinal jackets or orthoses, a wheelchair may help to improve the user's quality of life by extending their environment. Lightweight wheelchairs will assist the user with self-propulsion.

PERTHES' DISEASE
Background

This is a disease of the hip joint that affects children between the ages of 5 and 10.

Incidence

Eighty per cent of those affected are boys.

Clinical features

The femoral head becomes partly or wholly avascular and the cause is not known, though a number of theories have been reported. The child is generally well and the irritability at the hip, giving local symptoms of a limp and an ache at the hip, subsides fairly quickly. Pain is distinctly unusual. Abduction in flexion is the movement that is most restricted and X-rays show increased density of the head with an increased joint space.

Treatment

The following treatments may be used: traction, avoiding weight bearing with an orthosis, containment of the femoral head in the acetabulum with plaster splints or operations. The sequel to deformity of the femoral head is osteoarthritis.

Posture and mobility needs

Although these children are generally fitted with a non-weight-bearing caliper, they may need a basic wheelchair for school and social activities such as cubs or they may require a wider one to accommodate their orthosis. Older users may require a wheelchair to increases the distances they are able to travel.

RHEUMATOID ARTHRITIS (RA)

Background

RA is the most important inflammatory joint disease. Three per cent of females and 1% of males in the UK suffer with RA (Chamberlain 1988). The estimated incidence in a health district with a population of 250 000 is 4375, of whom, together with OA, 860 would be severe or very severe. The average age of onset is 40 years (Golding 1989). The course of the disease is variable and is characterized with exacerbations and remissions. For 50% of sufferers there is persistent activity with remission and no exacerbations leading to some deformity and for 10% the disease progresses relentlessly towards marked disability (Golding 1989).

Clinical features

There is symmetrical joint pain, stiffness, swelling before the age of 45 and as the disease progresses joints become eroded, lose cartilage, become unstable with muscle weakness and laxity. As a result, joint subluxation and dislocation can occur (Chamberlain 1988). The musculoskeletal system is affected and the symptoms commonly observed are:

- Painful, swollen and stiff joints. The hands and the feet are commonly involved early in the course of the disease and effusions are seen in the larger joints, especially the knee.
- Morning stiffness. The duration of the morning stiffness is a good index of the activity of the disease.
- Muscle wasting, especially around the affected joints.
- Deformity in the later stages.
- Subcutaneous nodules. These are present in approximately 20–30% and commonly on the back of the elbows.

Upper limbs

Hands and wrists. Here there is a loss of movement and an inability to flex the fingers or oppose the thumb due to pain and stiffness in the joint or fibrous adhesions in the flexor tendon sheath. Ulnar deviation is seen at the metacarpophalangeal joints, with hyperextension of the proximal interphalangeal joints and flexion of the terminal interphalangeal joints. This is commonly known as a swan neck deformity. There is also a weak grip due to flexion at the metacarpophalangeal joint and hyperextension of the interphalangeal joints.
Elbows. As the disease progresses there is increasing limitation of extension.
Shoulders. The shoulders become stiff and painful due to lesions of the rotator cuff or due to a capsulitis.

Lower limbs

Feet. Difficulty in standing and walking is experienced due to painful intertarsal and metatarsal phalangeal and interphalangeal joints being affected. Hammer toes develop where there is flexion at the interphalangeal joint and hyper-extension at the metatarsal phalangeal joints. The anterior metatarsal and longitudinal arches become dropped with spreading of the forefoot, progressive hallux valgus, painful heels and achilles tendinitis.

Knees. There is a progressive flexion deformity at the knees with lateral instability due to the laxity of the ligaments. Baker's cysts may be seen when there is involvement of the bursae of the gastrocnemius and semimembranous muscles.

Hips. These joints are affected late in the disease process and involvement causes a flexion and internal rotation deformity leading to problems in walking.

Spine. Instability of the cervical spine is due to the synovitis of the apophyseal joints which spreads to erode the ligaments, annulus fibrosis and cervical discs. Subluxation of the atlanto-occipital joint may lead to headaches, vertigo and parathesia in the limbs. Subluxation of the sub-axial joint may cause cervical root involvement, cord compression and hospital admission. Vertebral artery compression leads to drop attacks, ophthalmoplegia and occasionally cerebellar signs. The temporomandibular joints may also be affected.

Other systems. The skin and vascular system may be affected with hyperhidrosis (excessive sweating), palmar erthyema, leg ulcers and Raynaud's phenomenon. The eyes may also be affected with reduced tear secretions (Sjögren's syndrome), painful eyes and a loss of corneal opacity. The respiratory system may be affected with pleural effusions and fibrosing alveolitis. The nervous system may be affected with nerve compression, and mild or severe sensory and motor loss. Anaemia may be present which leads to tiredness and also leg oedema and infections may occur.

Functional activity

Functional activity may be assessed using the Brattstrom classification (Chamberlain 1988) or with the Stenbrocker's functional assessment scoring system. The Stenbrocker classification divides activities into four levels:

Class 1 – Can perform all activities
Class 2 – Moderate restriction of activities, performed with difficulty due to pain or limitation of movement
Class 3 – Marked restriction, limited activities of daily living
Class 4 – Incapacitated. Confined to bed or chair.

Treatment

Treatment aims to reduce pain, minimize joint disturbance and to improve function.

Drug therapy includes: non-steroidal anti-inflammatory drugs (NSAIDs) to control pain and stiffness, simple analgesia, steroid injections into joints to relieve inflammation, and gold, penicillamine and hydroxychloroquine which are thought capable of modifying RA. Regular monitoring is vital with monthly blood and urine tests as toxic reaction to the drug therapy may occur (Chamberlain 1988). Conservative treatment in the form of moving the joints through a full range daily and resting positions that do not encourage deformity should also be advocated with splints, orthoses and the modification of the environment.

Posture and mobility needs

The purpose of rehabilitation is to minimize disability and dependence and to provide joint protection. With this in mind load bearing should be avoided. For example, in rising from a chair or with assistance in holding the head up in the form of a collar (Chamberlain 1988). Users will find self-propulsion difficult, painful and detrimental to their condition. Powered wheelchairs are often used with the control joy stick in a position of comfort and with the minimum of exertion needed to access it. An attendant-controlled model may also be required for hospital appointments and for general outdoor use. Modifications that accommodate the deformity are often necessary; for example, extended backrests, supportive and comfortable backrest cushions, comfortable seat cushions that are shock absorbing and also pressure relieving, padded elevating legrests, extended footplates or footboards and padded or wider armrests to spread the load and avoid soreness over the elbows and the forearms when weight transfering. The seat to ground floor height may need attention to assist with transfers, standing and reaching surfaces with those with severe disabilities and the backrest angle may need to be increased if the hips are affected.

RICKET'S
Background

There are a number of types of ricket's documented but the commonest is the nutritional type where there is defective calcification of the growing bone due to a deficiency of vitamin D. In these cases there is also an inadequate exposure to sunlight which promotes synthesis of vitamin D in the body. The incidence is high in the West Indies and Asia and the condition is also seen in the UK with the immigrant and refugee populations.

Clinical features

Clinically the head is seen to be large and there is retarded skeletal growth with enlarged epiphyses. Deformity of the chest and curvature of the long bones are also seen.

Treatment

Nutritional supplements of vitamin D are given.

Posture and mobility needs

Wheelchair supply is sometimes necessary for these cases, especially if deformity is present. The modifications and models chosen will depend upon the findings at assessment.

SCOLIOSIS
Background

Scoliosis is the Greek for curvature. The term is used to describe any lateral curve. It may be associated with an exaggeration of the normal curve in the sagittal plane, a lordoscoliosis or a forward curve, or a kyphosis or backward curvature. Spinal deformities can be divided into structural and non-structural (Morley 1992).

Structural deformities

These occur where there is a loss of the normal flexibility of the spine and they do not correct anatomically or radiologically on side bending. In addition, the spine rotates about the vertical axis into the convexity of the curve, producing prominent ribs. The rib hump remains in forward flexion of the spine and is the basis of the forward bending test (Morley 1992).

Conditions that cause structural deformities are as follows:

Neuropathic causes

- Upper motor neurone – cerebral palsy, syringomyelia, spinal cord trauma.
- Anterior horn cell and lower motor neurone – spinal muscular atrophies, myelomeningocele, poliomyelitis, hereditary peripheral neuropathies, arthrogryposis.

Myopathic causes – muscular dystrophy, limb girdle dystrophy, congenital myopathies.

Other causes – congenital caused by failure of formation, idiopathic, genetic and metabolic diseases (Morley 1992).

Non-structural deformities

These deformities correct fully on forward flexion and are not associated with vertebral rotation on lateral bending. The commonest causes are: poor posture, which can be overcome with muscle activity, pelvic obliquity, which causes a compensatory curve which may be corrected by equalizing the leg length, or pressure over the nerve roots. All of these non-structural scolioses may become fixed with time and with growth if the underlying cause is not corrected (see Chs 3 and 9).

Clinical features

A full assessment is only a part of the whole

treatment as the child and the family must be involved in the treatment and understand the reasons for bracing and surgery, for example. At the physical examination, the deformity, aetiology and complicating factors should be recorded (Morley 1992). The spinal examination will include the level of the curve, the direction of the convexity and the presence of a kyphosis or lordosis, for example. The range of movement of the other joints should also be recorded and the individual's sitting ability, mobility and ability to transfer. It is important to encourage the individual to use the standing position for as long as possible to delay the development of the deformity. For those adults with chronic neurological disabilities such as multiple sclerosis, the need for good positioning when lying down is emphasized.

In *cerebral palsy* (see Ch. 9) approximately 40% of children have a structural deformity of more than 10 degrees and in many, especially the non-ambulatory suffering with quadraplegia and severe diplegia, this number is greater. Postural deformities, especially kyphosis, are common in the very young with loss of normal truncal reflexes. The curve is typically a long 'C' shape and it may impair walking and sitting ability (Morley 1992).

Rett syndrome affects girls after a period of normal development with subsequent global regression, with later manifestations of dystonia, spasticity, wasting and incoordination. Sixty-five percent of cases develop scolioses and 72% of all detected scolioses were apparent before the age of 8 years and after this age the curve increases rapidly. Hypotonia predominates in infancy followed later by spasticity more commonly (Morley 1992). The characteristic curve is a thoracolumbar curve which may be extended throughout the thoracic and lumbar spine into the pelvis, producing marked pelvic obliquity (see also Ch. 9).

In *myelomeningocele* cases (see Ch. 9), 75% develop a scoliosis. In the congenital deformities, the deformity is due to failure of formation or segmentation and is present at birth. The incidence of scoliosis is related to the level of paralysis and, generally, one can expect a 100% incidence of spinal deformity with defects at T12

and above, reducing to 25% at L5 (Morley 1992). The curve is progressive and does not respond to conservative treatment and early surgical intervention is therefore required. The congenital curves are more severe and never respond to bracing. In the paralytic types the curve is related to muscle imbalance and appears later.

In cases of *spinal muscular atrophy*, the scoliosis is more common in the less progressive types, that is, those children living into adolescence. The curves are collapsing and associated with respiratory problems. Orthoses are poorly tolerated with careful adjustment and compliance needed. If the opportunity to correct the deformity surgically is missed, rapid progress may occur with a loss of sitting balance and death from respiratory failure (Morley 1992).

With *Duchenne muscular dystrophy* the scoliosis usually develops after ambulation is lost. Early spinal bracing is used with the aim of increasing the lumbar lordosis in order to lock the posterior facets and to try to prevent lateral collapse. In these cases attention should be paid to good seating which should include a firm base, and a well placed backrest will reduce the tendency to asymmetry (Morley 1992).

Treatment

Conservative treatment is in the form of exercise programmes for the postural deformities, electrical stimulation, POP jackets, to spinal orthoses, seating and surgery for the more severe cases. The aim of POP jackets is for local correction of the curve maximally and to hold the position for 6–12 weeks and then to repeat with or without an orthosis for the young child with a mobile curve. Bracing is indicated if the curve is small, under 40 degrees, which remains flexible in a child with growth potential. In adults bracing is also indicated to slow down the downward progression. Seating is not a method of spinal control but a method to contain the child in an optimum position for function. Seating cannot alter the progress of the deformity. A rapidly progressive curve is likely to impair respiration and surgery can offer important benefits. Surgery usually takes place when the child is between 10 and 13 years of age and may be in the form of local fusion, anterior fusion, posterior fusion or both. However, surgery may not be indicated if cardiac function is poor and it is traumatic for both the child and their parents. The aim of the surgery is to improve the physical function through correction and stabilization (Morley 1992).

Posture and mobility needs

The needs of the user with a scoliosis vary, depending upon the severity of their condition and the total needs of usage for the equipment. The child with a minor deformity using a wheelchair simply for transportation may need modifications to ensure a symmetrical posture, such as pelvic/thigh pads and a harness. The more severely affected child may require a full seating system to assist with function, such as pelvic/thigh supports, thoracic supports, ramped cushion, pommel or kneeblocks, footstraps, chest harness and possibly head support. Such individuals spend a long time sitting and receive short periods of therapy. Adaptive seating should therefore reflect and reinforce therapeutic principles, encouraging the child to maintain his/her ability throughout the day and improve postural control. Seating should help to limit the progression of deformity whenever possible. If the deformity is fixed, then postural accommodation is required (Fearn et al 1992). The adult with a scoliosis may need a supportive custom moulded cushion for comfort. The armrest heights or a tray are critical for support, function and comfort. Even when wearing the orthosis or the POP jacket, inserts into the wheelchair seat may be required. If the user is sitting for a long period a pressure-relieving cushion may be required. Contoured cushions assist in distributing the body weight and therefore evenly distribute pressure (Sprigle, Chung & Brubaker 1990).

SPINAL STENOSIS
Background

In this condition there is cramping of the nerves and blood vessels in a constricted or narrow spinal canal. The condition may be congenital or acquired. The patient is generally middle aged.

Clinical features

Pain is generally felt in the gluteal region and the lower legs on one or two sides. After walking for 10–15 minutes, an ache is felt and the patient has to sit down to relieve the pain. Sitting brings relief and long standing periods should be avoided. Flexing the spine for 5–10 minutes relieves the pain by increasing the size of the canal.

Treatment

Mild symptoms may be controlled by the appropriate modifications of activities. For example, bicycling is better than walking. However, in more severe cases, surgical decompression of the canal may be necessary (Golding 1989).

Posture and mobility needs

These will be variable depending upon the severity and range from a basic model to a more complex prescription.

SYSTEMIC LUPUS ERYTHEMATOSUS (SLE)
Background

This is a generalized connective tissue disorder which mainly affects young females, with a female to male ratio of 9:1. It is commonest in the child-bearing years. SLE is characterized by skin lesions, arthralgia, system disturbance, leucopenia and many non-organic-specific antibodies. The disease is occasionally familial and is twice as common in negroes (Golding 1989).

It is a connective tissue disorder characterized by the following features of an autoimmune disease in addition to clinical similarities:

- high levels of immune globulins in the blood and tissues
- lymphoid and plasma cell hyperplasia
- usually good response to systemic steroids.

SLE is especially common in Asian and black teenagers (Golding 1989).

Clinical features

Joint pain is the most common feature of presentation in 50% of cases and it resembles RA in 90% of cases (Golding 1989). The systemic illness is, however, out of proportion to RA and there is also fever and malaise. Skin manifestations are seen in 75% of cases. They appear in areas that are exposed to sunlight, notably the 'butterfly' lesion on the face. The following clinical features may also be seen:

- alopecia and vascular lesions in the fingers or leg ulcers
- cardiovascular (pericarditis or endocarditis)
- renal disease
- pulmonary involvement (pleurisy or effusion)
- splenomegaly
- hepatomegaly
- ophthalmic lesions
- nervous system symptoms (migraine, depression, behaviour)
- neuropathy (isolated cranial nerve palsy, transverse myelitis leading to paraplegia, choreoathetoid movements)
- blood involvement
- gastrointestinal involvement.

Treatment

The initial treatment is to remove or avoid the precipitating factors such as the sunlight or drugs. Rest, NSAIDs, analgesia, corticosteroids, antimalarials, plasma exchange and immunosuppressive agents may be used (Golding 1989).

Posture and mobility needs

The time at which the user presents for a wheelchair may vary depending upon their social situation. It may be for a simple attendant-controlled chair to increase their environment or for a basic self-propelling model. When the wheelchair is used more frequently, the user will require pressure-relieving cushions and may require an extended backrest which is padded, padding on the armrests, and a light-weight model to assist with propulsion. The diameter of the handrims may also need to be increased in width to assist with comfort. In the later or more severe forms of the disease, powered models may be required. If the user is on steroid therapy, weight gain is likely with the subsequent need for changes in wheelchair seat size.

TUBERCULOSIS (TB) OF THE BONE
Background

This is a chronic illness that is slow to develop compared to other forms of TB. There is evidence of the disease elsewhere and the bones of the thoracolumbar spine, hips and knees are often affected.

Clinical features

There is pain which is worse at the end of the day and a pyrexia which is less marked. There is muscle wasting around the joint, swelling with possible effusion and deformity and a limp are common (Crawford Adams & Hamblen 1995). The abscesses are slow to form (Dandy 1994).

Treatment

Drug therapy in the form of systemic chemotherapy and also bed rest and splintage of the affected joints are prescribed. If the disease is advanced with destruction present, ankylosis of the bones is encouraged (Crawford Adams & Hamblen 1995).

Posture and mobility needs

These are various depending upon both the severity of the disease at presentation to the wheelchair service and the findings at the assessment.

TUMOURS
Background

Tumours can be either benign or malignant and

malignant tumours can be either primary in origin or secondary. They produce local destruction of the bone, often compressing nerves, especially in the spinal cord, and can interfere with the peripheral nerves (Crawford Adams & Hamblen 1995). Benign tumours include: osteoma, chondroma, osteochondroma and giant cell tumour. Malignant tumours include: osteosarcoma (generally seen in childhood or adolescence), chondrosarcoma of the bone (seen in middle age), fibrosarcoma of the bone (seen in young adults), Ewing's tumour (seen in children), multiple myeloma (generally seen in the years past middle age). Secondary tumours (metastases) are more common than primary tumours and are seen in later life.

Clinical features

Pain, swelling, pathological fractures, ill health, lethargy and neurological symptoms are the symptoms that will be found with tumours. In the later stages of malignant disease where secondaries are present, nausea, vomiting, dehydration, hypercalcaemia and weight loss are also seen.

Treatment

Tumours may be either left alone, excised if painful or with increasing size or the affected part amputated. Chemotherapy and radiotherapy are also treatments that are commonly used for this condition. The treatment will depend upon the type of tumour presenting, the age of the patient and its progress.

Posture and mobility needs

These will be various, depending upon the individual's needs, the type of tumour and the stage in its development. Young children may require a self-propelling model as they are getting over an excision or amputation. Older adults may require a model to enhance the distances they move in. If they are self-propelling, a lighter wheelchair may be required. For the user who has had an amputation, especially at a through hip or hemipelvectomy level, a custom-made cushion in the wheelchair is generally required to gain symmetry and comfort while sitting.

The individual with metastases generally requires a wheelchair in the later stages of the disease for outings and hospital appointments, for example, as they are so weak. Such loans, which are needed quickly and for relatively short periods, may be provided through the temporary loan service, the MacMillan Cancer nurse team or the district nurses. A soft cushion may be required to enhance comfort due to excessive weight loss.

REFERENCES

Apley G 1973 A system of orthopaedics and fractures. Butterworth, London

Ballard P A, Purdie D W 1996 The natural history of osteoporosis. British Journal of Hospital Medicine 55(8): 503–507

Chamberlain M A 1988 Osteoarthritis and spinal pain. In: Goodwill C J, Chamberlain M A (eds) Rehabilitation of the physically disabled adult. Croom Helm, London, pp 109–131

Crawford Adams J, Hamblen D L 1995 Outline of orthopaedics, 12th edn. Churchill Livingstone, Edinburgh

Dandy D J 1994 Essential orthopaedics and trauma, 2nd edn. Churchill Livingstone, Edinburgh

Disabled Living Foundation 1993 Wheelchair information. DLF, London

Dudley N J, McMahon M 1994 The changing pattern of wheelchair provision. Clinical Rehabilitation 8: 70–75

Fearn T A, Green E M, Jones M, Mulcahy C M, Nelham R L, Pountney T E 1992 Postural management. In: McCarthy

T G (ed) Physical disability in childhood. An interdisciplinary approach to management. Churchill Livingstone, Edinburgh, pp 401–450

Fenwick D 1977 Wheelchairs and their users. OPCS. HMSO, London.

Fisher S V, Gullickson G 1978 Energy cost of ambulation in health and disability: a literature review. Archives of Physical Rehabilitation 59(March): 124–133

Glaser R M, Edwards M, Barr S A, Wilson S A 1975 Energy cost and cardiorespiratory response to wheelchair ambulation and walking (abstract). Federation Proceedings 34: 461

Golding D N 1989 A synopsis of rheumatic diseases, 5th edn. Wright, Sevenoaks, Kent

Ham R O 1996 Annual Report. Newham Wheelchair Service, London

Ham R O, Richardson P 1986 The King's amputee stump board – Mark 11. Physiotherapy 72:124

Hildebrandt G, Voight E-D, Bahn D, Berendes B, Kroger J 1970 Energy costs of propelling wheelchairs at various speeds: cardiac response and effect on steering accuracy. Archives of Physical Medicine and Rehabilitation 51: 131–136

Jayson M I V 1996 Back pain. British Medical Journal 313: 355–358

Kettle M, Rowley C, Chamberlain M A 1992 A national survey of wheelchair users. Clinical Rehabilitation 6: 67–73

Kirby R L, Sampson M T, Thoren F A V, MacLeod D A 1995 Wheelchair stability: effect of body position. Journal of Rehabilitation Research and Development 32(4): 367–372

Morley T R 1992 Spinal deformity in the physically handicapped child. In: McCarthy G T (ed) Physical disability in childhood. An interdisciplinary approach to management. Churchill Livingstone, Edinburgh, pp 351–365

Sargent L 1996 Red Cross bridges the wheelchair gap. Therapy Weekly 16 May: 6

Sprigle S, Chung K C, Brubaker C E 1990 Reduction of sitting pressures with custom contoured cushions. Journal of Rehabilitation Research and Development 27(2): 135–140

Traugh G H, Corcoran P J, Reyes R L 1975 Energy expenditure of ambulation in patients with above knee amputations. Scandinavian Journal of Rehabilitation Medicine 5: 67–71

Wisbeach A, McCarthy T G, Fixen J A 1992 Osteogenesis imperfecta. In: McCarthy G T (ed) Physical disability in childhood. An interdisciplinary approach to management. Churchill Livingstone, Edinburgh, pp 331–350

9

Children with mobility problems

INTRODUCTION

There is little published information on the number of children who are wheelchair users in the UK. A national survey covering 89% of the wheelchair services in England taken during 1995 (National Prosthetic and Wheelchair Services Report 1993–96) found that on average 6% of wheelchair users were under the age of 19 with some services recording only 2% and others 14% in the lower age group. These figures exclude the large number of children using either privately or charity funded equipment. There is equally little information on the number of children seen in special seating clinics. Figures from Cambridge Health Authority (Royal College of Physicians 1995) found 6% of wheelchair users were classified as level 1 or 2 on the Chailey Seating Scale (Mulcahy 1986) (see Appendix 1); 29% of this group were under 18 years of age and 54 out of 62 (87%) had cerebral palsy. Figures recorded in the USA and Canada towards the end of 1989, on the number of seating systems issued in one year, included the following details:

- 46.3% were under 19 years of age
- 62.9% of all users were classified as cerebral palsy
- 37.8% of the group with cerebral palsy were under 19 years of age.

A seating survey carried out in Dundee in 1980 (TRES 1981), whilst not restricted to wheelchair users only, identified cerebral palsy as the second

155

largest group of people needing special seating. This group also presented some of the most severe postural problems (Bardsley 1993).

POWERED WHEELCHAIRS FOR CHILDREN

A later survey of marginal wheelchair users carried out in the Tayside area (Perks et al 1994) found that no one under 5 years of age was self-propelling. The Institute of Child Health, Wolfson Centre reported that providing powered wheelchairs to children as young as 3 years of age aided general development and increased individual confidence (Holt 1991). This work provided no details regarding diagnosis, though work carried out in the USA (Miller & Bachrach 1995) recommended provision of an electric wheelchair at about 2–3 years of age for children with osteogenesis imperfecta (brittle bones) or arthrogryposis (stiff joints). Children with these conditions are cognitively normal and have normal balance and motor control. However, it is felt to be inappropriate to apply the same criteria to children with cerebral palsy who were less likely to be able to manage the controls at such an early age. The report suggested that children with neuromotor disorders should be assessed at about 6 or 7 years of age when they have developed improved functional skills for handling controls. A group of children aged between 4 and 16 years old, with severe spastic tetraplegia and learning difficulties who were initially dependent upon others for both their mobility and daily living needs, learned to use powered wheelchairs with appropriately adapted controls after training for 2–3 hours each day over a period of time varying from 1 month to 36 months (Emmelot, van der Veldt & Mengerink 1992). At the end of their training, all the children selected for the scheme were able to cope independently in the home, school or a protected environment.

AN HOLISTIC APPROACH TO PRESCRIBING

There are many challenges when providing wheelchairs and seating for children. Correct seating in a wheelchair will influence posture and development of functional ability, social skills and self-esteem, whilst reducing postural deformity and pressure problems. Provision of any postural support should be part of an integral 24-hour postural management and development programme. Timely provision of appropriate equipment, including a wheelchair, will provide the child with the opportunity to participate in many daily activities whilst improving the quality of life for both the child and their family. The need of additional care for a disabled child, together with the social implications and attitudes of others, has a great impact on family life (Pimm 1996). Although appropriate equipment can improve life for the child and their family, it can in no way fully compensate for disability and, when prescribing, care should be taken not to raise the expectations of those concerned. A wheelchair should not be provided in isolation, but as part of an holistic and ongoing programme of rehabilitation, education and social integration.

Coordinating care and wheelchair provision

The needs of each child and their family must be fully understood and respected, bearing in mind age, ability, expectations, environment, life style and culture as well as the medical needs and prognosis. Most children with mobility problems are treated and cared for in a variety of settings by a number of people including doctors, teachers, psychologists, therapists and carers all of whom have their own views, ideas and expectations for the child generally based on their specialist knowledge and previous experience (Trachtenburg 1995). The wheelchair therapist, though not involved with the daily care, plays an important role in supporting those regularly working with the child by advising and providing wheelchair equipment which, if suitably selected, will not only enhance mobility but encourage the development of other skills. Communication between the various professionals and carers involved is frequently blurred and will depend upon personalities as well as geographical factors.

Many children, as well as attending a local school or centre, will be known to a specialist unit for some of their needs. The picture may well be complicated further when parents, anxious to do the best for their child or seeking a cure, will become involved with new methods or concepts of care and treatment, some of which may complement the existing programme, and others directly conflict with more traditional views.

The final prescription for a wheelchair may well reflect the anxieties and demands of the family as well as the needs of the child. Ideally all communication relating to the individual care programme should be channelled through a central contact person chosen by the family and someone in whom they have complete confidence. This ideal is rarely possible to achieve and professionals should be sensitive to the difficulties facing the family and the importance of integrating all aspects of care whilst ensuring that the views of both family and child are paramount. Before any decision is made regarding equipment, the wheelchair therapist should be certain that all the relevant information is received and recorded and all aspects of the child's everyday life, including social activities, education and transport issues, care, management and life style, are taken into account (see Ch. 6).

CHILDREN WHO NEED A WHEELCHAIR

Children needing mobility equipment, with or without postural control, can be divided broadly into the following groups:

- Those who can walk short distances but require a chair in order to travel further afield and who may or may not be able to self-propel.
- Those who have adequate physical and mental ability to learn to self-propel and, given the appropriate equipment, will achieve a degree of personal independence (Fig. 9.1).
- Those who have restricted upper limb func-

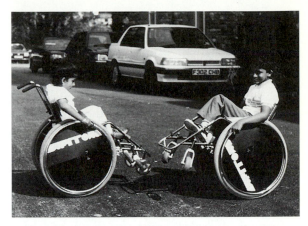

Figure 9.1 Children are able to self propel independently when prescribed appropriate equipment. Department of Health 1991 (with permission from Remploy Health Care and DoH).

tion though can learn to use a switch and control a powered wheelchair.
- Those who are unable to control or propel a wheelchair and are dependent on another person to push them.

Many children with a motor impairment that restricts their walking are also likely to require some form of postural support in their wheelchair or buggy. This should always be assessed in relation to other postural and mobility needs in order to avoid inappropriate prescription.

Disability groups of children requiring a wheelchair

Children with restricted mobility will have either a congenital or an acquired disability. Although many of the clinical and physical features demonstrated are similar in both groups, there are differences which need to be taken into consideration, particularly relating to psychological factors and the attitude, feelings and expectations of families and friends. Many children have multiple disabilities which will include impaired vision and hearing as well as learning difficulties or behavioural problems. Some 71% of children with cerebral palsy are reported as having impaired vision and hearing. These deficits can have an impact on selection of mobility equipment, particularly in the choice of head support for those wearing hearing aids or with restricted vision.

Congenital disorders

Cerebral palsy is the most common disabling condition of childhood and the one most frequently seen in wheelchair users under 16 years of age. Children with cerebral palsy have problems affecting movement and posture, as well as a range of other disabilities associated with damage to the nervous system. Spina bifida forms the second largest group of children with congenital disorders seen in the wheelchair service (see also Ch. 7). The degree of disability depends on the level of the defect in the spinal cord (see Ch. 4). A range of disabilities can be associated with this condition, including paralysis and loss of sensation as well as musculoskeletal abnormalities which affect walking and a tendency to pressure sores.

Less common congenital conditions seen within a typical wheelchair service will include a range of neuromuscular disorders such as muscular dystrophy, Rett syndrome and Batten's disease, as well as orthopaedic conditions including osteogenesis imperfecta (brittle bones) and arthrogryposis (stiff joints) (see Ch. 8) and possibly some rarer genetic disorders. Due to the relatively low number of children seen with some of these conditions, it can be difficult for the therapist to develop a particular expertise. However, specialist centres and national voluntary groups dedicated to the less common disabilities can usually provide information and advice and in some cases will have a regional or national consultant, therapist or field worker who will assist with assessment and provide support to the child and their family on broader issues. In many instances an early diagnosis is not always possible due to a delayed onset, such as occurs in Rett syndrome. Boys with muscular dystrophy are often over 3 years of age when clumsy walking signals the beginning of this progressive disorder and a diagnosis is first made. In these cases parents may view a wheelchair as confirmation of a situation they are reluctant to accept and great sensitivity will be required to persuade parents of the benefits a wheelchair can provide to the child.

All these conditions cover a wide range of disorders of varying complexity. Many of those less severely affected will learn to walk and only require a wheelchair on an occasional basis when going greater distances, for example on holidays or school outings. Others have complex problems which require a comprehensive assessment of medical, social, postural and mobility needs, often carried out over a period of time before a final prescription can be made (see Ch. 6).

Acquired disabilities

An acquired physical disability is commonly the result of an accident causing damage to the spinal cord or brain, or may be the result of an acute illness such as meningitis. The degree of permanent disability will depend on the site and severity of any brain damage but the overall picture will vary if other injuries are involved. For instance, following a road traffic accident a child may receive head injuries and brain damage but also have a tracheotomy, internal injuries or fractured bones. The degree of recovery expected cannot always be predicted until some months following the initial incident. This makes forward planning as well as assessment for equipment difficult.

EQUIPMENT FOR CHANGING NEEDS

Changing needs require a flexible approach. Whilst taking into account the anticipated course of the recovery, it is important that the correct equipment is available for immediate use so that essential rehabilitation time is not wasted or recovery delayed. Wheelchair services do not generally provide for short-term needs but may be willing to issue standard equipment. However, they are likely to have difficulty responding instantly to any request for highly specialized chairs. This is a situation where there needs to be close cooperation not only between the specialist unit and the wheelchair service but also with the purchaser, who should be kept informed of any needs that are not being met due to lack of resources. Many rehabilitation units and specialist centres hold a stock of suitable equipment including wheelchairs for short-term use with children who have rapidly changing or special, though temporary, needs. Wheelchairs with a range of adjustable features as well as static seats and accessories can often fit the need on a temporary basis. Designing and manufacturing highly complicated equipment can take a long time and it is not an efficient use of resources to order specialist systems for short-term use. There are a number of children's charities who are willing to provide funding to specialist centres, particularly where one piece of equipment can be adjusted and transferred or shared with other children. For home use, simple, practical equipment that can be easily handled will be better used, cared for and enjoyed by all concerned.

The design and range of equipment

In the UK wheelchairs were first issued free at source of need to children when the National Health Service was established in 1948. At this time and until the late 1980s, the design of children's wheelchairs was simply a scaled-down version of the adult government specifications (see Ch. 1). Emphasis was placed on stability and safety, making the wheelchairs more suited to less able children and restricting those with the ability and motivation to develop greater skills and independence. For this reason many children in this country had privately purchased wheelchairs generally funded fully or in part by one of the many children's charities.

Although there have been many models of children's wheelchairs available for some time on the private market, the first range of more attractive children's chairs was introduced into the NHS in 1987. Whilst more pleasing to the eye, the performance of these chairs was very similar to the earlier models and it was not until the early 1990s that the Remploy Teeny Roller (Fig. 9.2) became available on the NHS, then the Mini Meteor appeared in 1996, providing the option for a more active and attractive model with an adjustable wheel position. A wider range of

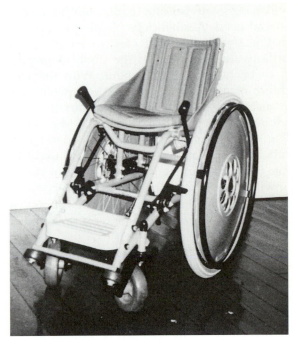

Figure 9.2   The teeny roller introduced for the younger child during the early 1990s.

models is now available in some services whilst an increasing range of lightweight wheelchairs with greater adjustability in all features can be purchased through the private market. Many families fund raise or seek financial help through charities such as 'Whizz Kidz' to purchase a more sophisticated and aesthetically pleasing model of chair to meet a specific need. In general, it is the families of the active and more able users who obtain their wheelchairs through charities whereas those with severely disabled children requiring continuing clinical support are more commonly seen by wheelchair services.

Meeting all needs

Children are not generally referred to the wheelchair service until they are over the age of 30 months. Until this time the paediatric therapist will provide the family with advice on positioning and the choice of suitable equipment. Few wheelchair services provide standard buggies for young children though the majority will assess, advise and endeavour to meet a special need. Aesthetically pleasing equipment, that is lightweight and easy to handle is the priority for the family if the disabled member is to be taken out and about. With the wide choice of attractively designed equipment now available, a commercial buggy which provides adequate support can generally be found (Fig. 9.3), though there are times when an unsuitable buggy has already been purchased. This can cause difficulties if the family is unable or unwilling to afford to change the model. If additional financial help is required, this should be discussed with the social worker or a voluntary group.

If further postural support is required, this should be kept discreet and to a minimum. Lightweight inserts incorporating pelvic and thoracic supports are available, or a polypropylene jacket, bead seat, body harness or waistcoat harness may be adequate, providing they are easy to fit and if the buggy is being used only for short periods of time (Fig. 9.4). Care needs to be taken with the fitting of any support as incorrect fitting of straps can cause discomfort and reduce

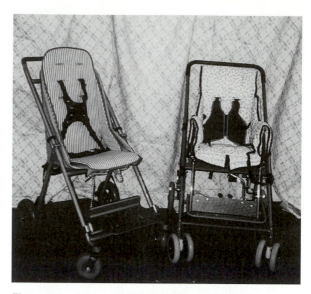

Figure 9.4   A range of lightweight harnesses and supports are readily available. The butterfly harness (left) and the waistcoat harness (right) provide greater support than a simple shoulder harness when correctly fitted.

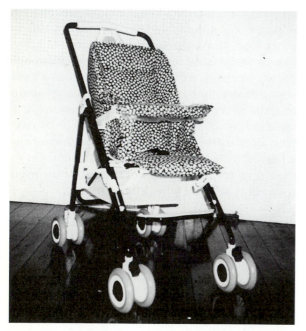

Figure 9.3   A suitable commercial buggy can generally give adequate postural support to a child under 3 years of age.

the effectiveness of the support. As the child grows and develops and spends longer periods of time in a buggy, the situation will need to be reviewed and increased postural support or a larger buggy or a wheelchair may be required.

Progressing from a buggy to a wheelchair can be a difficult period for most parents both from the emotional and the practical point of view. Larger buggies are available and may be the answer for some children, though these tend to be heavy and cumbersome and are not suitable as a main seating system or for children with complex postural problems. Providing these can create a dilemma for the wheelchair service as the cost can also be some ten times that of a child's wheelchair.

Children with the ability to self-propel and requiring only minimal postural support, will increase their mobility and independence by using a chair with adjustable stability and seat angle (Fig. 9.5). A child with good trunk and upper limb control can quickly become proficient and independent in getting up and down low steps and kerbs and over rough ground. A well-shaped and contoured base cushion will help to maintain pelvic stability. Additional postural

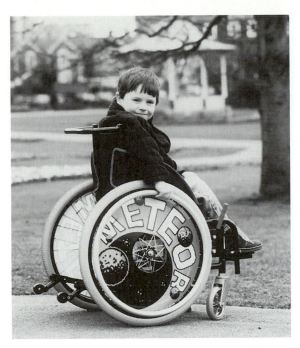

Figure 9.5   The Mini-Meteor provides greater mobility and independence for an able young child.

support for all those self-propelling should be kept to a minimum as thoracic pads can interfere with arm function and increase the effort required to propel the wheelchair. Some very severely handicapped children can become proficient in operating an electrically powered wheelchair and there is now an ever growing choice of controls and switches available to meet all needs.

Assessment is often arranged directly between the school and a specialist centre, particularly when other switches for communication or environmental controls are also being considered. The wheelchair service should be kept fully informed from an early stage of any plans or decisions which will eventually have to be funded from their budget or which affects their equipment. This will avoid any later misunderstandings or delay in the provision of essential equipment.

Twin buggy provision

Numerous unsuccessful attempts have been made to produce an acceptable twin buggy that will take a disabled child over 3 years of age, together with a younger sibling. Twin major buggies provide no support and are considered to be unsuitable for a young baby. Trials have been carried out by fixing two separate buggies together, but the width of the final result together with the imbalance between the heavier and the lighter child will make the buggy awkward to push and manoeuvre and impossible to get through shop doors or down supermarket aisles.

Custom made models or adaptations of a standard buggy where one child sits behind the other have had limited success, though again the imbalance of weight has proved to be a problem. The recent appearance of the heavier style Horacek and Max buggies appears to offer a partial solution, as they cater for a larger child and are sufficiently stable to carry a purpose-built baby basket hooked on to the pushing handle (Fig. 9.6). This, however, is an expensive and short-term solution, often suitable only for a few months and unlikely to be funded by most local wheelchair services, though it may be considered by charities such as STEPS who already deal with mobility problems for children.

In addition to the size of the older child, physical condition and temperament are also significant, as a child with uncontrolled spasm, a tendency to have fits or with behavioural problems can place the younger child at risk. To date this problem has not been successfully solved and mothers are advised to consider carrying the baby in a body sling for as long as is practical. In many cases the only solution is to have two buggies and two carers when both children need to be taken out together. In general, it has to be recognized that the greater the gap in age between a disabled child and the younger sibling and the greater the disability of the older child, the more difficult it is to solve this problem in a practical way. Other one-off adaptations have been made for mothers who are wheelchair users, to enable them to independently take their child out. ParentAbility is a group that provides support to mothers with a disability. This and other useful addresses for one-off manufacture and charities with specific information can be found at the end of this chapter.

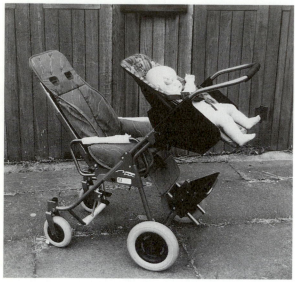
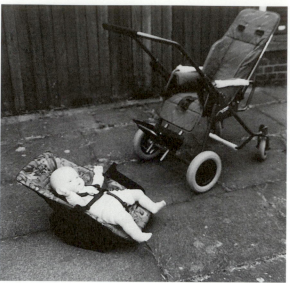

A   B

Figure 9.6   (A) A custom made adaptation for a commercial buggy enables a mother to carry her baby with a disabled older sibling. (B) The customized buggy can be separated for individual use. (Adaptation and photographs by Medical Engineering Resource Unit.)

POSTURAL MANAGEMENT AND SUPPORT

Postural management is the total approach to the facilitation of correct position in all postures (Fearn et al 1992). Muscular imbalance due to spasticity and persisting tonic reflexes in children with neuromuscular disorders (see Ch. 4) can quickly produce asymmetrical deformities and joint contractures (Sharrard 1967), particularly for children who spend long periods of time sitting. In spite of hypertonicity in the lower limbs, there is often hypotonus in the trunk (Trefler, Tooms & Hobson 1978, Bobath 1980) resulting in forward flexion and collapse of the upper body and head. Many children with this problem are unable to correct themselves as they lack the required righting or equilibrium reactions (see Ch. 2). The downward force of gravity reinforces this flexed posture. Early attention to any existing or potential postural deficit should be seen as a top priority when treating a physically disabled child. Clinical evidence has shown that early and persistent positioning of children

at risk of hip and spine deformities can radically alter a posture (Letts et al 1984, Scrutton 1989).

Teaching good postural habits should start as early as possible, as good posture not only improves physical function but gives a general feeling of well-being whilst encouraging healthy organic function, including respiration, bladder and bowel function and digestion. Correct positioning in lying, sitting and standing are of equal importance. The ability to change a position independently will reduce the likelihood of deformity, but many children with a neurological deficit are unable to correct their position. A large proportion of each 24 hours is spent in the lying position and children who lie with flexed hips and knees falling to one side without any form of postural support or correction are in danger of developing a windswept deformity with involvement of both the hips and the spine (see Ch. 4). Over a period of time shortening of the hamstrings and windsweeping, with possible dislocation of the hips, will seriously compromise the sitting position. A single approach to postural management is rarely effective and a 24-hour properly planned care programme, incorporating a variety of approaches, will influence the development of good postural habits and prevent or delay some of these deformities.

24-hour postural management

Although the wheelchair service will assess and prescribe postural support in the form of a cushion or seating system for use in a wheelchair, management of posture in all positions is a joint responsibility that needs a multidisciplinary approach. The programme should be an integral part of each child's care and daily activities. This should include:

- Correct positioning at all times and maintenance of movement in all joints.
- Regular supervised and purposeful activity, muscle stretching and maintenance of range of movement through physiotherapy and occupational therapy.
- Regular changes of position and equipment within the 24 hours.
- Regular review and reassessment of posture.

Also, if relevant and following full assessment:

- Provision of appropriate equipment with full instruction in use, e.g. lying board, standing frame, wheelchair with postural support, static seating, etc., as required.
- Medication to reduce or control spasticity and fits.
- Fitting of appropriate orthoses.
- Surgical intervention.

A period of daily standing should be encouraged as this will help to delay development of scoliosis and prevent shortening in the hip and knee flexors by maintaining length in all tissues. Attention must also be paid to good positioning of the feet, as the development of foot deformities frequently prevents a child continuing with a standing programme as they grow older.

Measuring postural ability

The evaluation of postural ability and the benefits achieved from a postural programme are generally based on visual observation by the therapist. Assessment may include reference to the seven levels of sitting ability developed at Chailey Heritage (Mulcahy 1986) incorporating work undertaken by Hare (Hallet, Hare & Milner 1987). Six levels of lying ability in both prone and supine and guidelines to standing ability have also been identified (Fearn et al 1992) and are a useful tool when assessing postural ability in a child (see Appendix 1). The Chailey sitting scale can be modified to include reference to the quality of posture (see Ch. 4).

A method of measuring windswept hip deformity, using a goniometer (Goldsmith et al 1992), can provide useful clinical information, but does not relate to functional ability. The results are useful for later comparison but the technique is time consuming and therefore not readily used by practitioners.

A sitting assessment scale that is used together with video film has been developed in Sweden (Myhr et al 1991). This provides more reliable information than individual observation, though again requires more time and regular access to a video camera.

Whichever method is used, it is essential to have some recognized way of monitoring and reviewing postural ability to ensure improvements are being achieved.

Alternative and complementary treatments

Initially a comprehensive assessment (see Ch. 6) is carried out to identify the most appropriate method of treatment required to prevent or correct postural deformities.

Daily physiotherapy and occupational therapy generally form the basis of any postural programme, though this may be carried out by a lay person. Other treatment may include some of the following detailed below.

Orthoses

Positioning of the feet and prevention of foot deformity is of particular concern (Carter & Edwards 1996) if standing and walking are to continue. Correct foot alignment can be maintained by stretching exercises, wearing supportive footwear and, if necessary, the fitting of a lightweight polypropylene ankle–foot orthosis (AFO) to maintain the foot in the necessary plantigrade position (Condie & Meadows 1993).

For spinal support, a well-fitted spinal jacket will allow correct forces to be appropriately applied to correct or delay development of a scoliosis (see Ch. 4). This will have a far greater influence on spinal posture than even the closest fitting custom made seat though, as with all intervention, there are advantages and disadvantages with wearing an orthosis. Apart from applying direct forces, a spinal jacket, if properly fitted to the body contours, can:

• Be worn for long periods of time, providing support and correction for up to 24 hours if required.
• Enable the child to use standard equipment with minimum additional support.
• Be worn under clothing and therefore is more aesthetically acceptable.

On the other hand, the disadvantages of using a spinal orthosis include:

• Contraindication for children with respiratory problems.
• Development of pressure problems and discomfort if not correctly fitted.
• Discomfort in hot weather or warm atmospheres.
• Limitation of all movement of the trunk and therefore restricts function including propelling a wheelchair.
• Perceived to be uncomfortable and therefore non-compliance or rejection by others, e.g. carers.

A hip abduction spinal orthosis (HASO) is sometimes recommended for management of the hips in cerebral palsy. Many of these children have involvement of all four limbs and may also be hypertonic, resulting in the twin problems of severe spasticity and deformity (Cooke et al 1989). These children also have little volitional movement and are therefore susceptible to the deforming defects of poor positioning (Sharrard 1967, Fulford & Brown 1976). A correctly designed HASO will control the range of hip abduction/adduction, hip extension/flexion and enable sitting, standing and lying (C J Drake 1994 unpublished lecture). However, this cannot be worn under clothing, is heavy and bulky in appearance and for handling, but holds the child in a good position and reduces the amount of seating support required. Problems may be experienced with wheelchairs when a child wears either a spinal jacket or some other form of postural support for only part of the day, as this necessitates a total change in seating prescription in order to provide adequate support and accommodate the child when out of the orthosis.

Surgical intervention

This is sometimes the choice selected for the prevention or correction of a deformity. A thorough physical assessment is first required as surgery carries a number of risks and complications for the child. For severely disabled children it may be useful for improving the sitting position. Surgery can be either superficial to the soft tissues or more radical involving the joints.

Segmental spinal instrumentation (SSI) using stainless steel Luque rods (Weiman, Gibson & Moseley 1983) is used to stabilize the spine for boys with Duchenne muscular dystrophy. It is important that the surgeon should set the spine in the appropriate position for sitting, as disturbance to sitting balance and loss of spinal flexibility can cause pressure sores under the buttocks. Dislocation of the hip can be corrected by hip surgery and also soft tissue release to tight adductors can noticeably improve the sitting position by widening the sitting base, though care should be taken as this could be contraindicated in some cases.

Early rather than later intervention of surgery tends to produce better results. However, all too frequently, because of its irreversible nature, there is a 'wait and see' attitude taken by parents and surgeons alike.

Medication

A range of drugs is available to control spasticity as well as seizures in children. Muscle relaxants such as diazepam or baclofen are commonly prescribed though may have side effects. In recent years there have been successful results from injecting botulinum toxin A directly into selected muscles and this has had some success when accompanied by regular physiotherapy.

Equipment in relation to principles and practice

Increased tone in the antigravity muscles, leg extensors and flexors in the arm results in an abnormal sitting position (Chapman & Weisdanger 1982). With these (CP) children, the pelvis is often tilted backwards due to tight hamstrings, the legs seem extended and internally rotated with extended knees and sometimes plantarflexed feet (Bobath & Bobath 1975, Levitt 1982). Some form of equipment may be required to maintain correct positioning and reduce loading on the spine. Seating designs and methods of positioning children with cerebral palsy are based largely on clinical practices that have been adapted as principles over time (Nwaobi 1986). Most of the research carried out on seating for children relates to children with cerebral palsy and considers the functional seating position. This is described as a position in which postural control allows the maximum degree of independent function when moving the arms and hands (Myhr 1994). In general, a good functional sitting position should include:

- a stable base providing balance and stability
- the pelvis in neutral or anterior tilt position
- the head in mid position with the line of gravity falling anterior to the 12th thoracic vertebra (Brunswic 1984) and over the supporting base which is formed by the ischial tuberosities.

A difference of opinion can arise when prescribing seating support systems. In general there can be conflict between:

- principles and practice
- support requirements and functional needs.

Frequently a compromise has to be found and this can only be achieved by setting priorities. Compromise is both an art and a skill. The art is to recognize the need for compromise, the skill is in determining the priorities (Pope 1996). The prescription will be based on the assessed need of the child, clinical expertise, theoretical knowledge, available equipment and resources. In all cases a balance needs to be achieved between providing support, comfort and encouraging development and function for the child, whilst considering the facility of care and handling for the family and others.

Information and training in the use of equipment

The degree of satisfaction and the success of a prescription will relate to:

- the depth and accuracy of assessment
- the understanding of the purpose and limitations of the prescription
- the training and information provided to all involved, both professionals and carer, in the use of the equipment
- good maintenance and care of all equipment.

The form in which information is provided is important, and both written and verbal information should use clear and simple terminology appropriate to the understanding of those being instructed, including parents, teachers and carers. An additional practical demonstration for both the key therapist and carer is invaluable with any non-standard equipment issued. They should then take responsibility for training all other handlers including volunteers, transport drivers, teachers and friends of the child, and also for monitoring day-to-day use. Regular review and provision of additional instruction may be necessary to ensure effective use and to correct any bad habits. A simple checklist prominently displayed or, if possible, an individual checklist attached to each chair (Fig. 9.7), can ensure correct use and satisfaction for all (see Box 9.1).

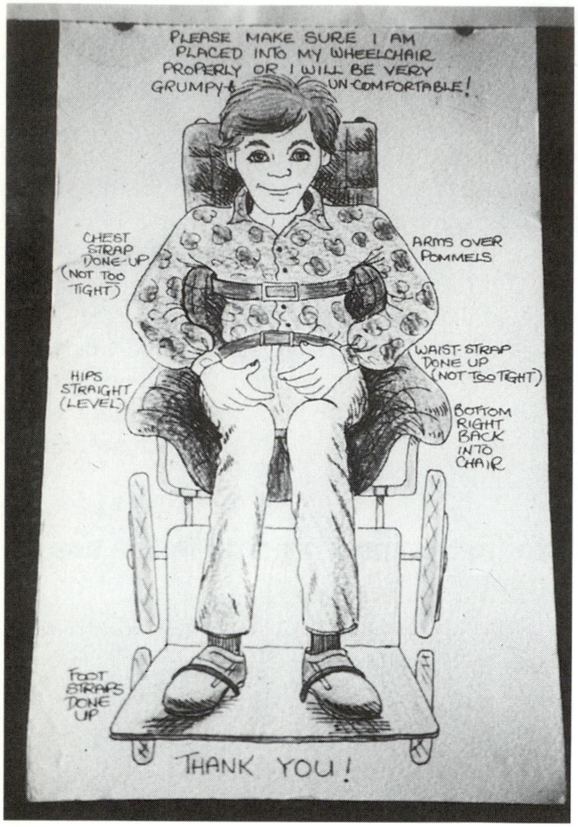

Figure 9.7 A simple illustrated check chart provided by a mother to assist carers to position her son correctly.

> **Box 9.1** Example of checklist for positioning a child in a wheelchair or seating system
>
> Use appropriate terminology for the occasion, e.g. hips rather than pelvis
> Provide the following basic details:
>   Name of child
>   Name and model of equipment
>   Details of accessories/seating insert provided
>   Name of contact person for help or information
>   Name of contact person for repairs to wheelchair.
>
> Preparation:
> - Check that all the parts of the chair are to hand and in working order, e.g. armrests, footrests, tray, headrest
> - Before placing child in the wheelchair, check: child has been toileted, is clean, correctly dressed, e.g. indoor/outdoor clothes
> - Check that the seat of the chair is clean
> - Check that brakes of the wheelchair are on.
>
> Positioning the child:
> - Speak to the child and explain what you are doing
> - Place the child in the chair as upright and symmetrical as possible, with the pelvis (bottom) against the back of the seat
> - Make sure the hips are level
> - Fasten the pelvic strap firmly
> - Place the feet on the footrest and fasten any foot straps
> - Fit the pommel or kneeblock into position if one is used with the system
> - Adjust the upper body and align correctly
> - Check clothing is smooth and comfortable
> - Adjust any thoracic (chest) support or fasten any harness or straps on the upper body
> - Adjust the head position and make comfortable
> - Fit the tray into position or any other accessories that need fitting
> - Check that the child is sitting comfortably and is happy in the seat and has all necessary belongings with him/her.

TRAINING SCHEMES FOR WHEELCHAIR USERS

Regular training in the use of the wheelchair will improve safety and help a child gain confidence and maximum independence. A RoSPA scheme is available nationally for wheelchair proficiency, though difficulties have been experienced when working with children who, though intellectually capable of following the scheme, were physically unable to complete the first section (see Ch. 14). For this reason some schools have set up their own programmes which encourage the children to use their chairs safely and increase their handling skills and independence (Holt & Baxter 1985).

TRANSPORTING A WHEELCHAIR

Transporting a child with a wheelchair and a seating system from home to school is an area of common concern. Safety requirements for transport will often conflict with the clinical and functional requirements, or make additional demands on a prescription. This can have financial implications which the wheelchair service may be unable or unwilling to meet. Funding responsibilities on this and other issues are discussed later.

The basic principles for transporting a child in a wheelchair include:

- Whenever possible the child should sit on the regular vehicle seat or in a recognized car seat with the wheelchair safely secured away from the passengers.

If this cannot be achieved, the following should be considered:

- All loose items, e.g. trays and preferably knee-blocks, should be removed; a head support should be fitted to the back of the wheelchair.
- The child should be independently secured into the wheelchair.
- It should be noted that straps provided with wheelchairs and seating are fitted with plastic buckles or fastenings. These are not car safety belts.
- The chair should be secured to the vehicle with recognized and approved fittings.
- A strap fitted with an approved fastening should be fastened across both child and chair.

Further information can be found in the MDD publication 'Transporting a child in a seating system' (MDD 1992).

Anyone involved in the regular transporting of either children or adults in wheelchairs would be advised to study the safety recommendations and guidelines that are available from the Department of Transport, Mobility Unit.

Apart from a few exceptions such as the Snug seat from the Hampshire Medical Company, children's seating systems are not intended for use as car seats. Safety seats specifically designed for the disabled child are not commonly available, though there is a growing range of commercially produced larger car seats and a wider choice of harnessing. The Disabled Living Foundation, a local motor accessory shop such as Halfords, or a motoring organization such as the AA may be able to provide information on the range available. Burnett body supports, or similar, vacuum seats can be used in some cases to support a child when travelling, but should be carefully fitted and secured to the child and then held with the car seat belt at all times. The local wheelchair service or a Disabled Living Centre should be able to advise or provide helpful information.

Manually lifting both child and their equipment into a family car is difficult and incorrect positioning may cause a back injury. The therapist should spend time providing instruction in safe lifting and handling procedures to everyone involved.

Banstead Mobility Centre, and other local mobility centres, can provide a range of information and advice on aspects of transporting disabled people of all ages. This includes car hoists, the purchase of suitable vehicles and methods of securing wheelchairs in or on a family car.

Information on travelling with a wheelchair user on public transport can generally be obtained from relevant information centres or can be found in the recent edition of the RADAR publication, 'Choosing a wheelchair' (Wells 1996), or the Department of Transport publication, 'Door to Door' (Department of Transport 1996).

FUNDING OF EQUIPMENT

Funding of children's wheelchairs and seating in the UK comes from different agencies which relate to the environment in which the equipment is to be used (Mandelstam 1994). As disabled people cannot divide their lives and their needs between health and social care (Living Options Partnership 1995), this creates unnatural boundaries and also grey areas which, in times of financial restraint, can be used as an excuse for non-provision with each agency placing responsibility on the next (National Prosthetic and Wheelchair Services Report 1993–96). This is particularly noticeable in the area of posture and mobility where the same equipment may be used for education, recreation and general mobility. Wheelchair services, like all NHS services, do not have an infinite budget, and as children have an ever increasing opportunity to participate in a wider range of educational and social activities including travel, expectations are raised and greater demands are made on the wheelchair service.

Professionals working in the field should be

careful not to raise the expectations of the children and their family and need to consider carefully the responsibilities of the NHS, local authorities, education authorities, charities and the families themselves before making requests for special equipment. There is a very thin line between need and want and although everyone is anxious that a disabled child should have access to as wide a range of activities as possible and make best use of all available opportunities, the budget holder is obliged to consider the interests of all users when allocating resources. Whilst every effort should be made to pursue funding for essential equipment, care should be taken to avoid situations where either statutory agencies deny responsibility for funding or where unnecessary time is wasted seeking funding from an inappropriate source. This may not only interfere with the child's progress and life style, but also cause frustration for all concerned. Lack of cooperation between services can easily create gaps in provision and reduce the effectiveness of both equipment and treatment that is provided. Any disagreements or failure to provide for assessed need should be taken up with the purchaser, who is in a position to allocate funding or to discuss joint funding with other agencies (Living Options Partnership with Department of Health 1995).

SHORT-TERM LOANS FOR MEDICAL NEEDS (see Ch. 8)

The majority of wheelchair services are funded to provide wheelchair equipment only to those with a permanent disability. There are times when children undergo elective surgery which then necessitates the need for a wheelchair for a limited period of time. This is common for children with recurring hip and spinal problems, including dislocation, congenital dislocation of the hips, Perthes' disease and other similar orthopaedic problems. Children who have an accident affecting mobility may also require a wheelchair on temporary loan. When there is a short-term need, the wheelchair service is not always able to provide equipment and an alternative source of supply is required, often at short

notice. All too often the search for a wheelchair is left to the parents of the child, causing additional stress at a time of acute anxiety.

A minority of wheelchair services are funded to meet this need or have an agreed arrangement with another agency. Others may be able to direct parents or professionals to an alternative source such as the British Red Cross, local disability groups, private suppliers, or charities particularly for standard equipment. STEPS, a children's charity particularly concerned with lower limb deformities, holds a limited supply of specialized equipment at some of their local centres, for use with children wearing full-length leg plaster casts, frog plasters, hip spicas or who have other special though temporary needs. Special equipment is not easily available and paediatric therapists who have regular need for this type of short-term loan are advised to make arrangements to meet this demand, either through their own unit or another reliable source. Setting up and funding a short-term loan service for medical need should be discussed with the health authority purchaser responsible for this area of provision. The wheelchair service should be involved or kept informed of any local arrangements funded through the health authority or any other agency (National Prosthetic and Wheelchair Services Report 1996).

PRIVATELY PURCHASED WHEELCHAIRS

Funding for private purchase of wheelchairs can be sought through a number of charities. In general, charities will assist with funding for equipment that cannot be provided through the statutory bodies. Charities specific to a particular disability, for example Muscular Dystrophy, Scope (previously the Spastic Society), can provide information on where funding can be obtained. 'Whizz Kidz' is one of the best known charities which provides a range of mobility aids. Generally, application for funding will need to be supported by an assessment carried out by an appropriately qualified therapist. NHS wheelchair therapists are not always able to provide this service due to existing demands on their time.

There are a few but growing number of independent centres for assessment and therapists based at some of the Disabled Living Centres are also able to provide an assessment service. Details can generally be obtained through disability information services such as DIAL and RADAR or from the College of Occupational Therapists.

Obtaining the correct equipment for mobility and independence is a top priority for children if they are to enjoy life with their families and develop their optimal level of ability. For those working in this field, it is important that they are constantly updating their knowledge and expertise in order to provide a quality service to the children and their families.

REFERENCES

Bardsley G 1993 Seating. In: Bowker P, Condie D N, Bader D L, Pratt D J (eds) Biomechanical basis of orthotic management. Butterworth-Heinemann, Oxford, ch 14, p 253

Bobath B, Bobath K 1975 Motor development in different types of cerebral palsy. Heinemann, London

Bobath K 1980 A neurophysiological basis for the treatment of cerebral palsy. Clinics in Developmental Medicine, no 71. Heinemann Medical, London

Brunswic M 1984 The ergonomics of seat design. Physiotherapy 70(2): 40–43

Carter P, Edwards S 1996 General principles of treatment. In: Edwards S (ed) Neurological physiotherapy. Churchill Livingstone, London, ch 5, p 87

Chapman C E, Weisdanger M 1982 The physiological and anatomical basis of spasticity: a review. Physiotherapy Canada 34: 125–136

Condie D N, Meadows C B 1993 Ankle–foot orthoses. In: Bowker P, Condie D N, Bader D H, Pratt D J (eds) Biomechanical basis of orthotic management. Butterworth-Heinemann, Oxford, ch 7, p 99

Cooke P H et al 1989 Dislocation of the hip in cerebral palsy: natural history and predictability. Journal of Bone and Joint Surgery 71B: 441–446

Disabled Living Foundation 1993 Wheelchair information. DLF, London

Department of Health 1991 Wheelchair training resource pack. Centre for Information for Department of Health, London

Department of Transport 1996 Door to door, 6th edn. HMSO, London

Emmelot C H, van der Veldt J, Mengerink G 1992 Independent operation of electrical wheelchairs by severely disabled children. Journal of Rehabilitation Sciences 5(2): 44–47

Fearn T A, Green E M, Jones M, Mulcahy C M, Nelham R L, Pountney T E 1992 Postural management. In: McCarthy G (ed) Physical disability in childhood, an interdisciplinary approach to management. Churchill Livingstone, London, ch 25, p 401

Frey J K, Tecklin J S 1986 Comparison of lumbar curves when sitting on the Westnofa Balans Multi-Chair, sitting on a conventional chair, and standing. Physical Therapy 66: 1365–1369

Fulford G E, Brown J K 1976 Position as a cause of deformity in children with cerebral palsy. Developmental Medicine and Child Neurology 18: 305–314

Goldsmith E, Golding R M, Garstang R A, MacCrae A W 1992 A technique to measure windswept deformity, a technical evaluation. Physiotherapy 78(4): 235–242

Green E M, Mulcahy C M, Pountney T E 1992 Postural management. Theory and practice. Active Design, Birmingham

Hallett R, Hare N, Milner A D 1987 Description and evaluation of an assessment form. Physiotherapy 73(5): 220–225

Holt K S 1991 Mobility aids and appliances for disabled children. British Medical Journal 302: 105–107

Holt K, Baxter H 1985 Safety with independence. The Pictor Wheelchair Proficiency Scheme. Physiotherapy 71(7): 315–316

Hulme J B, Gallacher K, Walsh J, Niesen S, Waldron D 1987 Behavioural and postural changes observed with use of adaptive seating by clients with multiple handicaps. Physical Therapy 67: 1060–1067

Lannert G, Ekberg O 1995 Positioning improves the oral and pharyngeal swallowing function in children with cerebral palsy. Acta Paediatrica 84: 689–692

Letts M R 1992 Principles of seating the disabled. CRC Press, London

Letts M R, Shapiro L, Mulder K, Klassen O 1984 The windblown hip syndrome in total body cerebral palsy. Journal of Pediatrics Orthopedica 4: 55–62

Levitt S 1982 Treatment of cerebral palsy and motor delay, 2nd edn. Blackwell Scientific, Oxford

Living Options Partnership 1995 The Power to Change. Commissioning Health and Social Services with Disabled People. Kings Fund Centre, London

Living Options Partnership with Department of Health 1995 The power to change. Report of a Conference 14 March 1995, DOH publ H35/001 4162

Mandel A C 1981 The seated man (homo sedens). The seated work position. Theory and Practice, Applied Ergonomics 12: 19–26

Mandel A C 1994 The correct height of school furniture. Physiotherapy 70: 48–53

Mandelstam M 1994 How to get equipment, 3rd edn. Jessica Kingsley publishers and Kogan Page for DLF, London

MDD 1992 Safety guidelines for transporting children in special seats. Medical Devices Directorate (now Agency MDA) Ref MDD/92/07 Blackpool

Miller F, Bachrach S J 1995 Cerebral palsy. A complete guide for caregiving. The John Hopkin University, Boston

Mulcahy C M 1986 An approach to the assessment of sitting ability for the prescription of seating. British Journal of Occupational Therapy 18: 367–368

Mulcahy C M, Pountney T E 1986 The sacral pad – description of its clinical use in seating. Physiotherapy 72(9): 473–474

Mulcahy C M, Pountney T E, Nelham R L, Green E M, Billington G D 1988 Adaptive seating for motor handicap: problems, a solution, assessment and prescription. British Journal of Occupational Therapy 51(10): 347–351

Myhr U 1994 On factors of importance for sitting in children with cerebral palsy. Department of Handicap Research, Goteborg University

Myhr U, von Wendt L 1991 Sitting assessment scale from improvement of functional sitting position for children with cerebral palsy. Development Medicine and Child Neurology 33: 246–256

National Prosthetic and Wheelchair Services Report 1996 Guidelines for partnership between the British Red Cross Society and NHS Wheelchair Services 1996. College of Occupational Therapists, London

National Prosthetic and Wheelchair Services Report 1993–1996 funded DOH project. College of Occupational Therapists, London

Nwaobi O M 1986 Effects of body orientation in space on tonic muscle activity of patients with cerebral palsy. Developmental Medicine and Child Neurology 28: 41–44

Perks B A, Mackintosh R, Stewart C P U, Bardsley G I 1994 A survey of marginal wheelchair users. Journal of Rehabilitation, Research and Development 31(4): 297–302

Pimm P L 1996 Some of the implications of caring for a child or adult with cerebral palsy. British Journal of Occupational Therapy 59(7): 335–340

Pope P 1993 Measurement of postural competency in the severely disabled patient. Booklets: Proceedings of a meeting, 17 May The Hare Association for Physical Ability. From Education Officer, HAFPA, Nottinghamshire

Pope P 1996 Postural management and special seating. In: Edwards S (ed) Neurological physiotherapy. Churchill Livingstone, London, ch 7, p 135

Royal College of Physicians 1995 The provision of wheelchairs and special seating. Guidance for purchasers and providers. Royal College of Physicians, London

Scrutton D 1989 The early management of hips in cerebral palsy. Developmental Medicine and Child Neurology 31: 108–116

Sharrard W J W 1967 Paralytic deformity in the lower limb. Journal of Bone and Joint Surgery 49B: 731–737

Stewart P, McQuilton G 1987 Straddle seating for the cerebral palsied child. British Journal of Occupational Therapy 50(4): 136–138

Trachtenburg S W 1995 Caring and coping. The family of a child with disabilities. In: Batshaw M L, Perrett Y M (eds) Children with disabilities, 3rd edn. Paul H Brookes

Trefler E, Tooms R E, Hobson D A 1978 Seating for cerebral palsied children. Inter Clinic Information Bulletin 17: 1–8

Trefler E, Tooms R E, Hobson D A 1978 A modular seating system for cerebral palsied children. Developmental Medicine and Child Neurology 20: 199–204

TRES (Tayside Rehabilitation Engineering Services) 1981 Body support systems for the severely disabled patient. Final Report to SHHD. K/RED/14/47

Weiman R L, Gibson D A, Moseley C F 1983 Surgical stabilisation of the spine in Duchenne muscular dystrophy. Spine 8: 776–780

Wells J 1996 Choosing a wheelchair. RADAR, London

FURTHER READING

Directory of Social Change 1996 A guide to grants for infants in need. Directory of Social Change, London (for information concerning grants)

Wells J 1996 Choosing a wheelchair. RADAR, London. (Contains wealth of information with addresses and further references on all aspects of wheelchairs including private purchase, charity contacts, etc.)

For information concerning grants:

- Refer to Directory of Social Change
- Contact Department of Transport Mobility Unit

10

Users with learning difficulties

BACKGROUND

Introduction

Before matters relating to wheelchairs and seating are addressed in this chapter, it is important that the reader is aware of the history, terminology and recent changes that have occurred relating to this group of users. People with learning difficulties were, for example, previously known as those with mental handicap.

History

In the UK until the mid 1800s, people with mental handicaps lived mainly at home if they survived birth and childhood. But in the 1850s the industrial revolution changed family life. Victorian society began to recognize the problem of mental handicap as society changed from being a rural one to an industrial one and with the introduction of universal education (Office of Health Economics 1978). Mental handicap became more visible. People not suited to live and work in the factories were moved to institutions, which were a cross between asylums and 'specialized education centres' for people with mental handicaps, physical handicaps and mental illnesses. The institutions varied and they gradually became long-term 'hospitals' caring away from the community. Mental deficiency emerged as a distinct problem and the Idiots Act was passed in 1886.

By the early 1900s, various government acts 'legalized' care out of the community. In 1913 the

Mental Deficiency Act was passed which established a separate system of care based on community support and segregated colonies. This was intended to be both protective and also as a way of limiting the population of such individuals, as mental deficiency was believed to be largely inherited (Chlebowski 1991). The colonies housed both the severely mentally handicapped and those with behavioural deviance seen either as drunkenness or moral incompetence, for example the birth of an illegitimate child.

Between the wars the numbers placed increased from approximately 5000 in 1918 to 50 000 in 1939. There was little differentiation at this time between mental handicap and mental illness and so they were both cared for in a medical environment with doctors and nurses. Some people with mental handicaps were living in the community in the 1920s and 1930s, this was generally with the assistance of voluntary organizations (Morris 1969).

Late in the 1940s and 1950s improvements in provision started the care in the community philosophy that is now in vogue (Chlebowski 1991). It was realized in the 1950s and 1960s through surveys, that many of the people who had been put into institutions and hospitals at the beginning of this century were in fact normal or of near normal intelligence and ability (Morris 1969). They were simply placed in these hospitals and institutions because there was a lack of alternative provision available for them at that time, to help them over their temporary crisis.

The Seebohm Report in 1968, the 1971 White Paper 'Better Services for the Mentally Handicapped', the Peter's Report in 1979, the Barclay Report in 1982 and the Short Report in 1985 were all influential in the thinking about care in the community (Chlebowski 1991). For example, some of the principles of the Department of Health and Social Security 1971 White Paper 'Better Services for the Mentally Handicapped' were that:

- The family with a mentally handicapped member have the same general needs for social services as other families as well as needs for special additional help.

- Such children and adults should not be segregated from the local community.
- Each person needs stimulation, social training, education, purposeful occupation and employment to develop to their maximum.
- Each individual should live with their own family as long as this is possible. But if they have to leave home, the links with home should be maintained and the alternative accommodation should be as homelike as possible.
- There should be close collaboration between the agencies providing services: the social services, health services, voluntary services and other services for the disabled (Department of Health and Social Security 1989a).

The 1970s therefore brought more integrated care for the mentally handicapped – care in the community rather than institutional care, the shift away from medical care to the emphasis on the social and educational needs of those with impaired mental abilities, the provision of a range of services in the community and the support of mentally handicapped people living in their own homes (Sines 1988a).

Terminology

Traditionally, terms like mental retardation and mental subnormality have been used collectively for three different phenomena: subnormal intelligence, reduced social and physical skills and deviant behaviour patterns (Office of Health Economics 1978).

Terms such as subnormal, feeble minded, educationally subnormal, moron, mildly retarded have all been used in the past for the mild mentally handicapped group and retarded, imbecile, idiot for the profoundly retarded group. Labelling individuals as idiots, imbeciles and feeble minded is objectionable, and the words defective or retarded are unacceptable to both parents and professionals alike (Office of Health Economics 1978).

Since the 1920s it has been customary to make the division between severely mentally handicapped people and the mildly mentally handicapped (Office of Health Economics 1978). The IQ test has been accepted for a long time as a crude indicator of intellectual ability (Department of Health and Social Security 1989a). Mild mental handicap relates to those individuals with IQs equivalent to 50–69 and such individuals are referred to now as people with *moderate learning difficulties*. Severe handicap refers to those people with IQs below 50 and today they are known as people with *severe learning difficulties* (Fraser & Green 1991). But the IQ is not taken on its own as a measure of mental handicap and there is no hard and fast dividing line in borderline cases. The diagnostic criteria will also include the concurrent deficits or impairments in adaptive behaviour, their ability to adapt to a normal independent life (Department of Health and Social Security 1989a), taking into consideration the person's age and if the onset of the impairment was before the age of 18 years. (When impairment occurs after the age of 18 years this is classified as dementia and includes brain damage after head injury, chronic psychosis and presenile dementias (American Psychiatric Association 1980).) The majority of those suffering with mild handicap have no clinical indications of nervous system damage or defect whereas those with severe handicap suffer some clearly demonstrable form of impairment, which may also include physical disabilities (Office of Health Economics 1978).

The present situation

Since the 1980s there has been a practice to move people with learning disabilities from more restrictive environments (i.e. hospitals) to less restrictive environments to promote 'normalization', a less intensive service and a more integrated environment in which to live.

Normalization

Individuals with learning disabilities are devalued by society because of the negative perceptions of their differences (Wolfensberger 1972, 1980). However, these disadvantaged people should lead culturally valued lives and it is this that led Wolfensberger to the concept of normalization which can be summarized as follows:

- A person's experience of behaviour and status is determined by the environment in which they live. Community housing should therefore reflect this.
- Full participation in the life of the community is both a right and a need of people who are at significant risk of devaluation.
- The objectives of community living are to enhance the quality of life experiences of those whose status has been significantly devalued (Emerson & Pretty 1987).

Such a change in philosophy needs to bring about change in the views of not only the people who work with learning difficulties but also the mainstream of society. People with learning difficulties have moved from the hospitals and the institutions to live in the community in small or smaller units and although there is physical integration in most areas, social integration in general has not occurred (Humphreys, Howe & Blunden 1982).

Today 'our goal is to see people with learning difficulties in the mainstream of life, living in ordinary houses, in ordinary streets, with the same range of choices as any citizen, and mixing as equals with the other, mostly non-handicapped, members of their own community' (King's Fund 1982).

When providing services to people with learning difficulties, staff should be aware that:

- Such individuals have the same human value as anyone else and the same human rights.
- Living with others in the community is both a right and a need.
- Services must recognize the individuality of people with learning difficulties (Towell 1988).

So people with learning difficulties should have the same basic rights, human value and wherever possible the same responsibilities as other members of society (Sines 1988b).

Nearly all British children with a learning difficulty now grow up in an ordinary family home, mostly with their natural parents, but also with foster parents or adoptive parents. Fostering for those parents unable to cope is proving to be a success both in the quality of the care provided and the value for money which it offers (McConkey 1991). Children with learning difficulties attend either special schools or integrated schools; after the age of 16–19 years, as adults, they often attend day centres or training centres, but these are rarely socially integrated into the local community and they are usually socially isolated from the community. Half the population, it is said, remains embarrassed to meet people with learning difficulties and avoids their company. However, it is the quality of the contact rather than the quantity of the contact that is important (McConkey 1991). Gradually, as those with learning difficulties become integrated into their community, attending events and centres with others, this will cease to be the case. The wheelchair and special seating supplied to such individuals is therefore very important and a vital piece of equipment in this process of integration and acceptance both visually and socially.

Priority in community care services is to support families caring for their handicapped offspring by providing short-term breaks, day care, counselling and advice on financial support (World Health Organization 1985). Such services are essential for the success of community care for those with learning difficulties, and wheelchair services need to be aware of the advantages for the family and carers, though follow-up or review can be delayed, while respite care of any nature is occurring. However, it should be noted that in some boroughs there are no respite facilities for people with learning difficulties (A Walker 1996 personal communication).

Advocacy

The Disabled Persons Act 1986 breaks new ground for the advocacy for people with learning disabilities. It gives people over the age of 16 the right to appoint someone to represent their needs regarding the provision of local social services. A vigorous and vocal advocacy movement is fundamental to successful care in the community. Without advocacy, people with learning difficulties will remain a people apart (Holland 1991).

The community care and community learning difficulty teams

Multidisciplinary care. People with learning difficulties can benefit from the help of many different agencies, which naturally leads to interorganizational and multidisciplinary co-operation from professional and carer alike for the benefit of the individual. The professional services are generally: the education service, with teachers and educational psychologists; the health service, with doctors, clinical psychologists and paramedical therapists; the local authorities, with social workers, care staff and the voluntary agencies.

Community teams for people with learning difficulties generally have a core staff comprising a social worker, a community nurse and a clinical psychologist. Other professionals join the team as and when required for the individual's needs. A key worker (though not necessarily from the team) is identified who acts as a contact point for the family and professionals alike. It is recommended that there is one community nurse trained in learning difficulties for a population of 25 000. In an average health district of 225 000, this amounts to nine nurses.

The Griffiths report 'Community Care: Agenda for Action' (1988), as did the report 'Caring for People' (Department of Health and Social Security 1989b), emphasized the social element rather than the health element of community care. A crucial person will be the care manager who coordinates the needs assessment and the multidisciplinary action planning with the individual person. The individual's needs are identified and it is important to emphasize that the appraisal of someone's needs can only be meaningful if people take the time to understand the needs of the person concerned in the total context of his or her life. One basic service principle is to provide care for people in such a way as to enable them to lead as independent and normal existence as possible. Services for integration must be judged against the quality of life they provide for their consumers within the framework of valued and community-based provision (Sines 1988c). The policy of integration should exploit naturally occurring opportunities rather than designing standard solutions to superimpose onto the local community. For example, local leisure facilities are used rather than hiring isolated venues. The realization of integrated community care depends upon the approach adopted by community support staff in preparing both the clients and the community into which they move. The community, as with all social systems, aims to preserve social order and avoid conflict through equilibrium. People with learning difficulties will be accepted if they observe the rules and the norms of the locality. Given time and the opportunity, the local community has the necessary skills and ability to adapt to change (Moore 1988). One measure of success of community care will be the extent to which people are accepted within their neighbourhoods and the only way that this may be achieved is by exposing each other to local services and sharing in the life of the local community (Sines 1988b). Again, wheelchairs and seating have a very important part to play if this integration is to work for the twentieth century.

In some areas of the country, more changes and innovative approaches to the care of this group of individuals have taken place. It is essential that the readers familiarize themselves with their own local practices in the health, social services and voluntary sector arenas.

PREVALENCE

The prevalence of learning difficulties (mental handicap) is: mild, 30:1000; severe, 3:1000; profound, 0.5:1000. Approximately 0.3:1000 will still be in and require 'health-care' environments (Minns et al 1989).

Between 2 and 3% of people per 1000 in the UK have IQs below 70. Of this total of approximately one and a quarter million, just over one in ten is severely affected. Of the estimated more than one million people who may be considered as having moderate learning difficulties, many live in the community without any special assistance. There are also approximately 160 000 with severe learning difficulties and a large number of these

are children who live at home with their parents (Office of Health Economics 1978).

The prevalence rate has not increased. The prevalence for Down's syndrome has, however, increased this century due to improved survival but still remains at less than 1%.

Although no significant variation in social class has been found in the severely disabled group, major differences in the pattern of mild mental handicap between socioeconomic groups has been found. Birch et al (1970) found that the prevalence of mild handicap was approximately nine times greater among children of unskilled manual workers than those with non-manual occupations. Studies have revealed a consistent pattern of material deprivation, poor housing facilities and substandard educational opportunities linked to large families and family instability (Office of Health Economics 1978). It has also been found that there is a close relationship between mortality in early life, low birthweight and mental and physical handicap. Of approximately 40% of babies born under 1500 grams who survive the first year, around half have some form of damage or defect resulting from conditions such as anoxia or hypoglycaemia (Office of Health Economics 1978). It is well known that at least 20% of women in the UK fail to seek medical care during the first trimester of pregnancy and this is especially common in the lower socioeconomic groups and ethnic communities.

CLINICAL FEATURES

Clinical varieties of people with learning difficulties have been categorized into eight groups (MacGillivary 1991a), which are described below.

Following infections

Examples are:

- Gastroenteritis at birth causing fluid loss and dehydration.
- Meningitis, an infection of the coverings of the brain.

- Congenital syphilis and the passage of the organism across the placenta in untreated pregnant women.
- Encephalitis, an infection of the brain substance following measles or rubella, for example.
- Congenital rubella syndrome contracted within the first 3 months of pregnancy.

Following injury or physical agents

Examples are:

- Pre-eclampsia and eclampsia in the last 3 months of pregnancy.
- Birth injuries, e.g. a difficult labour leading to anoxia.
- Rhesus incompatibility.
- Drugs taken by the mother in pregnancy and alcoholic mothers, leading to babies born with mental retardation and physical abnormalities.

Associated with disorders of metabolism

Examples are:

- Lipid disorder causing Niemann–Pick disease – a physical wasting and death often occurs before 2 years of age.
- Amino-acid disorder, e.g. phenylketonuria (PKU) which, if left to its natural course, always leads to mental impairment, often epilepsy and dwarfism. It can be controlled by a special diet during the first 3 years of life. All babies have been sceened for PKU since 1969 (Guthrie test) which affects 1 : 1000 births. Another example is maple syrup urine disease, where there is difficulty in feeding, breathing is irregular, there is limb stiffness and rapid deterioration.
- Carbohydrate disorders – gargoylism with dwarfism, hypoglycaemia.
- Endocrine disorders – (cretinism or retarded growth).
- Mineral and electrolyte metabolism, e.g. Wilson's disease, where there is rigidity in the limbs and muscle wasting.

Associated with brain disease

Examples are:

- Tuberous sclerosis, which is associated with severe mental handicap, epileptic fits and a butterfly rash on the cheeks and nose.
- Schilder's disease, which is associated with spastic paralysis, mental deterioration and muscular incoordinated limbs.

Associated with prenatal factors

Examples are:

- Hydrocephalus, where there is an increased volume of the cerebrospinal fluid within the skull.
- Microcephaly, where the cranium is less than 42.5 cm in circumference and spastic diplegia and epilepsy are common.

Association with chromosomal abnormalities

Some examples are detailed below.

Down's syndrome. Women aged 15–19 have a 1:2000 chance of giving birth to a Down's syndrome baby, whereas for women over 40 the risk is about 1:100. For mothers over 45 it rises to 1:50 (Office of Health Economics 1978). Down's syndrome presents with stunted growth, a small round head with flat face and occiput, eye defects, broad and clumsy looking hands and defects on the feet. The joints have an abnormal range of movement due to laxity of the ligaments and the more floppy they are, the worse the prognosis. The circulation is often poor, congenital heart disease is common and respiratory infections are also common as such individuals are usually mouth breathers. Dementia develops early in life and is generally seen in all those over the age of 40 years.

The patient mortality in the mentally handicapped was higher than in the general population 50 years ago but today the difference is relatively small. Longevity has increased by an average of 40 years in those with Down's syndrome and approximately 30 years in those with other handicaps. This increase is also bringing with it additional ageing, physical and mental disorders and therefore posing more problems to the carers, families and professionals alike. Cancer, diabetes mellitus, fractures and hepatitis B are also conditions commonly seen in this group.

Huntington's chorea. The disease is transmitted by the autosomal dominant gene and about half the offspring of the affected person can be expected to develop Huntington's chorea. It generally begins between 25 and 35 years of age but may develop as early as 3 or as late as 70 years. Neurological symptoms may be preceded by mood change, involuntary movements in the face, hands and shoulders, but abnormality of gait may be the first sign. Depression is common, as is suicide. Memory is well retained even when the disease is well established. The duration of the disease is 10–15 years with death before the age of 60 years, but it may be more slowly progressing.

Associated with prematurity

Some examples are detailed below.

Prematurity. Premature infants are likely to develop respiratory distress at birth, infants with a birth weight of less than 1500 g show an association between respiratory distress, mental handicap and neurological abnormalities and small for dates infants have been found to have an increased incidence of mental handicap (MacGillivary 1991a).

Cerebral palsy (CP). This is a permanent disorder of movement and posture due to a non-progressive defect of the brain occurring in early life. The incidence is about 1 : 500 live births. Mental handicap and CP are commonly found together, the same cerebral insult accounting for both effects. Neurophysiological pyramidal signs are commonly seen, such as hemiplegia, diplegia and quadraplegia, and some extrapyramidal signs such as ataxia and athetoid movements. Many are epileptic also. The more severe forms are associated with physical immobility and deformity and subsequent contractures (see Ch. 9).

There is an increasing tendency to mouth breathe, especially in the profoundly handicapped, causing the lips to become dry and fissured. Tooth grinding is also common in the profoundly handicapped (bruxism).

Unclassified

This is where there is no gross evidence of structural and biochemical abnormality but where there is a genetic contribution (e.g. Rett syndrome in 1 : 12 500 girls) or environmental contribution, or there are retarded parent(s). This group accounts for approximately 65% of all mental handicap cases. It has been found where the environment, genetic factors, parents of below average intelligence and social factors contribute: the cases are confined to social classes IV and V. Incidence is increased in the poorer areas of large inner cities with overcrowding, poverty, problem families, parents in debt and careless of property (MacGillivary 1991a). Both parents and siblings are often in need of special education.

EPILEPSY

The incidence of epilepsy increases with the severity of the mental and physical handicap and it is likely that at least one-third of individuals with severe or profound disability suffer with epilepsy (Fischbacher 1991).

There are two main categories of epilepsy. Primary or idiopathic, where no cause can be found for the seizures, and secondary or symptomatic, where a probable aetiological factor is discovered either prior to birth (infections, effects of X-rays, genetic defects), at the time of birth (anoxia, physical trauma to the cranium) or postnatal (metabolic disturbance such as hypoglycaemia, and infections such as meningitis). In addition to the aetiology, there also appears to be some type of trigger to provoke a seizure, for example flickering lights in photosensitive epilepsy, emotional stress, a noise, infections, hormonal fluctuation, drugs or alcohol.

In the early 1980s, the International League Against Epilepsy drew up a classification of the seizures into partial and general.

Partial seizures

These are generated locally in the brain and the effects will depend upon the part of the brain affected.

Simple partial seizures. Consciousness not impaired.

Complex partial seizures. Consciousness impaired.

Motor partial seizures. Movement of muscle groups will be seen when the motor cortex is affected.

Sensory partial seizures. Sensory or psychological seizures occur when the mortor cortex is not affected. For example, speech, thought difficulties, numbness, tingling, dreams, sensations of sight, hearing, smell, and taste may be experienced.

Partial seizures. Secondarily generalized.

Generalized seizures

Absence seizures. Previously called petit mal, with brief periods of unawareness, abrupt onset and recovery. These chiefly occur in children and young adults. Slight twitching of the face or limb muscles may be seen.

Myoclonic seizures. These are sudden spasmodic contractures of muscles and are most common in infants, notably extension of the arms and flexion at the waist – the 'salaam attack'.

Clonic or tonic seizures. These are major generalized seizures where the tonic or clonic phase is absent.

Tonic-clonic seizures. This is classically the grand mal seizure. There is a prodromal period where vague symptoms lasting as long as 24 hours occur. This is followed by an aura – some physical or psychological sensation, which is often unpleasant, which is the start of the seizure itself. The tonic phase follows where the patient becomes unconscious with strong muscle contractures which may involve the jaws, constriction of the respiratory movements and tightening of the abdominal muscles, which may lead to urinary or faecal incontinence. This lasts approximately 30 seconds to 1 minute. The clonic phase follows and lasts approximately 1–2 minutes, where

there is repetitive jerky movements of the head and limbs often with frothing of the mouth. There is then a phase of unconsciousness which lasts a variable length of time.

Note that if another tonic phase follows the clonic phase, status epilepticus results, which is a serious medical emergency as it can be life threatening and lead to brain damage.

Atonic seizures. These are also known as drop attacks. There is a sudden loss of consciousness and postural control, leading to a fall and an almost immediate return of consciousness. Injuries may occur to the head and face and leather 'helmets' are worn.

Unclassified seizures

Here seizures do not appear to fit into any of the categories (Fischbacher 1991).

Treatment

Anticonvulsant medication is the main treatment for epilepsy and this is generally long term so use of the correct drugs and the correct amounts is important. The main drugs commonly known and used are: carbamazepine, nitrazepam, phenytoin, phenobarbitone and diazepam.

The carer has a key role in the management of the person with epilepsy, as they are present when the fits occur and observe the occurrence and all the manifestations. It is advisable to ask carers about the nature of the epilepsy when assessing for mobility aids.

When an attack does occur it is important that the person is protected from injury. No other active intervention is recommended today (Fischbacher 1991).

Driving and quality of life

A person suffering with epilepsy who has been free of daytime seizures for a period of 2 years is not debarred from holding a driving licence. This enlightened legislation accepts a degree of risk and this should be the norm in order to permit a reasonable quality of life (Fischbacher 1991).

MENTAL ILLNESS

Although mental illness and learning difficulties are often grouped together under the broad term 'mental disorder', care must be taken to distinguish them (Department of Health and Social Security 1987). Mental illness can occur at any time of life and with treatment it can often be cured. However, mental illness does not generally show itself until the adolescent stage is reached, which is different when compared to mental handicap, which presents itself early. Learning difficulties cannot be cured in the same way, although with the right training, education and care, an improvement in the person's general development can be achieved (Department of Health and Social Security 1987). The lower the IQ in the individual, the more difficult it is to recognize mental illness, but any type of mental illness is possible.

Treatment

Intervention programmes

Most programmes for this group involve encouraging and promoting the early development of those abilities and skills that normally emerge in the first few years of life, the foundation blocks for subsequent learning (Wishart 1991). For example, in the Portage programme, teaching is mainly carried out by the parent under the supervision of a 'home visitor' – a health visitor, speech therapist or psychologist, for example. The teaching is focused on the child's developmental level and a few new activities or skills are added as appropriate. The preschool model is also aimed at developmental progress, maintaining the motor and cognitive skills of the child. It should be noted that educational integration has come about because of parental pressure rather than the success of early intervention programmes.

The developmental processes of the handicapped child differ qualitatively as well as quantitatively from the normal development process. It is not simply a slowed down version of the normal development process (Wishart 1991). It is possible to supplement the mentally handi-capped child's experience in ways that will encourage and promote the maximum gains from whatever level of cognitive functioning is available to the child, which will encourage the child to make full use of his or her abilities however limited these may be (Wishart 1991).

Drugs

A variety of drugs are used with this group. Sometimes drugs are used to calm individuals and reduce stereotypes but only in combination with behaviour management problems. The treatments include:

- Sedatives to assist with sleep.
- Anticonvulsants to treat epilepsy.
- Antispasmodics to control disorders of movement and muscle tone which can occur as an unwanted effect of major tranquillizers.
- Tranquillizers to calm the patient and reduce tension, agitation and anxiety.
- Antidepressants to elevate mood in psychiatric illness rather than environmental factors.
- Others, for example lithium, to reduce mood fluctuation in illness (MacGillivary 1991b).

EDUCATION
Children

It was the Warnock Committee's report 'Special Educational Needs' (1978) which marked the critical change in the official philosophy of the state system of special schools from having an emphasis on the pupil's disabilities to an emphasis on their special educational needs. The aims of education as stated in the report are to increase knowledge, to encourage development of independency and self-sufficiency.

The children with the greatest degree of developmental delay often spend much of their lives asleep and may hardly be aware of their surroundings. Therefore their awareness is increased in the form of activities to stimulate their senses of vision, hearing, movement, taste and smell. Children whose disabilities are less profound will spend time developing such things as: communication skills, forming relationships with other people, making decisions and improving their personal ADL skills (Mackay 1991). Some pupils with severe learning difficulties do learn to read and write, but for the majority the emphasis is on the development of communication, social and self-help skills, practical problem solving and leisure pursuits (Mackay 1991).

The degree of difficulty the child has with learning is determined formally by a process known as 'recording' in Scotland and 'statementing' in England and Wales. The child is assessed by a professional team of varying sizes depending upon who is working with the child and if the child is at school or not. Often the team meet to discuss their findings and a Record (or statement) of Needs is then produced. The education officer draws up a final Record of Needs, taking into consideration the team's opinions but not necessarily all their recommendations (Mackay 1991). Unlike the USA, annual reviews of needs are not compulsory in the UK but they do often take place annually. There is, however, a compulsory Record of Needs which is carried out in the pupil's last 2 years at school. This is a record of their achievements, the plans for the final period of schooling and the preparation for life after school.

Adult

Although the school leaving age was raised in 1972 to 16 years, many people with learning difficulties stay on at school until they are 18, 19, or even 20 in some cases. Provision of where to go to next is often a problem. Each individual is unique and will develop at different rates. Development should continue to be monitored through the Individual Programme Plan (IPP), which is a written plan of action containing practical and realistic goals and the strategies for achieving these relating to different areas of an individual's life (Guinea 1991). IPP meetings should be held regularly so that the key people involved with the individual can meet and discuss how to build on the strengths of the individual and meet the identified needs. Such meetings are generally facilitated by the key worker.

There are five accomplishments from the principle of normalization and goals should be set in the following areas:

- Community presence – sharing community life.
- Choice – for the individual in all aspects of their life (informed choice).
- Increasing competence – performing a variety of skills and activities.
- Respect – valued place in a network of people and community life.
- Community participation.

Communication

Although the spoken word is more adaptable, less conspicuous and socially acceptable, systems have been developed to assist with communication and some of these methods are used with people with learning difficulties. Unfortunately, only a few members of the public also use signs or symbols, which cuts off people with such handicaps from communicating with the general population (Stansfield 1991). Many staff and teachers are, however, trained in such methods.

Communication methods used with this group may include signed English, key word signing, signal systems and static systems.

There are two major British signed English systems, the Paget Gorman sign system (PGSS), an artificially designed language which is almost the exact translation of English, and BSL (SE) signed English which follows the English word order and adds sign markers to indicate changes in syntax (Jones & Cregan 1986). There are also several American systems (Stansfield 1991).

The Makaton vocabulary may also be used, where the key words are signed, accompanied by grammatical spoken English. Facial expressions and body language are used to increase intelligibility (Walker 1986). SE can be used as a supplement to Makaton, giving greater potential for this group.

Static systems include the written word and symbols. The written word has limited value as those people who can read and write can often also communicate verbally. However, symbols methods are used and these include the Blissymbolics, which is a form of written Esperanto.

Some of the symbols are pictures but the majority are abstract symbols. Although to be used in full, Bliss does require a higher level of cognitive functioning, but a few symbols may be used successfully for the more cognitively impaired (Stansfield 1991).

Non-verbal communication

The place of non-verbal communication and body language in communication has been recognized and acknowledged for a long time. Social behaviour, dress code and the distances between people in conversation are all recognized and often differ with different cultures. It is important that people with learning difficulties are helped to assimilate the cultural rules as much as they can, especially if they are to become more integrated into the community's society (Fraser 1991). Individuals with learning difficulties often want to get closer and touch more often than is generally accepted and this may cause problems with the general population (Fraser 1991). However, others find close proximity frightening and often use body language as a protective barrier.

Some people with Down's syndrome develop complex gestures to describe what they cannot through speech. Their body language may also be 'closed' and more restrictive when they are with a stranger than with someone they are familiar with (Leider 1981).

Challenging behaviour

The term 'disturbed behaviour' has now been replaced by 'challenging behaviour', which is said to more truly reflect the nature of the behaviour and has moved away from the problem being within the individual towards those who are providing a service for them.

Common behaviour problems in the mentally handicapped include: aggression, stereotype behaviour, antisocial conduct, self-mutilating behaviour, mood disturbance and withdrawn behaviours (Fraser 1991). After eliminating medical causes, medication, depression and psychosis, causes are sought in the environment and in the way the individual is handled. Such behaviour may also be a 'frozen stage' in the person's development.

Staff therefore look for the cause of the behaviour. Such questions would include: Is there an antecedent which triggers the behaviour? What does the individual do and how often with what severity? What happens after the behaviour has occurred? By observing challenging behaviour, triggers, the setting or events and what happens after the behaviour, factors may emerge that can be changed to subsequently alter behaviour.

Art and music therapy and the creative process are exciting and effective therapeutic instruments which help in the growth of the individual. It is possible for the client to attain a new skill after months or even years of lack of progress.

Art therapy is an enabling process in its creativity, producing a sense of identity, expression and personal growth. The aim of art therapy is to create opportunities for positive lasting change and growth.

The aims of music therapy are:

- communication (feelings, vocalization, eye contact, socialization)
- awareness (self and others, body awareness, relationship building)
- motor skills (increasing control of involuntary movements, meaningful use of hands, relaxation, reaching, grasping, gross and fine movements)
- utilization of hearing, sight
- increasing concentration
- decreasing self-mutilation
- reducing anxiety
- increasing motivation
- expressing their character (Montague 1991).

POSTURE AND MOBILITY NEEDS

The needs for mobility from the wheelchair service for this group range from the simplest attendant-controlled wheelchair to complex seating systems to accommodate deformity. The disability of adult users with learning difficulties includes those seen previously in the paediatric group with mild and severe handicap, but the interaction with the parents, foster parents or carers is less intense, as the greatest amount of developmental potential has been reached. The social situation has been resolved and is established, the disability is accepted and the care programme or package has been drawn up and agreed. There are good multidisciplinary team links and the professionals' needs from the equipment are also well defined.

In the late 1980s and early 1990s, when many of the larger institutions started to close, many complex seating supports and systems and mobility cases began to be seen by the local wheelchair services. Although such cases had been issued with wheelchairs and seating systems in the larger institutions, their review, potential and social needs were often absent or lacking. The equipment needs were also different, being 'passive' and institutional mobility items rather than the independent, functional, manoeuvrable, easy to use, socially acceptable items required today. Many of the seating systems were paid for by the individuals themselves from their mobility allowance, as it was rarely being spent for outings or transportation at that time.

Today the majority of individuals with learning difficulties are living in the community either with their parents, or in foster care or in smaller staffed housing units. The carers are familiar with the individual's programme plan and needs, whether at home or at a day centre that they may attend, and this also applies to the equipment they are requesting for their activity level, social interaction, safety and independence.

Assessment

The assessment of the user should take place in the individual's home or the day centre which they attend regularly. Here the staff caring for the individual with knowledge of the individual and the individual's programme plan will be able to input into the needs for the equipment and the needs of the specific carers. It is these carers and care staff who are with the individual 24 hours a day and not the professionals. The professionals involved with the user should join in the assess-

ment, identifying postural and behavioural needs and to also inform the wheelchair staff of the current therapy programmes that are being used for the user that may alter future equipment requirements. Wherever the assessment takes place, other carers or staff should also be involved in the assessment needs, even if this is by telephone after the event, to ensure the prescription for equipment meets everyone's needs. Although this is time consuming, staff whose opinion is not sought often come up with requirements that cannot be accommodated easily once the equipment has been issued. Knowing the future plans for the individual user will also assist in the mobility planning requirements. If the user spends time or an increasing amount of time in foster care, the future plans should be clarified with staff before major decisions are made that may need to be altered. Everyone involved with the user should be heard.

Postural needs

The user with postural deformities will need to be physically assessed, as with paediatric cases. This physical assessment may well also have been carried out by the occupational therapist or physiotherapist treating the user and information gained in such cases is invaluable. Developments, changes, deformities and dislocations should all be identified and any future operative procedures planned and noted. Attention will be paid to the pelvic, thoracic, hip, knee and head positions, deformities and functional and postural needs.

For the severely disabled user with learning difficulties, a total contact system which accommodates their contractures and allows as much function as possible is used. Such systems will include the Matrix, Odstock or Derby mould. In some homes and with some individuals, Jay seating systems may be successful, but this is very much dependent upon the needs of the carers, if they want to fold the wheelchair and the time they have available for removing the system and generally caring for it. Allowance for the positioning of slings for hoists should be

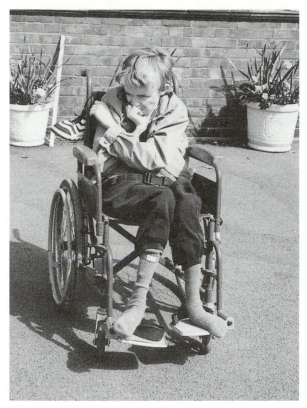

Figure 10.1 A typical complex seating problem in this group of users.

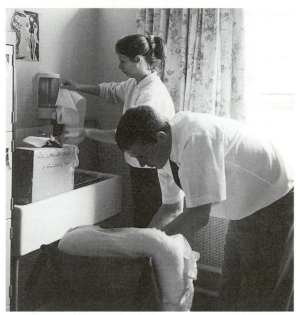

A

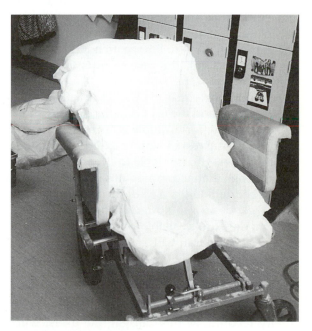

B

Figure 10.2 (A) Plastering the cast for a total contact Odstock system. (B) The plastered cast.

noted and the time and method of transfer used by the carers. Whichever system is chosen by the therapist to best meet the user's needs, it is important that the parents or carers are shown illustrations of the systems, if not a system itself, before the work is started. Rejection is found to be higher when full involvement of all those concerned is not sought. The needs of the home, parents, centre, transportation, care staff and the robustness and safety aspects of the system should all be considered before a system is finally selected.

The user's size and weight is obviously different from that of a child, and this has be to taken into account when choosing the wheelchair or chassis as weight limitations apply. However, the needs are often the same as with children as the equipment is used for posture, function, feeding, resting, mobility, social integration,

pushing outdoors and for transportation. The size and weight of the user and the equipment chosen has implications for the carers who seek manoeuvrability, ease of pushing, easy access with hoists and slings, clamping facilities for coaches or vehicles and access into black cabs, for example. Community integration is the key point and it is the care staff who often have much to comment upon with the appearance of the equipment they use and society's reaction to it in the community setting. Visual appearance, design and user and carer choice when it is available, are therefore important considerations with this group of users. Also, the needs of one 'home' setting will be different from another, depending upon the style of care adopted, the immediate local environment and the individuals concerned. For example, Barrett models are popular for their 'sleek look' by some homes but when tall male care staff are employed often telescopic handles are required for ease of pushing. For some homes, Odstock systems are popular as they are regarded as 'fitting in' with the homely furniture better than a matrix system ever would. The activities and outings of the homes are also very variable and can range from short trips to the local park, day trips to France, to holidays at UK 'Centre Parcs' and 'Butlins', to trips to Florida, USA.

Postural inserts may be required if there is a gross scoliosis and the user is in the chair for long periods of time, for example a Burnett mould or an Odstock backrest or simply a lumbar insert.

For the user who is unable to sit at right angles, a wheelchair that accommodates a greater angle should be tried. Often a 15 or 25 degree backrest with a good seating surface proves successful. Such models are available on special orders or through the Bencraft CELT range.

The head position of the user is often a concern and support for comfort, function, social participation and feeding need to be considered. The head should not be tilted backwards, known as gravity feeding, as this can gag the users, who may choke on the food and develop an inhalation pneumonia. When drinking the head must not be tipped back as this opens the airway. It is important to offer a variety of positions and a tilt in space facility may be used to alter the position of the individual for different periods in the day. Whichever type of headrest or backrest extension

is chosen, it should be able to come off separately from the rest of the unit to assist the carers during the day so that people do not become increasingly stiff and deformed. It is important that residents are involved in activities and outside events, and the wheelchair and seating system is a key to this.

General needs

Some general needs for this group of users range from buggies and attendant wheelchairs for children with Down's syndrome to basic adult models of wheelchair (both self-propelling and lightweight) in order that they keep up with their parents or school peer group. It is important to issue equipment that is age related and to ensure that the user is safe in it. Often seat belts that fasten at the back to stop the user releasing them are required. Powered models are often issued to learning difficulty users. Time should be taken for training in the locality the chair is to used and alterations may be required to the joy stick and the control box. The safety of others is a key requirement.

As the parents of the user with learning difficulties become older and their own health deteriorates, a lighter chair may be required to assist the parent. Such issue may be refused by some wheelchair services on their local criteria but the health needs of these parents need to be taken into consideration as they will become the in- or outpatient requiring treatment in the future and the user may even need other care staff who are fitter to push the individual, another expense to the services. It is an issue for debate on a wider scale with other providers than simply for the wheelchair service.

Different needs for care staff have already been mentioned but should not be overlooked as it may make the difference between outings and no outings for the user. The equipment's appearance and 'modernness' should not be overlooked, especially when community integration and acceptance is the current philosophy. Staff need to feel comfortable and 'proud' when they are taking the user into the community, to clubs, pubs and to shopping centres. Listening to the parents and carers will ensure their needs are met whenever possible and compromises should be fully discussed.

Safety is another consideration that should not be overlooked. This applies to weight allowances for the equipment and chassis, user safety in the equipment and the transportation of the equipment whether by community transport systems or in Dial-a-Ride. Wheelchair service staff should liaise with such services to ensure safety practices are known and applied. Models of wheelchair issued should be the variety that the transportation services are able to clamp. For example, the Carters Action 2000 is a problem in this respect.

Footstraps, harnesses, butterfly harnesses and vests may all be issued to meet postural and safety needs. They should be easy for care staff to apply and as 'foolproof' as possible. For example, chest harnesses often have to be fixed at the lower insertions to ensure that the straps are not simply pulled up at the top and left in a position where they are near to the user's neck.

Attendant models are generally used for ease of use and also for safety, so that the individual user does not put their fingers into the moving spokes. If a self-propelling model is chosen, spokeguards are available either from the manufacturer or the approved repairer. Wide thoracic padded straps may also be required in the thoracic position for safety when being taken out 'into the community'. Trays, especially 'U' shaped trays, are often provided for functional use and again safety features such as 'metal collars' on the tubes to a set position may be required. The width of the tray should be the minimum required for function to allow for doorways, smaller rooms, etc.

For the epileptic users, belts and harnesses that are easily released may be required by staff or parents. The quick release seat belt type is usually chosen.

If the position of the feet is difficult to accommodate on the footplates with straps, then a footboard may be selected. With very contracted knees this can be used with the greatest amount of plate posteriorly or when the knees are held in extension with the plate facing outwards. A surface that is both non-slip and easy to clean is advisable to assist the staff, as food, powder, etc. can often be a problem.

When accommodation of contractures, comfort and pressure relief are required, a seating insert such as the Spenco seat infill may be used successfully. If pressure areas do develop, the district nurse should be asked to liaise with the care staff regarding any treatment required. Where there is abduction or adduction at the hips, cushions with various size pommels or raises and inserts may be chosen for positioning and ease of use for the care staff. Some users will wish to cross their legs when in the wheelchair, a position of habit. Ensuring the wheelchair is wide enough to accommodate such movements rather than not allowing it to occur due to space restrictions will make the user happy. Whichever cushion is chosen, whether for postural needs, comfort or pressure relief, it is important that the wheelchair therapist asks about continence history and takes into account the needs of the staff or carers in maintaining the cushions or cleaning the covers. Where staff or carers change often, cushions that indicate the correct position in the wheelchair, are light and easy to manage, should be the first chosen by the therapist.

The biomechanical principles of posture and seating (see Chs 3 and 4) and the paediatric considerations (see Ch. 9) should also be noted when prescribing for this group. Taking time to truly listen to all concerned, the parents, professionals and carers alike, before recommending a system, wheelchair or management method is the only way forward for successful practice.

REFERENCES

American Psychiatric Association 1980 Diagnostic and Statistical Manual, DSM iii. APA, Washington, DC

Birch H G, Richardson S A, Baird D, Horobin G, Illsley R 1970 Mental subnormality in the community. Williams and Wilkins, Baltimore

Chlebowski V 1991 Social services. In: Fraser W I, MacGillivary R C, Green A M (eds) Hallas' caring for people with mental handicaps, 8th edn. Butterworth-Heinemann, Oxford, pp 202–214

Department of Health and Social Security 1971 White paper. Better services for the mentally handicapped. HMSO, London

Department of Health and Social Security 1987 Mental handicap: progress, problems and priorities. HMSO, London

Department of Health and Social Security 1989a Mental handicap: progress, problems and priorities. HMSO, London

Department of Health and Social Security 1989b Caring for people. Community care in the next decade and beyond. HMSO, London

Emerson E, Pretty G M H 1987 Enhancing the social relevance of evaluation practice. Disability, Handicap and Society 2: 151–162

Fischbacher E 1991 The management of epilepsy. In: Fraser W I, MacGillivary R C, Green A M (eds) Hallas' caring for people with mental handicaps, 8th edn. Butterworth-Heinemann, Oxford pp 123–131

Fraser B 1991 Communication and behaviour disorders. In: Fraser W I, MacGillivary R C, Green A M (eds) Hallas' caring for people with mental handicaps, 8th edn. Butterworth-Heinemann, Oxford, pp 87–93

Fraser B, Green A M 1991 Changing perspectives on mental handicap. In: Fraser W I, MacGillivary R C, Green A M (eds) Hallas' caring for people with mental handicaps, 8th edn. Butterworth-Heinemann, Oxford, pp 1–7

Guinea S 1991 Individual programme planning. In: Fraser W I, MacGillivary R C, Green A M (eds) Hallas' caring for people with mental handicaps, 8th edn. Butterworth-Heinemann, Oxford, pp 64–75

Griffiths Report 1988 Community care: agenda for action. Department of Health, London

Holland M 1991 Advocacy. In: Fraser W I, MacGillivary R C, Green A M (eds) Hallas' caring for people with mental handicaps, 8th edn. Butterworth-Heinemann, Oxford, pp 271–276

Humphreys S, Lowe K, Blunden R 1982 Long term evaluation of services for mentally handicapped people in Cardiff. Mental Handicap 16: 23–26

Jones P G, Cregan A 1986 Sign and symbol communication for mentally handicapped people. Croom Helm, London

King's Fund 1982 An ordinary life: comprehensive locally-based residential services for mentally handicapped people, 2nd edn. King's Fund Centre, London

Leider I 1981 Strategic communication in mental retardation. In: Fraser W I, Grieve R (eds) Communicating with normal and retarded children. John Wright, Bristol, pp 113–129

McConkey R 1991 Community integration. In: Fraser W I, MacGillivary R C, Green A M (eds) Hallas' caring for people with mental handicaps, 8th edn. Butterworth-Heinemann, Oxford, pp 283–302

Mackay G 1991 The school years. In: Fraser W I, MacGillivary R C, Green A M (eds) Hallas' caring for people with mental handicaps, 8th edn. Butterworth-Heinemann, Oxford, pp 34–40

MacGillivary R 1991a Diagnostic categories and clinical conditions. In: Fraser W I, MacGillivary R C, Green A M (eds) Hallas' caring for people with mental handicaps, 8th edn. Butterworth-Heinemann, Oxford, appendix 2, pp 362–383

MacGillivary R 1991b The use of drugs in mental handicap. In: Fraser W I, MacGillivary R C, Green A M (eds) Hallas' caring for people with mental handicaps, 8th edn. Butterworth-Heinemann, Oxford, appendix 3, pp 384–394

Minns R A, Brown K, Wong K, Fraser W 1989 Neurodevelopmental study of profoundly mentally handicapped children in hospital care. Journal of Mental Deficiency Research 439–455

Montague J 1991 Music Therapy. In: Fraser W I, MacGillivary R C, Green A M (eds) Hallas' caring for people with mental handicaps, 8th edn. Butterworth-Heinemann, Oxford pp 167–172

Moore K 1988 Towards integration in the local community. In: Towards comprehensive services for people with mental handicaps. Chapman & Hall, London, pp 79–107

Morris P 1969 Put away. Routledge and Kegan Paul, London

Office of Health Economics 1978 Mental handicap: ways forward, No 61. White Crescent Press, Luton

Sines D 1988a Introduction. Setting the scene. In: Sines D (ed) Towards integration. Comprehensive services for people with mental handicaps. Chapman & Hall, London, pp 1–5

Sines D 1988b Maintaining an ordinary life. In: Sines D (ed) Towards comprehensive services for people with mental handicaps. Chapman & Hall, London, pp 28–36

Sines D 1988c Towards comprehensive services: its nature and design. In: Sines D (ed) Towards comprehensive services for people with mental handicaps. Chapman & Hall, London, pp 165–198

Stansfield J 1991 Communication. Augmentative and alternative systems of communication. In: Fraser W I, MacGillivary R C, Green A M (eds) Hallas' caring for people with mental handicaps, 8th edn. Butterworth-Heinemann, Oxford, pp 76–86

Towell D (ed) 1988 An ordinary life in practice: developing community based services for people with learning difficulties. King Edward's Hospital Fund, London

Walker M 1986 Line drawings for the revised Makaton Vocabulary. MVDP, Camberley

Warnock Committee Report 1978 Special educational needs: report of the committee into education of handicapped children and young people. Cmnd 7212, HMSO, London

Wishart J 1991 Education and training. In: Fraser W I,

MacGillivary R C, Green A M (eds) Hallas' caring for people with mental handicaps, 8th edn. Butterworth-Heinemann, Oxford, pp 27–47

Wolfensberger W 1972 The principle of normalisation in human services. National Institute on Mental Retardation, Toronto, pp 13–25

Wolfensberger W 1980 The definition of normalisation – update, problems. In: Flynn R, Nitch K (eds) Normalisation, social integration and community services. Baltimore University Press, Baltimore, MD

World Health Organization 1985 Mental retardation: meeting the challenge. WHO, Geneva

11

Elderly users

INTRODUCTION

In the populations of the western world, longevity is increasing with improved disease control, nutrition, style of living and advances in health care. In the sixteenth century, elderly people were those over the age of 35 years. More recently, elderly people were described as those over the age of 65 years, the retirement age for men. With the increase in the number of elderly people in western societies, this age description has increased to 75 years. Although retirement may be a cut-off point in a description related to the elderly, some people do not retire at 65 years and some retire as early as 55 years. Life expectancy has increased in the UK and now stands at 78 years for women and 73 years for men (1987–89), a considerable increase from 70 and 66 years respectively in 1950–52 (HM Government Actuary's Department).

Historical background

It is now more than 50 years since the Act was passed that abolished the Poor Law Institutions, poor house infirmaries or 'workhouses' that the elderly associate so readily with disgrace and degradation. There was overcrowding, long stays, high dependency, fear of admission, minimal prospects of discharge, basic nursing care and regular medical input (Garrett 1987). Medical care and management was isolated from the mainstream of medical activity and it was not until the National Health Service (NHS) took responsibility for these infirmaries and the work of the pioneer of modern geriatric medicine, Majory Warren, that practice began to change.

Sadly many of the redundant institutions were later passed on to the NHS and converted into geriatric (derived from the Greek *geras* – old age and *iatros* – physician) units which produced negative reactions from many elderly people who remembered them as 'institutions' and all the grim reminders of the past were recalled (Garrett 1987).

For more than three centuries after the Poor Law Act was passed in 1601, the needs of the elderly came under the same classification as the sick and destitute of any other age group. Their support was initially under the responsibility of the parish where they lived and later central government under the Poor Law Amendment Act of 1843. The poor were obliged to enter institutions and the conditions in them are well documented by authors such as Charles Dickens. The Royal Commission of 1905, led by Lloyd George, marked the beginnings of the Welfare State in the UK with weekly pensions, the National Insurance Act and, finally, the inception of the NHS and the National Assistance Act which secured health, pensions, benefits and accommodation for the elderly (Garrett 1987). Today the elderly are cared for predominantly in the community outside hospitals.

The physical, psychological and social factors of ageing

Physical, psychological and social factors have a wider range in people over the age of 65 and the elderly present with multiple pathology. The major diagnoses that affect the elderly are: cardiovascular disease, Parkinson's disease, dementia, arthritis, osteoporosis and advanced stages of other diseases. The main physical disabilities experienced by the elderly are those of locomotion, personal care and dexterity.

With the elderly there is a loss of physical reserve due to ageing or previous chronic disease, multiple pathology combining together to produce disability, polypharmacy, mental vulnerability due to depression or confusion, low

expectations by the patient, staff or family. Some disability occurs in 12% of people aged 65–69 and 80% of those over 80 years. Two-thirds of the 200 000 wheelchair users in England and Wales in 1977 were people over the retirement age (Fenwick 1977) and 75% of users were found to be over 60 years of age in a more recent study (Kettle & Rowley 1990).

Physiological aspects of ageing

Ageing brings with it a number of physiological changes that result in reduced physical activity, lessening of coordination and an increased reliance on seating devices and wheelchairs. In a 1980 survey in the Dundee district of Scotland, of the seating needs of disabled people, the elderly were found to dominate the results (Bardsley 1993). The major factors that bring them to the attention of the health services are the various changes that take place in their bodies. These are described briefly below.

Musculoskeletal system. Between 20 and 70 years, there is a 5 cm (2 inch) height reduction in the spine as the fluid in the vertebral discs is reabsorbed. The bone mass is reduced, the muscle fibres atrophy, being replaced with fibrous tissue, and the joints enlarge. All these changes lead to slower voluntary movement, reduced mobility and postural changes. Falls and minor accidents are increasingly common in the elderly and as their movements and reactions are slower and their sight and dexterity reduced, incidents such as catching legs and ankles on the wheelchair footplates are regular occurrences.

Excretory systems. There is a loss of tissue elasticity and a reduction in the amount of subcutaneous tissue which leads to wrinkling of the skin which is so familiar in the elderly. These factors also make the elderly more vulnerable to the development of pressure sores. The epidermis thins, the blood vessels become more fragile and haemorrhages from these cause the purpura seen commonly on the skin of the elderly. The sweat glands atrophy with a reduction in perspiration, and the nails thicken. Greying of the hair is due to the loss of its pigment and the hair also becomes thinner. There are changes in the kidneys and bladder, which is most noticeable at night when almost three-quarters of all elderly people are required to break their sleep.

Gastrointestinal tract. The flow of saliva is reduced and there is lessened motility, with slower oesophageal and gastric emptying with a tendency to constipation because of the lack of muscle tone and reduced mucus secretion. The elderly body is less efficient at handling drugs due to the slowing of gastric and intestinal mobility and the absorption rate also slows down. Malnutrition is also a problem with the elderly, especially males over 75 years, who are bereaved, living alone, housebound and suffering from dementia (Pushpangadan & Burns 1996).

Cardiovascular system. The blood vessels become less elastic as collagen is laid down in vessel walls. To compensate for this peripheral resistance, the blood pressure rises and this will take longer to return to normal following exercise or stress than in younger individuals. The cardiac output drops by 40%, that is, there is more energy expenditure for a less efficient result. Women benefit from the protective effects of oestrogens against atheroma and live a less hazardous life style than men, for example they are exposed to a lesser extent to wars, smoking, alcohol, reckless driving and homicide.

Respiratory system. The lungs become less elastic in the elderly and the vital capacity is reduced by 25%. Coughing and expectoration is more difficult also. Many elderly users suffer with chronic respiratory diseases and require supplementary oxygen therapy. Portable cylinder holders are often requested to be attached to the back of the wheelchair. (It should be remembered that this adds weight to the model and the carer should be informed of this. Also, the model should be checked for stability whenever anything that is heavy is added to a chair.)

Nervous system. Generally a higher threshold of stimulation is required in the elderly for stimulation of the senses, for example external temperature, taste buds, smell, hearing and vision (Garrett 1987).

The biological age of the individual relates to the body changes of ageing such as grey hair and musculoskeletal changes. The social age relates to the social role of the individual interacting with society. There are changes and developments throughout life and the individual's experience of adapting to earlier changes influences his/her responses to the present and the future.

Psychological and cognitive aspects of ageing

Psychologically and cognitively it becomes more difficult to perform simple tasks, a factor which begins from the age of 30 years, and the effort is greater and the motivation less. Short-term memory is reduced and the elderly find it more difficult to perform new tasks. Elderly wheelchair users, for example, often forget how a wheelchair operates, how the cushion should be inserted or how to have the wheelchair repaired. Compliance with medication is also a common problem, but there are aids available to assist with dosages, dose and time reminders, large print labels, bottles that are easier to open and metered dose inhalers (Corlett 1996). The reaction time is reduced and more time is taken to make decisions which can affect tasks. There is also a general stiffening of the body and this again reduces the reaction time. The elderly do have experience on their side and this is an advantage when they are able to use previously learnt skills. When training is necessary, it is better to train on tasks that are put into context rather than tasks that are meaningless (Haynes 1984). The individual's level of intelligence remains the same as it always was but if the tasks of daily life are taken away from someone, the brain activity lessens and the intelligence level is dulled. It is therefore important to keep the elderly as independent as possible, both physically and mentally.

Social aspects of ageing

People become more not less varied as they age. The elderly are not an homogeneous group but old age is built upon the framework of the individual's earlier life. With retirement, the social aspects of the workplace are lost, income is reduced, the individual can feel that they are not useful to the country any more and they can become less and less involved with other people and become increasingly isolated (Haynes 1984). In the UK, as the elderly migrate to certain coastal and rural retirement communities and the families of those elderly living in the inner city move away, support systems break down and loneliness can develop. Social roles and new activities should be encouraged.

Financial aspects

Older people make up the largest low income group in the UK (Teale 1996) and over half of the pensioner households depended on the state pension for at least 75% of their income in 1991. Low income benefits are available to the elderly and are based on the individual's income and savings, rather than their National Insurance contributions. For example, the basic state pension for a single person is £61.15, which is 20% of the average adult wage. A couple's pension increases by £36.60 to £97.75, which is 32% of the average adult full-time wage (1992–93). However, many elderly people have savings, receive good pensions or have supportive families. For such individuals they may choose to buy their own chair and simply use the NHS wheelchair service for advice and as a source of information (Research Institute for Consumer Affairs 1996). (Further details of the other benefits available are given in Box 11.1.)

Transportation

Reduced or free fares on the local transport system, with a bus pass for example, and Black Cab schemes, are offered by some local borough councils for pensioners and on coaches, air flights and trains, various reductions are available at off-peak times (Department of Transport 1996) (see also Ch. 13).

Box 11.1   Financial benefits

The benefits available include:

- Income Support, a safety net to bring people on low incomes to a minimum weekly income and where the savings are less than £8000 currently
- Help with council tax and housing where eligibility depends upon age, income, savings, disability, number of people in the family, for example
- The Social Fund, where lump sum payments are made towards specific expenses, for example cold weather payments, community care grants towards cookers, beds, funeral expenses and budgetary crisis loans
- Health-related costs such as free prescriptions to people of pensionable age, and those receiving Income Support are also entitled to free dental treatment, sight tests and help towards the cost of glasses

Individuals with disabilities are also entitled to other benefits. These include:

- Attendance Allowance, which is payable to people with a physical or mental disability who need supervision or help with personal care. Although paid to the disabled person, they usually use it to pay the carer or to pay for community services such as bathing. It is paid at two rates, the lower rate for help in the day or night (£32.40) and the higher rate (£48.50) for help both in the day and at night. The medical condition requiring help has to remain for 6 months for the allowance to be paid

- Disability Living Allowance is initially claimed by individuals before they are 65 years but payments continue until the age of 75. There are two components: Mobility payments at two levels (£12.90 or £33.90) and Care payments at three levels (£12.90, £32.40 and £48.50). The level of payment received depends upon the disability. An Invalid Care Allowance (£36.60) is paid to those carers who are unable to work because they are looking after someone who receives Disability Living or higher rate Attendance Allowance
- Invalid Benefit (£57.60) is payable to someone who is unable to work for at least 28 weeks because of sickness or disability and is payable for 5 years after pensionable age
- Severe disablement allowance is paid to disabled people who have not paid enough contributions to qualify for the severe disablement allowance. The basic rate is £36.95 (Teale 1996)

Help with residential or nursing home fees is again linked to savings or capital and currently when this falls below £16 000 assistance is available, either by topping up or with no contribution

The Disabled Persons Transport Advisory Committee (DPTAC, a statutory body) has recommended improvements in the design of buses and these include lower steps, split level steps, 'kneeling buses', non-slip floors and specially adapted buses for wheelchair users where assistants are available to help (Roper & Mulley 1986). Some of these buses operate semi-fixed routes and are flexible, allowing users to alight near to or at their homes. From February 1989, all new London taxis were licensed if they could carry a wheelchair. Such vehicles have wide door frames, wider angle of opening and ramps and the rear seat tips backwards to increase the space in the cab. The ramps are generally the two-track variety and it should be noted that some of the larger tyres on outdoor models are too large to travel on the ramps safely. From January 2000 all London taxis are to meet this requirement and such schemes are developing throughout the country. However, wider doors can actually make access harder for those who have a mobility problem but do not use a wheelchair, as the distance from the door to the seat is greater.

Dial-a-Ride is the door-to-door service for mobility impaired people and it is accessible to wheelchair users. It is a system which is operated and managed locally to provide cheap and suitable transportation for the disabled person. A number of journeys are funded by the local borough annually (Buchanan & Chamberlain 1978). Dial-a-Ride is available in most cities for those unable to use public transport and the service is booked in advance. The Shopmobility scheme is available in some shopping precincts for those with mobility problems. The scheme may be linked to Dial-a-Ride in some places and also needs to be booked in advance (Department of Transport) (see also Ch. 13).

Local community transport is also available for outings, excursions and for transportation to day centres and clubs, for example. Mainline stations are becoming increasingly wheelchair accessible, with disabled toilets, and parking and ramps are available to assist users on to trains. On trains and tubes, seats or seating areas nearest to the door have been allocated for wheelchair users and the disabled on the new stock, but on some old stock, wheelchair users have to travel in the guard's van.

All airlines who are members of the International Air Transport Association (IATA) have devised a special form called INCAD (incapacitated passenger handling advice form) which gives details of the person's travel plans and personal requirements. The GP is required to complete Part 2 of the form. Frequent travellers may choose to complete the FREMEC (frequent traveller's medical card) form which is issued by the medical department of the airline. Disabled travellers board the aircraft first and disembark last. Narrow wheelchairs are available on aircraft to access the toilets (Roper & Mulley 1986).

Community care

There is now considerable emphasis on care in the community and therefore a shift from institutional and residential care to community care. Since the implementation of the Community Care Act in 1993, the needs of older people and their carers are now formally assessed and ideally suitable services are then provided (Barodawala 1996). The reforms have meant that voluntary and private organizations are now increasingly being asked to provide residential care, day care and home-based services.

Most elderly people live independently in private or rented accommodation. However more of the 'oldest old', that is less than 1% of the elderly population in total, live in residential care or hospitals. Of these 'oldest old', 29% of people aged over 85 compared with only 1.1% of those aged between 65 and 74 years live in residential homes (Laing & Buisson 1993). It is this section of the population that is growing the most rapidly (Andrews 1985) and especially the number of women (Hodkinson et al 1988).

Sheltered housing, residential and nursing homes

Individuals who are unable to cope with living on their own in the community, may move into one of the three types of care accommodation:

sheltered housing, residential care or a nursing home.

Sheltered housing may be organized through the local authority, a joint venture with a housing association, or privately. This type of housing is in short supply (Wanklyn 1996). In this accommodation, the individual lives in a self-contained flat, bungalow or house with cooking and bathing facilities. The developments usually contain 20–40 properties. The individuals have to be able to look after themselves and each of the units may have a residential warden overseeing the units. The units may also have some type of alarm call system and many include day centre or communal facilities for the residents and their guests.

If the individual requires a greater amount of assistance for the activities of daily living, then a residential home may be required. Here individual or two- or four-bedded rooms are found and assistance is available from care staff for bathing, toileting and meals. They may be private, voluntary or run by the local authority. Each has to be registered with the local authority if they are caring for four or more elderly or dependent people and they are inspected twice a year (Wanklyn 1996).

When nursing care is necessary, the individual will enter a nursing home. These are generally privately run and at least one qualified nurse has to be on duty at each shift. To be licensed as a nursing home, all such homes are inspected twice a year by the health authority to ensure good and adequate standards are in place. Although the majority of homes are privately run, many of the residents who have assets of less than £16 000 (1996) are funded or part funded by the social services.

The British Geriatric Society states that a home should provide:

- personal choice in food, clothing, form of address, social activities, daily routine and a GP
- privacy
- an easily accessible complaints procedure
- an advocacy system for residents
- personal control of finance and medication where possible

- access to a full range of diverse activities
- access to community, health and social services
- an individualized care plan (British Geriatric Society 1990).

In all residential accommodation for the disabled elderly, and especially for those in wheelchairs, there should be suitable access with ramps, wide doorways, adequate space in the hallway, sockets, switches and surfaces at waist level and toilets and bathrooms that are suitably converted or designed (Wanklyn 1996).

Statutory and voluntary support

The new community care arrangements were introduced in 1993 and since this time the social services have become more responsible for assessing need, designing care plans and securing delivery of the appropriate services (Renwick 1996).

Many of the elderly who require support while living alone in the community access this through the social worker and local social services department. Such support includes: meals on wheels, frozen meals, luncheon clubs, day centres, housing and adaptations, outings, respite care and holidays, community transport, care workers, home care, equipment for daily living, telephones and personal emergency alarms in case of falls, for example. From the health service such support as liaison, district and palliative (Macmillan or Marie Curie) nurses, health visitors for the elderly, physiotherapy, occupational therapy, optical, dental, chiropody, nutrition and dietetic services (Pushpangadan & Burns 1996), equipment for nursing purposes, day hospital, bathing assistance and continence services are available.

Apart from the statutory services, the voluntary sector in the UK also contributes enormously to support in the community with help groups, for example the Cross Roads attendant scheme, the Red Cross equipment loan services, the WRVS support groups, clubs such as the Stroke Association, the Multiple Sclerosis group and Age Concern, the listening library for the visually impaired, CRUSE for the bereaved and Help the Aged, to name but a few.

Changes in society and the built environment (Fig. 11.1)

Changes in society in the numbers of elderly, disabled people and the increase in time for leisure has increased disabled people's horizons and mobility. For disabled people to access the wider horizons, the built environment and transportation has to accommodate the less able-bodied individuals. A recent survey in Liverpool found that over a quarter of GP premises were inaccessible to patients using wheelchairs (Ratoff, Heyes & Haddleton 1993). However,

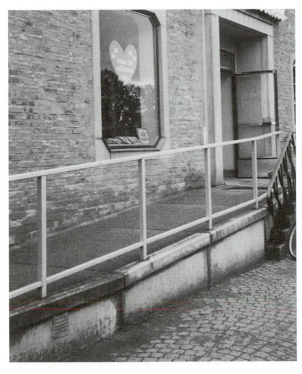

A

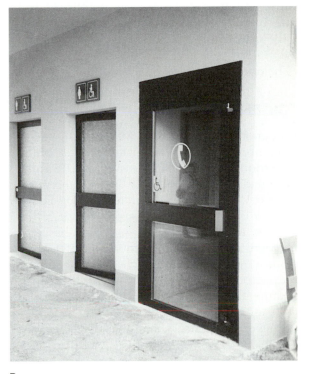

B

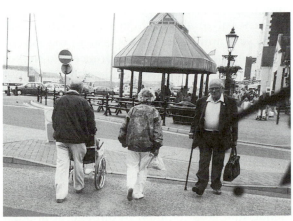

C

Figure 11.1(A–C) Changes in the built environment which assist the disabled user.

many improvements have occurred over the last decade, many as a direct or indirect result of legislation. Since 1985, the law has stated that new public buildings should be accessible and guidelines were published in 1987 and 1991 by the Department of the Environment. Ramps have been provided as an alternative to steps or as an addition to steps in many public places and kerbs have been dropped at major road junctions. More controlled crossings have been established and central reservations have divided many busy roads. Supermarket doors are automatic and have flush thresholds for easy access (Buchanan & Chamberlain 1978).

INCIDENCE

In common with most of the west, the UK has an ageing population. In 1961 just under 12% of the population were aged 65 or over, by 1994 this figure had increased to 16%. Overall, the numbers of those aged 60 and over has risen by a third since 1961 to 12 million. The proportion of the over 60s who are aged 80 and over has also increased, from 11% in 1961 to 19% in 1994 – that is four million people (Church 1996). The ethnic minority population in the UK has a younger age structure than the white population and only 5–10% of the ethnic populations are currently aged over 65 years. Those who came to this country in the 1950s and 1960s aged between 20 and 30 are now reaching retirement age and so the numbers of ethnic elderly will therefore increase in the next two decades (Ebrahim 1996).

CLINICAL FEATURES

Some general features of ageing will be discussed first and then specific medical conditions associated with the elderly will be highlighted.

Incontinence

Urinary incontinence is common in old age, affecting approximately 10–20% of females and 7–10% of males living in their own homes and a higher percentage living in nursing and residential homes. The consequences of urinary inconti-

nence are both medical and social, with higher rates of depression and social isolation among people who are incontinent. A thorough assessment is essential so that the appropriate management can be planned. This includes a social and environmental assessment, advice on fluid intake and diet, prevention of constipation, bladder retraining, pelvic floor muscle exercises, advice on appropriate aids, help with catheterization and counselling (Pushpangadan & Burns 1996).

Incontinence results from a combination of:

- urinary urgency
- the time and ease to get to the toilet.

Common factors causing incontinence which are reversible include faecal impaction, senile atrophic vaginitis and prolapse and urinary infection.

Urinary incontinence is usually associated with either:

- Detrusor instability where the treatment includes bladder drill and pelvic floor exercises and sometimes drugs.
- Ineffective voiding, for example due to bladder outflow obstruction (e.g. prostate stricture) or an underactive or autonomic bladder (e.g. CVA, peripheral neuropathy). Treatment may include intermittent catheterization.

When issuing wheelchairs and pressure-relieving cushions, an individual's bladder habits and state of continence are vital information for the therapist to seek to ensure the correct equipment is issued. Such factors may include: the material of the cushion's cover; its washability; the number of covers issued; the skin of the wheelchair user and its tolerance to different materials, especially if few clothes are worn; use of continence aids or catheters (especially when ramped cushions are recommended); method of toileting; the angle or position that may be necessary for urinating, and use of fitted or incontinence pads.

Mental illness

Mental illness is common in old age. It is often associated with physical illness and social problems which are commonly due to deprivation or traumatic life events and responds well to antidepressant drugs (Wattis 1996).

Loneliness

It has been said that one in five old people are lonely sometimes and that one in ten are lonely very often, which is almost one million old people (Forbes 1996). Those most affected are the very old, widows or widowers, those people isolated by disability and old people who are caregivers who may also feel isolated. A lack of money limits the individual's opportunities and many of the elderly are either on low incomes or are reluctant to spend any money. Loneliness is found to be less prevalent in rural communities than in densely populated urban areas.

There are two kinds of loneliness. External, where the loneliness is brought about by life circumstances, for example a bereavement, and internal loneliness, where it relates to a personality type. Signs of loneliness are verbal outpouring, prolonged holding of one's hand or arm, drab clothing and certain body language such as tightly crossed arms (Forbes 1996).

Frequently the elderly users of the wheelchair service may call the wheelchair service administrator for a 'chat' or the approved repairer service for a 'repair' simply to see a familiar kind face in the form of a technician (Fig. 11.2). If this occurs regularly, therapists should look into the situation further.

By giving people the opportunity to help others it helps them to retain an active involvement in their own lives and the elderly may need encouragement to participate in such helping activities. For disabled people the telephone is a useful aid. Loneliness can also be relieved by activities outside the home such as day centres, luncheon clubs, adult education classes, community activities (details of which are available from the Council for Voluntary Services), the local churches or religious centres, courses run by the University of the Third Age, locally organized outings and local support groups which may or may not be related to the individual's disability. Befriending schemes are also organized by the

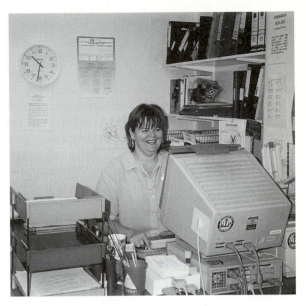

Figure 11.2 The wheelchair service administrator who often deals with the lonely elderly user on the telephone.

local community care scheme, the church and the local branch of Age Concern. (Addresses are given at the end of this book.)

Depression

Although depression is no more common in younger adults than older adults, when it does occur in the elderly, it is likely to be more severe and it is more likely to need hospital admission due to the elderly living on their own in many cases. Individuals suffering with depression are slow in functional activities and need to be given time to complete tasks (Wattis 1996).

Delirium

Many elderly also suffer with delirium which presents with confusion and an acute physical illness such as heart failure, chest or urinary infection. It should not be confused with dementia which does not have an acute onset. Delirium may be best managed at home as long as there is adequate social support (Wattis 1996).

Dementia

Dementia is an acquired global condition with intellectual deterioration, memory impairment and personality disorganization in the presence of unimpaired consciousness. The syndrome is irreversible and leads to impairment of the following: thinking, orientation, comprehension, calculation, learning capacity, language and judgement. The cognitive impairments are often accompanied or preceded by deterioration in emotional control, social behaviour and motivation.

Dementias are common and affect around 8% of people over 65 years, that is 1 in 12. Prevalence rises rapidly with age from 2 to 3% in the 65–69 age group, to 5% in the 75–79 age group and to 20% in the over 80s. The main diagnoses are Alzheimer's disease, vascular dementia and a combination of the two. More females present with Alzheimer's disease and more men with vascular dementia. Reversible dementia may be due to vitamin B_{12} and thyroid deficiency, space-occupying lesions and alcohol-related dementias (Wattis 1996).

Mild dementia may be missed, and in diagnosing dementia the risk factors such as family history, vascular and hypertensive disorders and the nature of the onset (rapid or slow) are taken into account. A sudden onset suggests delirium, a stepwise deterioration suggests vascular dementia and a gradual progression Alzheimer's disease.

Presenile dementia is a progressive disease where the language and visual perception are affected (Wattis 1996).

Alzheimer's disease

Alzheimer's disease is a physical disease which causes a progressive decline in the abilities to remember, learn, understand, communicate and reason. It is the most common type of dementia and was first described by Alos Alzheimer, a German neurologist, in 1907 (Alzheimer's Disease Society 1996). One in three Alzheimer sufferers have a similarly affected first degree relative and the causes are thought to be dietary with the influence of aluminium, repeated head injury and hereditary factors.

The clinical features include memory loss where new information is not stored in the long-term memory, with the result of items being mislaid or conversations being repeated. Gradually the long-term memory is lost and the patient confabulates to compensate and gradually becomes aphasic. Language can be hindered with expressive dysphasia, which leads to distress as people think the patient cannot understand. Praxia, the inability to perform coordinated motor tasks, develops and various types of agnosia, the failure to recognize sensory stimuli which may result in familiar faces and objects not being recognized and used correctly. There are also perceptual problems such as the depth and distance of steps which can often lead to falls. Dysphasia is normal but there is an inability to access names of objects, for example. Physical changes also occur, which include weight loss, weakness, a stooped posture, abnormal gait, a decrease in the mass of the internal organs (i.e. heart, liver, kidney), which can result in bronchopneumonia and death. Wandering, physical aggression, repetition, shouting, inappropriate behaviour, sexual disinhibition and other behavioural problems may develop as the dementia advances.

Vascular dementia

Vascular dementia is characterized by a stepwise deterioration with patchy infarcts which lead to various deficits in intellectual functioning. Hypertension, heart disease, smoking and alcohol consumption are all risk factors. The patient presents with headaches, vertigo, numbness, tinnitis, insomnia, a lack of appetite, general fatigue and loss of concentration, memory and depression.

Other dementias include Pick's disease, Creutzfeldt–Jakob disease, cortical Lewy body disease, dementia of the frontal lobe and 20–80% of all people suffering with Parkinson's disease have dementia.

It is also important that other medical and physical reasons are eliminated. For example, tumours, subdural haematoma, myxoedema, hypoglycaemia, renal and hepatic disease, vitamin deficiencies, alcoholism and infections.

Box 11.2 The ten-item abbreviated mental test

Ask the patient:

1. Their age
2. The time
3. Give an address such as 42 West Street for recall at the end of the test. Ensuring that it has been heard is important
4. Current year
5. Name of hospital (or place being seen)
6. Recognition of two people
7. Date of birth
8. Year of First World War
9. Name of present monarch
10. Count backwards from 20 to 1.

To assess the cognitive state, the modified abbreviated mental test (AMT) score is often used (Box 11.2) (Hodkinson 1972, Young 1996). This test is reliable and correlates well with cognitive function. If the score is less than eight then a problem is identified. With dementia, the written hand writing is small and if boxes are drawn they are not square but flattened.

Most old people with dementia never enter psychiatric institutions.

Diseases of the cardiovascular system

Peripheral vascular disease (PVD)

Artherosclerosis and its complications account for half the deaths in the developed world and it is the commonest reason for amputation (Ham & Cotton 1991), cardiac disease and stroke. The cause is unknown but there are established risk factors: smoking, diabetes, hypertension, lack of exercise, hyperlipidaemias and social deprivation. Reduction in dietary fat and body weight are thought to be effective and the control of hypertension reduces the number of strokes.

Artherosclerosis is a generalized disease and it may affect limbs, the heart or brain separately or together. Lipid substances and cholesterol are deposited underneath the intimal lining of large and medium sized arteries causing an atheroma (Greek for porridge) plaque which gradually causes fibrosis and narrowing of the artery, a stenosis. The vessel wall also becomes fibrosed.

The plaques themselves may cause no trouble but if they are strategically placed, serious sequelae may follow. For example, in the carotid artery bifurcation, the cerebral or retinal area may be affected with transient ischaemic attacks and this may be followed by a permanent stroke. At the site of the renal artery, the plaque and stenosis may lead to renal hypertension and in the limbs, plaques may occlude the vessels, leading to intermittent claudication (pain in the calf on exercise), rest pain (pain from tissue ischaemia) and eventually gangrene if there is no time for intervention (Ham & Cotton 1991). If this occlusion builds up gradually, the collateral circulation is developed locally to compensate for the blocked arteries. With emboli, such time is not available and ischaemia is acute and if intervention does not occur within 6 hours, ischaemia of the tissues and gangrene follow.

Operations for the relief of arterial disease. If conservative treatment fails then wherever arteriosclerosis affects the arteries, surgical procedures have been developed. These are described below.

Sympathectomy. By ablating the sympathetic chain at the appropriate level to the lesion, either chemically or surgically, the venules and arterioles are denervated and the blood flow to the capillaries and hence the tissues is improved with the dilatation of the arterioles that follows. Approximately 40% of sympathectomy procedures are found to be effective and in general it is used to relieve rest pain and minimal gangrene.

Arterial reconstruction. The techniques of bypass, patch grafts or balloon angioplasty are all used to overcome the arterial constriction and to increase the blood flow or vessel lumen to the affected parts (Ham & Cotton 1991).

Amputation. The most common causes of amputation are arteriosclerosis (58%), diabetes (22%), trauma (6%), malignancy (3%) and congenital deformity (0.8%) (Ham, Luff & Roberts 1989). The objective of limb amputation is to remove sufficient diseased and gangrenous tissue to permit the stump to heal and to retain as much limb length for prosthetic (artificial limb) fitting on suitable patients. Today in a general hospital practice there should be approximately as many amputations at the transfemoral as the transtibial level, with the preservation of the knee joint which is so important for walking. Hemipelvectomy and hip disarticulation levels, although possible for arterial disease, are generally performed with a diagnosis of malignancy or trauma. In amputation for vascular disease, healing is paramount and nursing care and equipment is designed to assist this process, for example the wheelchair stumpboard (Ham & Richardson 1986).

Following lower limb amputation, the patient will be rehabilitated on an early walking aid to assess them for the potential for a prosthesis. If they are unable to manage this they are unlikely to be refered for a prosthesis (which costs at least £1000) and will continue their rehabilitation as a wheelchair user.

Venous ulcers

Ulcers due to venous disease, varicose veins or as a result of deep vein thrombosis (DVT) are common, costing the NHS £400–£600 million a year. They affect 1% of the population and 4% of the population over the age of 75 years, with an incidence of approximately 150 000 in the UK. Venous disease causes failure of the calf muscle pump to clear the blood from the leg because of damage to the veins or valves in them. Failure to clear blood from the legs results in waterlogging of the tissues and ulceration, which is relieved by recumbency or pressure bandages, with possibly a surgical operation to the varicose veins. However, some ulcers become chronic and may encircle the lower leg and cause misery, pain, social isolation and discharge (Ham & Cotton 1991). Treatment with compression bandages for a 12-week period heals 80% of ulcers but the management is costly as it takes up a great deal of the district nurse's time.

Coronary heart disease

There is a high prevalence of coronary heart disease in the more developed countries and it affects at some time 50% of the population (Jackson 1988). It may present clinically as angina pectoris, coronary thrombosis, myocardial

infarct or heart failure. Today there is less heart valve disease as there is less rheumatic fever in the population. One in five males are likely to have symptoms by the age of 65 and the incidence increases especially in middle aged and younger men (Hazleman 1980). The factors disposing to coronary heart disease are: diet, cigarette smoking, lack of exercise, obesity, stress, hypertension and diabetes (Bloom 1995a). Smoking is responsible for 25% of coronary deaths in those under 65 years and 80% of those under 45. Those with diabetes and hypertension are at greater risk (Jackson 1988).

There are three forms of restriction: chest pain, breathlessness and/or fatigue and syncope (fainting). The treatment is initially conservative but coronary bypass grafts and valve replacement may be necessary where there is residual restriction. The aim of rehabilitation is to return to a full physical, social and mental level of activity.

Angina pectoris. This is a clinical symptom produced by a reduction in blood supply to the muscles of the heart. The cause of angina is atherosclerosis of the coronary arteries, high blood pressure and, less commonly, aortic aneurysm, severe anaemia and aortic stenosis. The chest pain is brought on by effort or emotion and is felt behind the sternum and frequently radiates into the right arm (Bloom 1995). It is relieved by rest and drugs, notably sublingual glyceryl trinitrate, may be used to increase the blood supply to the heart. Patients under the age of 65 will be assessed on a treadmill and regular moderate exercise is encouraged but exertion that brings on the pain should be avoided (Bloom 1995a–e). Treatment includes an improved diet with less fat, weight reduction and stopping cigarette smoking. Beta blocking drugs may be used or bypass surgery if necessary (Jackson 1988).

Coronary thrombosis. When there is a thrombosis in the major coronary branches, sudden death occurs. If it occurs in the smaller branches, then the tissue in the region supplied dies and this is called myocardial infarction (MI). The dead tissue is replaced with a fibrous scar which if small may hardly interfere with the function of the heart. If, however, the scar is larger then the heart function is impaired and heart failure may follow (Bloom 1995a).

Myocardial infarction. The treatment of MI has changed radically from 6 weeks' bed rest in the last decades, to early ambulation and return to work. This change has occurred due to the dangers known of bed rest and the risk of thromboembolism and the recuperation powers of the heart. The advantages of early mobilization are also psychological, reduced muscle wasting and less risk of loss of physical performance.

In the first few weeks at home physical and mental rest is advocated. Walking is a recommended exercise with hills and the cold being avoided. Patients tire easily and the day should be planned so that fatigue is avoided. Anxiety and depression are common after discharge in both the patient and the spouse. There is a lack of self-confidence and an increased chance of permanent unemployment if the patient is away from work for longer than 10 weeks.

The outcome of MI is related to the individual's personality (their coping ability and the comprehension of illness), social background (their work, housing, finances, response of the family) and the family strengths and weaknesses (e.g. if they are married, divorced, strength of spouse) (Jackson 1988).

The usual time for most people in suitable occupations to return to work is 6 weeks and the sedentary jobs are the easiest to return to. After MI, 90% return to work and 65% to their original occupation. Tiredness, dyspnoea and chest pain should be avoided. Those not returning are often close to retirement or have been previously persuaded to retire by a doctor, employer or friends. Neither the patient's age nor the presence of angina have any overall effect on the return to work but recurrent infarction and physical signs of severe cardiac damage associated with invalidism does. The quality of the work or activity is unimpaired but the patient tires easily. Returning to car driving after 4 weeks is possible except for those who drive public vehicles and in some working environments (Hazleman 1980).

Heart failure. Chronic heart failure is usually a result of longstanding heart disease which eventually affects the heart by severe strain over a long period. The heart usually enlarges, the muscle hypertrophies to overcome the added strain. If the strain is only on the left side of the heart, it results in left ventricular failure (LVF). Later the right side becomes affected and this is known as congestive cardiac failure. The right atrium becomes distended, leading to stasis of the venous system with leg oedema developing (Bloom 1995a). If the problem of heart failure is due to the valve, a valve replacement will be considered. If the problem is due to heart muscle disease, vasodilator drugs may be used. Diuretics to remove the volume of fluid and relieve breathlessness, and digoxin, are used.

Cardiac illness does not just affect the individual, it is a family problem (Jackson 1988). Although many younger individuals return to a near normal way of life, for the elderly, cardiac conditions are often added to their previous multiple pathologies. Although they may function satisfactorily in the house, they may remain fragile and with limited exercise tolerance and so come to the wheelchair service.

Blood disorders

Anaemia. Anaemia is defined as a haemoglobin of less than 11.5/100 ml in women or less than 12.5/100 ml in men (Bloom 1995c). It is a condition of diminished oxygen-carrying capacity of the blood due to a reduction in the numbers of red blood cells or in their content of haemoglobin. The symptoms include general tiredness, shortness of breath on exertion, giddiness, headache, pallor, palpitations, oedema of the ankles and in the elderly occasionally angina pectoris. The causes of anaemia are either due to failure of red blood cell production in the marrow or a loss of red blood cells through haemorrhage. Both causes lead to iron deficiency in the body. Following investigation for the cause of the anaemia, iron therapy will be given (Houston et al 1968a, Bloom 1995c).

Sickle cell anaemia. This is an hereditary abnormality in the red cells which is practically confined to negroes and inherited as a mendelian dominant gene. There is an abnormal haemoglobin in the red cells which causes the cells to assume a sickle shape at the lower end of the physiological range of oxygen tension and to increase the blood viscosity, which tends to promote capillary thrombosis. The sufferer presents with chronic anaemia and sometimes in acute crisis with thrombotic episodes and the treatment is transfusion in cases of severe anaemia (Bloom 1995d, Houston, Joiner & Trounce 1968a).

Metabolic disorders

Obesity

This is a serious disease which results from eating more food than is required and is common in prosperous communities. Although the common cause for 90% of cases is gluttony, hypothalamic disorders or as a consequence of severe emotional stress may also be causes. The condition obesity is defined as a weight of 20% or more above the acceptable range, based on sex and height. It can also be quantified by the Body Mass Index (BMI). The Index is calculated from the body weight in kilograms, divided by the square of the height in metres. Readings greater than 30 indicate obesity, readings between 25 and 30 overweight and between 19 and 25 as normal. The weight gain is proportional to the dietary excess but once obesity is established it may be maintained by quite small amounts of food intake. Fat can be removed by eating less food than is required.

Obesity is not only a social stigma in western countries but it is also a hazard to health (Bloom 1995d). Obesity tends to run strongly in families due to an hereditary tendency.

The effects of obesity are widespread. Extra effort is required for all activities and extra blood and energy for the metabolism of fat. This increases demand on the heart and lungs and may cause heart failure. With the insulating effect of the extra fat it is difficult to lose body heat. Joints and ligaments suffer from the extra weight and osteoarthritis is common in the knees. There is difficulty with personal hygiene in the obese individual, which leads to skin conditions such as fungus infections and keratinized skin. Certain diseases predispose themselves to obesity, for example diabetes, hypertension, gall bladder disease, gout, heart disease, hyperlipidemia, colon and breast cancer and atheroma (Bloom 1995d, Houston et al 1968b).

The problems for the wheelchair service are numerous. Larger models have to be ordered which take time to be made as specials, are heavier to handle and are more expensive than the standard models. Although the standard NHS models are available in heavy-duty versions which take up to 18 stone (115 kg), often larger non-standard chairs with greater weight capacity up to 32 stone (203 kg) are required. These often cost four times the price of a standard chair. Extra weight also has implications for the user and the carer in manoeuvring, lifting and pushing it. These factors should be emphasized to the user and carer alike.

Diabetes mellitus

Diabetes mellitus is a common disorder characterized by an excess of glucose in the blood. It occurs in all parts of the world and in all age groups. It is diagnosed in the first instance in 50% of patients over the age of 50 years. It is a breakdown of the body's insulin-glucose economy. When it occurs in middle age, the symptoms may be mild and may pass unnoticed in the early stages. When it occurs in children or young adults, the symptoms are more severe.

Hyperglycaemic patients present in three ways:

- Acute onset with polyuria, rapid weight loss and thirst. If treatment is not begun a coma will develop.
- Gradual onset which is more commonly in the middle aged with less intense symptoms of polyuria, thirst and nocturia. Weight loss will occur over a few months.
- Symptoms and organs in which complications develop – affecting the eyes (cataract or retinitis), peripheral nerves (neuritis), kidneys, or blood vessels (gangrene, intermittent claudication or coronary artery disease) (Bloom 1995e, Houston, Joiner & Trounce 1968a).

Treatment is either in the form of insulin injections or subcutaneous pumps and diet management for the insulin-dependent diabetic and tablets and/or a dietary regime for the non-insulin dependent diabetic.

Malignant tumours or cancer

Cancer is the second leading cause of death in the western world, the most common being lung cancer in men and breast cancer in women. Cancer is an abnormal growth and proliferation of cells resulting in distinctive morphological alterations of the cell and tissues. The TNM (tumour node metastases) staging procedure is widely adopted and gives details of the size of the tumour (e.g. T 1 2 3 4), nodal involvement (e.g. N 1 2 3) and the presence or absence of metastases (e.g. M 0 1). Knowledge of these staging characteristics enables therapists to plan realistic goals because the stage of the cancer is strongly correlated with survival (Fulton 1994).

The treatments for cancer include surgery, chemotherapy, radiotherapy and a combination of these. Chemotherapy and radiotherapy aim to disrupt and kill the abnormally high rate of cell division. Before the 1970s, the standard initial approach was radical surgery when cancer was diagnosed. Today less radical surgery occurs and it is carried out in combination with other treatment methods.

Some wheelchair services do not issue long-term loans to cancer patients but refer them to the loan service. Others issue them as they would other users and also prioritize the delivery. Each service has its own established operational policy that it follows.

Diseases of the respiratory system

Respiratory conditions are frequently chronic and disabling. It is estimated that a quarter of males between the ages of 50 and 59 have chronic bronchitis (Moxham 1988). Smoking is an important aetiological agent in chronic bronchitis, emphysema, lung cancer and ischaemic heart disease. Smoking causes a cough, aggravates asthma and increases the individual's suscept-

ibility to chest infections. The aim of therapy is to reduce disability by tackling recurrent infections in the case of chronic bronchitis, airways obstruction in cases of chronic bronchitis and emphysema, breathlessness, hypoxia and poor exercise tolerance.

Chronic obstructive airways disease (COAD)

In chronic bronchitis and emphysema, the air flow is reduced due to reduced elastic recoil of the lung, hypertrophy and oedema of the bronchial wall mucous membrane, excess mucus in the airways and the contraction of bronchial wall smooth muscle. Airways obstruction therefore increases ventilatory work at the same time as reducing ventilatory capacity. Although chronic obstructive airways disease (COAD) was conventionally thought to be irreversible, the majority of patients show signs of improvement with therapy to relax bronchial smooth muscle, commonly salbutamol and terbutaline administered in an aerosol (Moxham 1988). Chronic bronchitis is a disease of long chronicity, characterized by a cough, sticky sputum and increasing dyspnoea.

Emphysema

Emphysema is a condition of the lungs where there is pathological enlargement of the distal air spaces (the alveolar sacs) either from chronic dilatation or from destruction of the walls. It occurs with longstanding disease of the bronchi, namely chronic bronchitis or chronic asthma or a combination of the two. It may also be related to occupational causes. Lungs with emphysema lose their elasticity and therefore expiration requires muscular effort and there is alveolar hypoventilation. The main clinical feature is dyspnoea, initially after exertion and gradually the patient is only able to walk a few steps. Quite frequently the breath is exhaled through pursed lips. The rate of progression of the condition is variable from slow to rapid, often precipitated by an infection or the weather conditions (Bloom 1995b, Houston, Joiner & Trounce, 1968c).

Asthma

In asthma there is bronchial spasm and the secretions are sticky, leading to wheezing and difficulty in breathing. The cause is complex and several factors contribute to its development:

- Heredity. When asthma starts in childhood there is more likely to be a history of an allergic disorder in the family, for example hay fever, asthma, urticaria and migrane.
- Allergy to various substances which may either be inhaled or absorbed. For example pollen, dust, plant spores or face powder.
- Infection such as respiratory tract infections as a complication of chronic bronchitis, for example.
- Psychological influences play a part in nearly all asthmatics. Anxiety, frustration or tension at home often underlie the tension of the bronchi.
- Reflex factors. The bronchi are supplied by the vagus nerve and various stimuli may induce attacks by a reflex mechanism, for example cold air, exertion or a heavy meal (Bloom 1995b, Houston, Joiner & Trounce 1968c). An attack usually starts suddenly and may last for about 1 hour. A severe attack that lasts for more than a day is known as status asthmaticus.

Treatment consists of drug therapy to produce bronchial dilatation used either at the time of the attack or between attacks. Steroids may be used for chronic asthmatics.

Oxygen therapy. People with COAD often receive oxygen therapy, which has been found to help survival and avoids hospital admissions. It has been said that oxygen therapy may be prescribed without careful assessment and many of those who would benefit from it may not be receiving it (Moxham 1988). It is an expensive drug to administer and although it may be supplied in oxygen cylinders, more commonly now it is administered though an oxygen concentrator. Many patients use oxygen in their homes to relieve breathlessness after activity as oxygen therapy reduces the respiratory rate. Portable oxygen cylinders weighing 2 kg have sufficient oxygen in them to last approximately 30 minutes (Moxham 1988). During acute exacerbations of COAD, oxygen therapy is necessary to avoid hypoxia.

Wheelchair users who use oxygen cylinders often ask the wheelchair service to supply an attachment to hold the cylinder.

The use of oxygen cylinders with powered chairs has been debated due to the potential fire risk. This risk has been investigated and the following is recommended:

- The cylinder should be either a D or E cylinder of pressurized oxygen.
- The cylinder should be securely attached to the wheelchair and protected so that the stem and regulator cannot be broken off.
- The user or carer should not smoke.
- When using oxygen, never replace or charge the batteries.
- Do not drape the oxygen line near any moving parts of the wheelchair, especially the powered recliner.
- The oxygen tubing should be checked daily.
- The oxygen source should be turned off when it is not in use (Anon 1992).

People with COAD often become depressed and during acute episodes of respiratory infection or during the night when respiratory activity is diminished, they may become hypoxic and confused (Nichols 1980). Families and carers need support, reassurance and explanations about this. Unemployment may follow when the condition becomes worse and this can cause tension in the household.

Disabled people often gain weight with less exercise which increases the resting respiratory work and severe obesity affects the chest wall mechanics. Depression and severe breathlessness are positively correlated (Morgan et al 1983) and when the respiratory disease is advanced there is weight loss and muscle atrophy which also affects the respiratory muscles.

Pneumoconiosis

Prolonged exposure of certain types of dust may cause irritation of the lungs from the constant inhalation of the particles of dust. The result is a dense diffuse fibrosis throughout the lungs. People that are affected may include coal miners (anthracosis), stone workers and potters (silicosis) and asbestos workers (asbestosis) (Bloom 1995b). Asbestosis, for example, is a dust disease of the lungs caused by the inhalation of asbestos fibres, which largely consists of magnesium silicate, causing a progressive diffuse fibrosis of the lungs, particularly the lower lobes. The chief symptoms are dyspnoea, a chronic cough and sputum. Carcinoma of the bronchus is a common complication and malignant mesothelioma of the pleura also occurs (Bloom 1995b, Houston, Joiner & Trounce 1968c).

Pulmonary tuberculosis

Infection in a patient for the first time with the tubercle bacillus is called primary tuberculosis. Reinfection after the primary lesion is called post-primary tuberculosis. In most western countries the infection is caused by the human bacillus. In less developed countries the disease may be caused by milk infected with the bovine organism.

The human bacillus is spread almost exclusively by droplet infection and lesions other than in the lung are uncommon. The risk of infection is much increased by proximity, either by overcrowding or by exposure, and the risk may be increased by malnutrition, overwork and a lack of sleep. The rate of infection has decreased steadily since the turn of the century but in some inner city areas where there are large numbers of immigrants, many who have never had any immunization, overcrowding and poverty, the rate of TB is again rising. TB can affect many parts of the body, glands, meninges, bones, kidneys and joints (Bloom 1995b).

Most patients are symptomless but there may be haemoptysis. The disease is well advanced by the time the symptoms have developed. Classically the symptoms are chronic ill health, cough with mucoid sputum, low grade fever, anorexia, tiredness, progressive weight loss and night sweats (Houston, Joiner & Trounce 1968c).

Many elderly people have respiratory conditions which limit their mobility. Generally such users require a basic chair, attendant or self-propelling, to increase their quality of life and social interactions.

TREATMENT
Assessment

When assessing the elderly user, the recent and relevant past medical history, the reason for referral, recent admissions to hospital and relevant drugs should be noted. When physically assessing, the following should be noted: the joint ranges and muscle strength of the relevant limbs, head, neck, back and hand function, the respiratory and nervous system, balance, any gait with the mobility aid used and the method and technique of transfers. Continence, pressure areas or areas at risk, assistive aids such as glasses, shoes, hearing aids should be noted and if there has been any previous use of a wheelchair. The psychological assessment should include the mental state, depression or anxiety, communication and comprehension and orientation (Smyth 1990, Squires & Taylor 1988, Wagstaff & Coakley 1988). The social assessment should note the local support systems in place, for example family, friends or carers, the type of acccommodation and access, the statutory and voluntary support received, the hobbies or occupation, transportation methods and the activities or routines that are carried out regularly. Obviously not all this information is necessary for every case but these details highlight the information that may need to be collected to help with the wheelchair prescription criteria.

Communication

It is important to listen to the elderly users carefully, speaking slowly and clearly with courtesy, and to 'reflect' the conversation to ensure the listener has grasped the correct meaning. The phrases should be simple, may need to be broken down and may need to be repeated. The questions should be in a logical order, though a rigid format and rapid topic changes should be avoided. Jargon should also be avoided and by asking the user questions about what you have said, their memory can be checked. Backing up verbal information with written information is useful as a reminder to the user and is also of benefit to the family or carers.

It is important that you always approach the user from the front or to one side and have eye contact with them (see Ch. 5). Some form of physical contact is usually appropriate and this is generally a handshake. Before sitting down in the home to communicate at the same level, always ask the user if you may sit down, 'Here?' for example. Sometimes the most obvious chair belongs to another member of the household and this may be the dog! It is advisable to acknowledge the elderly user by their title and to only use first names when they wish you to. This ensures no one's differences are overlooked. Cultural and gender differences should always be noted in the area in which you work and often local texts are available to help. Privacy, respect and dignity should be routine for all users but especially for the elderly. The interaction will be improved if the non-verbal communication between the therapist and the user is satisfactory. This includes: gestures, facial expressions, tone of voice, dress, posture and proximity, listening and the use of silence, for example (Smyth 1990, Squires & Taylor 1988). The quality of the interaction does not depend solely on the knowledge base of the professional but on the interaction itself.

POSTURE AND MOBILITY NEEDS

Most people spend a third of their lives sitting. The older we get, the more we sit. Wheelchair use increases with age and the numbers have been found to increase from the age of 50 with the greatest use in the 70–79 age group (Smith, McCreadie & Onswath 1995). The wheelchair and seating needs of the elderly have increased significantly in the last 20 years. Such needs may range from a simple attendant or self-propelling wheelchair, a powered indoor or indoor/outdoor wheelchair, to a wheelchair with a good cushion to improve posture or some form of thoracic postural support, to a complete seating system. In general, the elderly require functional mobility in the simplest form available for their needs and they are generally in a hurry!

Wheelchair locomotion has been found to use up to 9% more kilocalories per minute than normal ambulation (Traugh, Corcoran & Reyes 1975) and therefore is not only safe but also requires almost the same amount of energy as walking (Fisher & Gullickson 1978) and less energy expenditure than prosthetic or crutch usage (Deathe 1992).

The demand for better seating grows, especially among the significant percentage of very elderly people who spend much of their waking time in a seated position (Bardsley 1993). This is especially true in nursing homes (Redford 1993). For those using the chair for a number of hours each day, a good sitting posture will help to decrease fatigue, improve both the cardiac and respiratory function, assist with feeding and the user's overall general care. With the self-propelled chair a cushion that distributes the weight evenly over the buttocks and thighs is important and the ability to move the footrests for standing is important for safety especially. Uncomfortable or cumbersome wheelchairs have a negative effect on the individual's life. It can also say something about the individual's taste, interest and self-image (Smith, McCreadie & Unsworth 1995).

A wheelchair is not just a chair with wheels but is actually wheels with a seat (Lewis 1975). There are more and more elderly people using wheelchairs for disabilities arising from both acute and chronic conditions (Bradey et al 1986). As an 'orthosis' it is an energy-saving, independence-giving substitute for lost muscle power which allows the disabled elderly increased participation in life and less reliance on carers (Cornwell & Kavanagh 1996, Crewe 1979, Kamenetz 1969). However, the elderly occasional user may not be eligible for a wheelchair from some NHS wheelchair services and in others there may be long waiting lists (Cornwell & Kavanagh 1996). Local dealers may also loan wheelchairs at a small cost for such people and especially for holidays.

In the elderly users, strength and coordination are reduced and chronic health problems persist, but in general the majority of the elderly do not have major deformities. Features such as the chair's weight, ease of folding, handling and of propulsion are key issues, as are the possibility of, and need for, safe transfer methods. Simple movements such as getting into and leaving the chair are important for the elderly user and their carer.

Some wheelchairs have inflatable tyres, especially self-propelling models, and the brakes work by a plate pressing against the tyre. If the tyre is flat the brake will not function effectively and propelling and steering the wheelchair will be difficult and more energy will be needed. In a recent study, a third of elderly users were found to have inadequately inflated tyres (Howorth et al 1983). Another study found that users in the community did not maintain the tyre pressure of 45 lbf/in^2 (p.s.i.) (= 310 kPa) as recommended by the manufacturers. The authors noted the effort needed for this was considerable, especially with a hand pump, and they also noted the benefits of the solid synthetic tyres commonly found now on attendant-propelled wheelchairs (Henriksen, Hunter & Warren 1994).

The addition of a puncture-proof insert (Penn et al 1989) or replacing the pneumatic tyre with a foam-filled tyre will assist both the elderly users and the carer in aspects of maintenance, safety and ease of manoeuvrability. It is important that the replacement has a tread to grip outdoor surfaces especially in wet conditions.

Nursing and residential homes

In a New York study looking at wheelchairs and seating in a nursing home, it was found that there was a lack of a coordinated approach to wheelchair management which decreased the personal independence amongst users, increased the costs, inhibited safety control measures and contributed to deterioration in the user's physical condition (Epstein 1990). The problems of issue to nursing homes are often discussed and debated in wheelchair services in the UK. Some services supply wheelchairs to specific, named

individuals living in the homes or continue to maintain the original chair issued if the user moves to such a home. Others supply only if the chair is used three or more times a week for outings and other services do not supply to these individuals at all, as the cost of equipment for care is part of the community care assessment. The issue of equipment for nursing care use only and issue for independence for the user adds to the debate. Often wheelchairs in these homes are poorly looked after by the staff, many of whom change frequently, and users are too often pushed about without footrests being used, for example. The supply, review and maintenance issues of wheelchairs in nursing and residential homes are negotiated locally and follow no national standard. If wheelchairs are issued to the individual user from the local service, then it is important that regular review sessions take place at the homes, for example every 6–8 weeks, to ensure that all the residents' and carers' needs are being met and any physical changes are accommodated. Equipment that is no longer required should be regularly removed to ensure that all items in use are correct and in a safe working condition. Many homes have restricted storage space, so again regular reviews assist all concerned.

Poor seating leads to poor posture, which results in the patient sliding or leaning to one side of the wheelchair. Conventional wheelchairs with soft hammocks or sling-type seats and backs have been found to contribute to a kyphotic lumbar posture (Harms 1990). In contrast, firm padded seats or cushions contoured to fit the body were found to be both more comfortable and acceptable. They help to eliminate pelvic obliquity and posterior pelvic tilt and in turn reduce the risk of skin breakdown. For older people, flat or slightly contoured surfaced cushions, filled with good quality foam and covered with a two-way stretch waterproof cover which is easily cleaned, possibly covered with a towelling cover for ease of laundering, is best to ensure correct posture, positioning and pressure relief. If the cushion is contoured it is important that arrows or words indicate the correct way to place the cushion in the chair as there are many staff changes involved in the care of such individuals. Staff should be trained to check the shape of the cushions regularly to ensure that the foam has not 'bottomed out' (see also Ch. 12). However, nursing homes do not generally give the proper attention to seating equipment for their residents because of the expense and because staff are unaware of the critical role of posture in the well-being of the elderly (Redford 1993). Appropriate seating equipment will help to improve respiratory and cardiac function, improve posture, the function possibly, the general well-being of the residents and in general help to facilitate most aspects of care in the unit (Redford 1993).

Typically, a resident sitting in a wheelchair with a sling seat presents with a faulty posture due to the biomechanics of the wheelchair seat and back. The sling seat and backrest of a conventional folding wheelchair make correct posture and stability difficult to maintain. The hard frame is commonly used for position and postural control (Chung & Brubaker 1991). The middle of the sling seat when open is lower than the sides and as the upholstery stretches the hammock effect becomes worse. Users will shift their position for comfort which will either involve taking more weight on one buttock causing pelvic obliquity, or slipping forwards, commonly called sacral sitting (Krasilovsky 1993). Use of a firm-based cushion or a cushion with a crescent insert or included within it, help to eliminate this problem.

Bilateral amputation

As the majority of amputations in the west are for vascular disease in the elderly population, it is now increasingly common to see amputees who have lost both their legs. The time from losing the first limb to losing the second varies from 6 months (Ebskov 1986) to 5 years (Dormandy & Thomas 1988). Patients who become bilateral amputees must be taught bed mobility, arm exercises, balance re-education, transfer techniques and wheelchair mobility.

For the user who has bilateral transfemoral amputations, a wheelchair with an extended wheelbase or wheels set back (1 in, 2.5 cm) should be prescribed for safety reasons and stability (see Ch. 3). This will increase the turning circle slightly but removing the footrests indoors may help some users. However, as the rear propelling wheels are set back, these users, and especially women, are at risk of developing shoulder problems such as a frozen shoulder as the range required to propel is increased. Safety in manoeuvres and positions, transfers and the heights of surfaces for transfers are very important in increasing the user's confidence and subsequent quality of life.

Users who are preparing to receive a prosthesis may require a stumpboard as well as a footrest so that they can be interchanged as necessary. Comfort in pressure-relieving cushions that also assist with transfers are also important with this group of wheelchair users. Powered wheelchairs may be considered in the correct environment and with a suitable user can increase their horizons and quality of life.

Family or carer needs

Caring by families and friends is the backbone of community care. There are approximately six million carers in the UK today. The Carers (Recognition and Services) Act 1995 came into force on 1 April 1996. The Act amends the National Health Service and Community Care Act 1990 in order to create a new duty on local authorities to assess the needs of individual carers (those providing a substantial amount of care on a regular basis) and to enable (though not oblige) the authority to provide appropriate services for carers (Travers 1996). These reforms have meant that voluntary and private organizations are now increasingly being asked to provide residential care, day care and home-based services under contract to social service departments (Barodawala 1996).

Carers face physical, emotional, social and financial problems. They need recognition, information and support from the health professionals with whom they and the person they care for come in contact (Travers 1996).

Such support is in the form of an appropriate

wheelchair and information from the service about mobility and transport matters. It is important to include the needs of the spouse, child or carer when prescribing a wheelchair for the elderly user. In a recent survey this was found not to be the case (Smith & McCreadie 1994). This may include taking into consideration a number of different needs and requirements and compromising in some cases on the equipment issued. Car space, the health of the attendant, the condition of the user, how often and the amount of time the chair is used, where it is used, the capability and interest or involvement of the carer are all considerations in the issue of this equipment. Often there is a need to talk to more than one member of a family, or carer, to ensure the needs are being met.

The majority of wheelchair services will only supply the standard models of state wheelchair to this group of users as they are generally less frequent users than the younger disabled groups and require a wheelchair for an average of 20 months (National Prosthetic and Wheelchair Services Report 1993–1996). However, for many carers and family who are often also approaching 'old age', the extra exertion and effort of propelling a wheelchair is much greater than they imagine. It is also not generally at the time of life when extra physical activity is sought and many spouses may have medical conditions such as osteoarthritis, cardiac conditions, diabetes or a neurological condition. However, this is the situation for many spouses and their families in the western world today. Lighter wheelchairs are often asked for and in some services they are issued. However, it is generally not simply the extra few pounds or kilograms of the wheelchair that are the problem but the weight of the wheelchair user themselves and the general strength or health of the attendant that are the combined problem. A decade ago the standard wheelchair from the British government was 42.5 cm (17 in) wide. Today wheelchair services hold 45 cm (18 in), 47.5 cm (19 in) and 50 cm (20 in) wheelchairs in their main stock as the nation is becoming both taller and larger. Heavy duty wheelchairs, especially in areas of deprivation where disability is high, for those users over

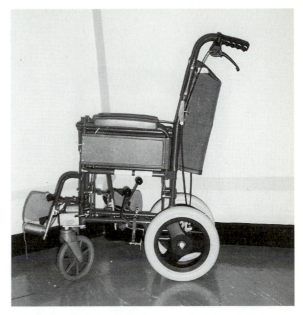

Figure 11.3 A wheelchair with attendant brakes on the handles.

108 kg (17 stone) are becoming increasingly the norm. This extra weight is an increasing problem for the attendant who may also be elderly. Power packs may be a solution for some, attendant-controlled outdoor powered wheelchairs the solution for others, but the weight of the user remains a problem for all concerned.

For some confused users, attendant brakes may be necessary to avoid the user putting them on when the carer is pushing (Fig. 11.3).

Type of accommodation

Many elderly people, especially in inner cities, live in accommodation that is rented and is possibly old in the facilities it has to offer. Space is at a premium with furniture, belongings and pets for example. In some cases the wheelchair equipment has to be as narrow as possible for internal use and so often a glideabout is requested. This is similar to a commode but with a complete seat (Fig. 11.4).

The access into and out of the accommodation may need to be altered, both at the front and at the rear, and in older flats there may be a step in the hallway or corridor. Storage for the wheel-

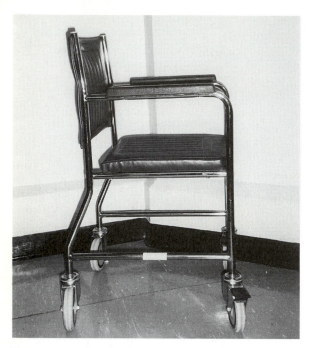

Figure 11.4 A glideabout chair.

chair if the user lives in a flat may be a problem if a shed, cupboard or a lift are not available. Space in the flat or house may be another problem, especially for the disabled who also require other items of equipment for their activities of daily living. Carpeting or floor coverings may not help the manoeuvring of the wheelchair. Powered chairs need to have access to electric circuits that are modern and safe to use and ventilation for charging is another consideration (see Ch. 13). Access to the facilities may also be a problem, especially if there is a toilet outside or one upstairs.

Amount of use and models of loan services

In some wheelchair services in the UK, the amount the user intends to use a wheelchair influences whether they will receive one from the state. For some areas supply is only when the items will be used for more than 3 days each week; in other areas this question does not arise. Most wheelchair services have a loan service or

access to one for their users. Such loan services range from:

- A small number of wheelchairs being identified from within the service for temporary use with or without a charge for the loan. These chairs will be administered from within the service's staffing and budget.
- In other areas, the loan service will be run by the local British Red Cross medical equipment loan service who have 900 outlets for such equipment throughout the country. A nominal charge may be made for the loan.
- In other services, local voluntary organizations loan out wheelchairs to the local residents with no charge but the two services work very closely together.

For example, in the London Borough of Newham, the wheelchair service has a contract with Newham Association for Disabled people (NAD) to assist in the temporary loan of wheelchairs by updating their stock with financial grants when possible, repairing the chairs throughout the year, updating some stock annually and assisting financially with the administrative costs of the service. The use of this loan service has increased by 15–19% each year for the last 3 years, reflecting the increased demand for wheelchairs generally.

Many private suppliers also loan wheelchairs and ask for both a deposit and a small charge. Shopmobility schemes in town centres should also be considered (Wells 1996) (see also Ch. 13).

Training

A number of wheelchair services issue simple equipment items following the request being completed by an approved assessor, who has attended either a local or regional wheelchair training course, without seeing the user further. In such cases the user will be issued with a wheelchair manufacturer's handbook and may or may not receive further training in the use of the chair. The approved repairer's technical staff, in the majority of services, also demonstrate to the new user the features of the particular model and how the equipment works when they deliver the wheelchair to the user's home. This contact between the technician, user and the service is vital to both the user and the service staff in the future, as the technician will report on physical changes, equipment misuse, environmental and carer changes he or she sees when he is called to repair or exchange a chair (Fig. 11.5).

In other services, potential users and their carers will attend the service to be shown how to use the wheelchair and for their questions to be answered. Few services in the UK have the staff time to train the carer in the environment in which they are going to use the wheelchair. Often local voluntary groups assist with this task and therapists train local carers, for example at day courses or training sessions at the voluntary groups' meetings.

Information about the equipment and a practical demonstration should be carried out by each wheelchair service either by the therapist, an assistant, a rehabilitation engineer or the technician from the approved repairer. Today all equipment should have printed instructions with it as people remember very little, especially if they have a cognitive problem and have a number of carers (see Ch. 5). A problem often arises with reconditioned equipment. Here locally developed booklets should be used or a supply purchased from a manufacturer.

The users and attendants should also be warned of the safety precautions in using wheelchairs to avoid accidents. In a recent survey wheelchair-related accidents were found to be relatively common (Dudley, Cotter & Mulley

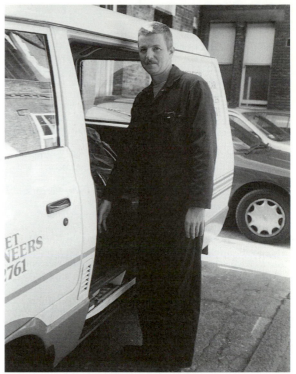

Figure 11.5   The approved repairer's technician, the wheelchair service's frontline man.

1992). Keeping the wheelchair in a good state of repair, using the correct restraining straps in vehicles, education of the attendants in the use of the chair, especially the tipping levers, the use of spoke guards if necessary, a lap strap to reduce the number of falls out of a wheelchair and the use of dropped kerbs and ramps will all help to reduce the number of accidents.

REFERENCES

Alzheimer's Disease Society 1996 Alzheimer's disease – what is it? Information sheet 1. Alzheimer's Disease Society, London

Andrews K 1985 Demographic changes and resources for the elderly. British Medical Journal 209: 1023–1024

Anon 1992 Safe use of supplemental oxygen with powered wheelchairs. Health Devices 21(8): 291

Bardsley G 1993 Seating. In: Bowker P, Condie D N, Bader D L, Pratt D J (eds) Biomechanical basis of orthotic management. Butterworth-Heinemann, Oxford, pp 253–280

Barodawala S 1996 Community care: the independent sector. British Medical Journal 313: 740–743

Bloom S R (ed) 1995a Diseases of the circulatory system. In: Toohey's medicine. A textbook for students in the health care professions, 15th edn. Churchill Livingstone, Edinburgh, pp 77–114

Bloom S R (ed) 1995b Diseases of the respiratory system. In: Toohey's medicine. A textbook for students in the health care professions, 15th edn. Churchill Livingstone, Edinburgh, pp 115–148

Bloom S R (ed) 1995c Diseases of the blood. In: Toohey's medicine. A textbook for students in the health care professions, 15th edn. Churchill Livingstone, Edinburgh, pp 235–258

Bloom S R (ed) 1995d Metabolism and vitamins. In: Toohey's medicine. A textbook for students in the health care care professions, 15th edn. Churchill Livingstone, Edinburgh, pp 279–298

Bloom S R (ed) 1995e Diabetes mellitus. In: Toohey's medicine. A textbook for students in the health care professions, 15th edn. Churchill Livingstone, Edinburgh, pp 299–314

Bradey E, Colman P, Crinklaw Wianko D, Wagman J 1986 A validity study of guidelines for wheelchair selection. Canadian Journal of Occupational Therapy 53(1): 19–24

British Geriatric Society 1990 Policy statement no. 4. Private and voluntary homes. British Geriatric Society, London

Buchanan J M, Chamberlain M A 1978 A survey of the mobility of the disabled in an urban environment. RADAR, London

Chung K-C, Brubaker C E 1991 Seating and wheelchairs. Current Opinions in Orthopaedics 2: 824–829

Church J 1996 Social Trends 26, Central Statistical Office. HMSO, London

Corlett A J 1996 Aids to compliance with medication. British Medical Journal 313: 926–929

Cornwell M, Kavanagh J 1996 The role of the wheelchair in the mobility chain. British Journal of Therapy and Rehabilitation February: 69–74

Crewe R A 1979 Wheelchair choice or the biomechanics of wheelchair selection. British Journal of Occupational Therapy 42: 272–274

Deathe A B 1992 Canes, crutches, walkers and wheelchairs: a review of metabolic energy expenditure. Canadian Journal of Rehabilitation 5(4): 217–230

Department of Transport 1996 Door to door. A guide to transport for disabled people. HMSO, London

Dormandy J A, Thomas P R S 1988 What is the natural history of a critical ischaemic patient with and without a leg? In: Greenhalgh R M, Jamieson C W, Nicolaides A N (eds) Limb salvage and amputation for vascular disease. Saunders, London, pp 11–26

Dudley N J, Cotter D H G, Mulley G P 1992 Wheelchair related accidents. Clinical Rehabilitation 6: 189–194

Ebrahim S 1996 Ethnic elders. British Medical Journal 313: 610–613

Ebskov B 1986 The Danish amputation register 1972–1984. Prosthetics and Orthotics International 10: 40–42

Epstein C F 1990 Wheelchair management: developing a system for long term care facilities. Journal of Long Term Care Administration 8: 1–12

Fenwick D 1977 Wheelchairs and their users. HMSO, London

Fisher S V, Gullickson G J R 1978 Energy cost of ambulation in health and disability: A literature review. Archives of Physical Medicine and Rehabilitation 59: 124–133

Forbes A 1996 Loneliness. British Medical Journal 313: 352–354

Fulton C D 1994 Physiotherapists in cancer care. A framework for rehabilitation of patients. Physiotherapy 80(12): 830–834

Garrett G 1987 Health needs of the elderly, 2nd edn. The essentials of nursing series. Macmillan, London

Ham R O, Cotton L 1991 Limb amputation: from aetiology to rehabilitation. Chapman & Hall, London

Ham R O, Richardson P 1986 The King's amputee stump board – Mark 11. Physiotherapy 72: 124

Ham R O, Luff R, Roberts V C 1989 A five year review of referrals for prosthetic treatment in England, Wales and Northern Ireland 1981–1985. Health Trends 21: 3–6

Harms M 1990 Effect of wheelchair design on posture and comfort of users. Physiotherapy 76: 266–271

Haynes N 1984 A first course in psychology, 3rd edn. Nelson, London

Hazleman B 1980 Rehabilitation after a heart attack. In: Nichols P J R (ed) Rehabilitation medicine. The management of physical disabilities. Butterworth, London

Henriksen P A, Hunter J, Warren P M 1994 Wheelchair tyre pressure: a community survey and an investigation of the effect of low pressure on physiological energy expenditure during self propulsion. Clinical Rehabilitation 8: 36–40

Hodkinson E McCafferty F G, Scott J N, Stout R W 1988 Disability and dependency in elderly people in residential and hospital care. Age and Aging 17: 147–154

Hodkinson H M 1972 Evaluation of a mental test score for assessment of mental impairment in the elderly. Age and Aging 1: 233–238

Houston J C, Joiner C L, Trounce J R 1968a Disorders of the blood. In: A short textbook of medicine. Unibooks, English Universities Press, London

Houston J C, Joiner C L, Trounce J R 1968b Diseases of metabolism. In: A short textbook of medicine. Unibooks, English Universities Press, London

Houston J C, Joiner C L, Trounce J R 1968c The respiratory system. In: A short textbook of medicine. Unibooks, English Universities Press, London

Howorth E, Powell R H, Mulley G P 1983 Wheelchairs used by old people. British Medical Journal 287: 1109–1110

Jackson G 1988 Cardiac disability. In: Goodwill C J, Chamberlain M A (eds) Rehabilitation of the physically disabled adult. Croom Helm, London, pp 193–211

Kamenetz H 1969 The wheelchair book, Mobility for the disabled. Charles C Thomas, Springfield, Illinois

Kettle M, Rowley C 1990 Report on the wheelchair survey. DSA (90) 18. HMSO, London

Krasilovsky G 1993 Seating assessment and management in a nursing home population. Physical and Occupational Therapy in Geriatrics 11(2): 25–38

Laing and Buissan 1993 Care of elderly people, market survey 1992/3. Laing and Buissan, London

Lewis J 1975 Five tips for successful wheelchair fitting. Patient Aid Digest November–December: 18–20

Morgan A D, Peck D F, Buchanan R, McHardy G J R 1983 Effects of attitudes and beliefs on exercise tolerance in chronic bronchitis. British Medical Journal 286: 171–173

Moxham J 1988 Respiratory disease. In: Goodwill C J, Chamberlain M A (eds) Rehabilitation of the physically disabled adult. Croom Helm, London, pp 212–223

National Prosthetic and Wheelchair Services Report 1993–1996. DoH funded project. College of Occupational Therapy, London

Nichols P J R 1980 Chronic bronchitis. In: Rehabilitation medicine. The management of physical disabilities. Butterworths, London, pp 262–269

Penn N D, Belfield P W, Young J B et al 1989 No more flat tyres: a trial of a tyre insert for wheelchairs. Clinical Rehabilitation 3: 149–150

Pushpangadan M, Burns E 1996 Community services: health. British Medical Journal 313: 805–808

Ratoff L, Heyes J, Haddleton M 1993 Does you don't have access? Health Service Journal 29 April: 32–34

Redford J B 1993 Seating and wheeled mobility in the disabled elderly population. Archives of Physical Medicine and Rehabilitation 74: 877–885

Renwick D 1996 Community care and social services. British Medical Journal 313: 869–872

Research Institute for Consumer Affairs 1996 Powered wheelchairs, scooters and buggies, 2nd edn. Research Institute for Consumer Affairs, London

Roper T A, Mulley G P 1986 Public transport. British Medical Journal 313: 415–418

Smith C, McCreadie M 1994 A heavy load: survey of carers of wheelchair users. Health Service Journal April: 32–33

Smith C, McCreadie M, Unsworth J 1995 Prescribing wheelchairs: the opinions of wheelchair users and their carers. Clinical Rehabilitation 9: 74–80

Smyth L 1990 Practical physiotherapy with older people. Chapman & Hall, London

Squires A J, Taylor M 1988 Assessment of the older patient. In: Squires A J (ed) Rehabilitation of the older patient. Chapman & Hall, London, pp 64–78

Teale C 1996 Money problems and financial help. British Medical Journal 313: 288–290

Traugh G H, Corcoran P J, Reyes R L 1975 Energy expenditure of ambulation in patients with above knee amputations. Archives of Physical Medicine and Rehabilitation 56: 67–71

Travers A F 1996 Carers. British Medical Journal 313: 482–486

Wagstaff P, Coakley D 1988 Physiotherapy and the elderly patient. Chapman & Hall, London

Wanklyn P 1996 Homes and housing for elderly people. British Medical Journal 313: 218–221

Wattis J 1996 What an old age psychiatrist does. British Medical Journal 313: 101–104

Wells J 1996 Choosing a wheelchair. RADAR, London

Young J 1996 Rehabilitation and older people. British Medical Journal 313: 677–681

Special issues

SECTION CONTENTS

12

Pressure management

INTRODUCTION

Most of us will have experienced sitting on hard and uncomfortable seats for long periods and are aware that sustained pressure can cause discomfort. Maintained for longer without relief, pressure concentrations may also lead to tissue breakdown. The sores that develop are known by different names such as bedsores, ischaemic ulcers, decubitus ulcers and, for the purpose of this chapter, we will put them under the heading pressure sores and hence recognize pressure as a fundamental causative factor. Pressure sores are generally preventable through sensible pressure management based on an understanding of the causes of pressure sores, risk factors and methods of redistributing pressure.

Scale of the problem

There is no doubt that pressure sores can cause considerable pain, suffering, loss of dignity and psychological harm to the individuals who experience them. The time and cost of treating pressure sores also places a significant burden on carers and the health service.

Reports on the prevalence of pressure sores vary considerably according to the population studied. Studies in Lincoln in 1989 and North Derbyshire in 1991 concluded that pressure sores were present in 16% and 9.6% respectively of hospital patients and both studies agreed on a prevalence of 6.7% in community patients (Department of Health 1993).

It was estimated in 1981 that the average cost of treating a pressure sore in the UK was £25 900. More recent estimates of the total cost to the health service in England of treating pressure sores vary from £180 million to £321 million. These calculations do not include the cost of litigation: one claimant who suffered a pressure sore was awarded damages of £100 000 in 1987 in recognition of the physical and psychological trauma (Touche Ross 1993).

Although the majority of pressure sores reported in the above studies are perhaps linked to time spent in bed, there can be no doubt that many are attributable to time spent sitting in a wheelchair seat when full body weight is supported over a relatively small area for long durations.

Pressure sore development

Skin tissue is made up of a microstructure of materials such as collagen, elastin and reticulin in a viscous ground substance and the survival of this structure depends largely on the plight of the cells living within it. The living cells in turn rely on a regular supply of oxygen and nutrients via blood vessels and also clearance of waste products via lymph vessels. These blood vessels and lymph vessels have non-rigid walls so that when the pressure on the outside of the vessel exceeds that of the fluid on the inside, the vessel collapses, stopping the flow of fluid through the vessel. An occluded blood vessel will cause the cells to be deprived of oxygen and nutrients, resulting in local anoxia which eventually leads to ischaemia, cellular necrosis and hence ulceration of the tissue. Where a lymphatic vessel is occluded there is likely to be a build up of toxic metabolites which, combined with the ischaemia, will accelerate tissue damage (Krouskop 1983).

Beneath the epidermis and dermis lies subcutaneous fat, connective tissue, muscle and eventually either bone or body cavity. When sitting, the sites on the body which are at most risk of developing a pressure sore are those sites where relatively thin layer of tissue cover a bony prominence such as at the sacrum, ischial

tuberosities, greater trochanters, elbows and heels. This is because the pressure experienced by the blood and lymphatic vessels is likely to be concentrated more over the bony prominence as the tissue is compressed between the bony prominence and support surface. Other areas of tissue away from the bony prominence will deform more readily and achieve a more even distribution of pressure.

Grading of pressure sores

A pressure sore is sometimes defined as an area of tissue damage which persists after the removal of pressure and which is likely to be due to the effect of pressure on the tissues. This may vary from persistent discoloration of the intact tissue to the creation of large cavities within the subcutaneous tissue exposing the underlying bone. Most methods of grading pressure sores involve dividing them up into four categories based on the level of tissue damage (Table 12.1).

FACTORS CAUSING PRESSURE SORES

Before considering various pressure management techniques, it is important to understand the factors which predispose an individual to the development of a pressure sore. These factors can be divided into extrinsic factors, related to the individual's immediate environment and intrinsic factors, related to their medical or physical condition.

Table 12.1 Grading of pressure sores (Department of Health 1993)

Grade	Level of tissue damage
I	Discolorations of intact skin, including non-blanchable erythema, blue/purple and black discoloration
II	Partial thickness skin loss or damage involving the epidermis and/or dermis
III	Full thickness skin loss or damage or necrosis of subcutaneous tissues, but not through the underlying fascia and not extending to the underlying bone, tendon or joint capsule
IV	Full thickness skin loss with extensive destruction and tissue necrosis extending to the underlying bone, tendon and joint capsule

Extrinsic factors

Direct pressure

At this stage it may well be worth reminding ourselves of a few basics about pressure.

$$\text{Pressure} = \frac{\text{Force}}{\text{Area}}$$

Pressure is equal to the force applied divided by the area over which the force is applied. Obviously a larger force applied to the same area will result in a larger pressure. Alternatively, the same force applied to a smaller area will also result in a greater pressure. Therefore for two people of the same weight the one with the smallest area of contact with the seat surface is likely to experience the greatest pressure at the support interface.

Although we talk about pressure as the main cause of pressure sores, it is important to remember that assuming that the person is not floating or falling in space we cannot remove pressure from the support interface altogether. Under static conditions the weight of an individual (which will correspond to the force applied in the equation above) will remain constant and must be supported by the seat on which they are sitting. Therefore we must try to spread that force over as large an area as possible to keep the pressure at any site to a minimum. Alternatively, we could try to actively redistribute the support so that greater pressure is taken where the tissue is pressure tolerant and less pressure is taken at any sites considered to be at risk.

An average size person weighing 70 kg (about 11 stone) sitting on a firm seat may be supported over an area of about 600 cm². Assuming that one-quarter of the weight is taken through the feet and that the remainder is distributed evenly over the limited area of the seat, the resulting pressure in the tissue in contact with the seat would be in the region of 65 mmHg. In reality the distribution will not be even and the pressure under the ischial tuberosities will be significantly higher. An obvious question that should be asked is at what pressure is vessel occlusion and anoxia likely to occur?

Studies have shown that the pressure resulting in anoxia varies considerably from one site on the body to another and from one individual to another. Pressures as low as 40 mmHg were found to be sufficient to cause anoxia in some elderly subjects (Bader & Gant 1988), whereas as much as 540 mmHg was required to produce complete anoxia at soft tissue sites of younger subjects (Seiler & Stahelin 1979). Generally it is recognized that anoxia may occur in tissue covering bony prominences when subjected to pressures in the vicinity of 30–150 mmHg (Bar 1989). Miller & Seale (1985) showed that a decrease in lymphatic drainage occurred when pressures exceeded 60 mmHg.

In addition to direct pressure there is another way that tissue can be stressed to cause vessel occlusion and anoxia.

Shear stresses

Shear stress is caused by a force which acts on the tissue in a direction parallel to the plane of the support interface. For example, if you recline a backrest with the seat base remaining level, gravity will act on the occupant, increasing their tendency to slide anteriorly. Without friction the occupant would slide out of the seat. With friction holding the occupant of the seat in place, however, there will be shear stresses acting on the tissue at the support interface causing it to distort. The top layers of skin may remain stationary with respect to the seat surface due to friction whilst the deeper layers can move, causing blood and lymphatic vessels to stretch and distort. Hobson (1992) reported a 25% increase in surface shear force with a backrest reclined by 20 degrees.

Shear stress can also occur when there is a steep pressure gradient with a high pressure area immediately adjacent to a low pressure area, for example in tissue covering a bony prominence which is under load.

Bennett et al (1979, 1981) found that the direct pressure level capable of disrupting blood flow could be reduced by half in the presence of moderate shear stress. They concluded that it was the combination of direct pressure and shear that is particularly effective at producing vessel occlusion.

Although pressure and shear can cause occlusion of blood and lymph vessels and produce anoxia, this on its own is not enough to cause a pressure sore.

Duration of pressure

It is the duration for which pressure is applied, and hence anoxia sustained, that determines the degree of ischaemia which will eventually lead to ulceration. Various research workers (Kosiak 1959, Reswick & Rogers 1976) have looked at the relationship between the magnitude of pressure and duration that the pressure is applied and found that in order to cause tissue damage an inverse relationship exists between the two variables. This relationship is shown in Figure 12.1.

The graph in Figure 12.1 shows how combinations of pressure magnitude and duration which can be plotted to the left of the curve are acceptable, whereas those combinations that can be plotted to the right of the curve will potentially cause irreversible tissue damage. The curve therefore represents a limit of tissue tolerance. It would appear from the shape of the graph that large pressures can cause tissue damage after only a short period but also that relatively small pressures can cause damage after being applied for a relatively longer duration.

Temperature

As the temperature of the soft tissue increases so does the metabolism of the living cells within its structure. Fisher et al (1978) suggested a 10% increase in metabolism with each 1°C rise in temperature. The cells act like chemical engines and their metabolic demand for fuels (i.e. oxygen and nutrients) therefore increases dramatically with temperature and if deprived of this fuel due to vessel occlusion the cell will die sooner. An increase in temperature would therefore have the effect of shifting the tissue tolerance curve in Figure 12.2 to the left.

Conversely it has been shown that the ability of tissue to withstand ischaemia is increased by lowering the temperature (Romanus 1976). This would correspond to a shift in the tissue tolerance curve to the right.

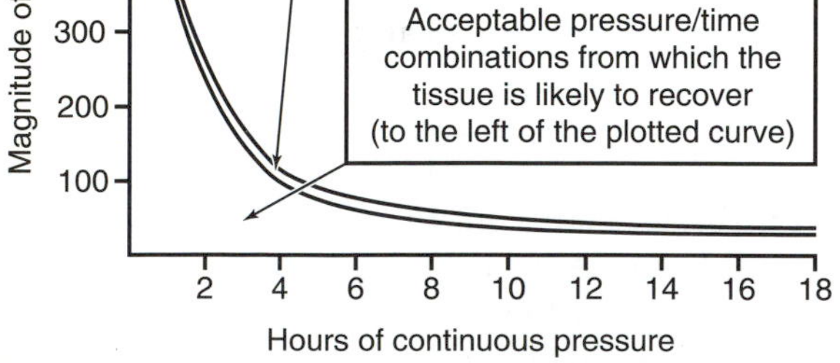

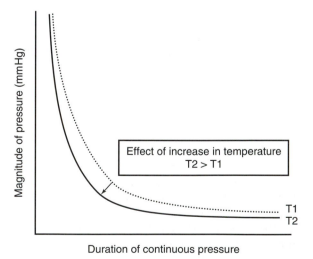

Figure 12.1 Tissue tolerance guideline. Shows transition from acceptable to unacceptable loading of tissue in terms of both the magnitude and duration of pressure application.

Figure 12.2 Effect of increase in temperature on the tissue tolerance curve. Shows exaggerated shift of the curve explained in Fig. 12.1 to the left due to an increase in temperature. For a given magnitude of pressure the time necessary to bring about tissue damage is reduced.

Intrinsic factors

Motor deficit

Following the consideration of the importance of the duration of pressure in causing a pressure sore, it would seem sensible to assume that if individuals can lift themselves or adjust their position periodically to relieve the pressure in the tissues at the support interface, it is likely that this will help to delay the onset of tissue damage.

Studies have confirmed that intermittent pressure relief of tissues allows increased pressure tolerance (Ferguson-Pell et al 1980, Krouskop et al 1983) and that reduced frequency of spontaneous movement has been linked to a higher incidence of pressure sores (Exton-Smith & Sherwin 1961).

Reduced mobility is something which affects all wheelchair users. However, it is the reduced ability to adjust position within the wheelchair that exposes the tissues to prolonged pressures and increases the risk of pressure sore development.

Sensory loss

Most people adjust their position either consciously or subconsciously, prompted by messages from pressure, stretch and pain receptors in the skin, muscle and tendons. Any sensory loss is likely to reduce the incentive to adjust position and therefore potentially increase pressure sore risk.

Muscle atrophy

Wastage of muscles is likely to reduce the blood volume in the tissue and reduce the area available for supporting weight. In particular, where there is atrophy of the gluteal muscles the ischial tuberosities become more prominent (Dhami et al 1985) and take a greater concentration of pressure when sitting.

Posture

Postural deformity is often linked to the development of pressure sores. As sitting posture changes, the surface area for weight bearing is often reduced and pressures experienced over bony prominences increased. For example, an established pelvic obliquity on a standard seat will cause increased pressure over the lower ischial tuberosity and possibly over the greater trochanter on the same side, if the obliquity is severe enough.

Another common site for a pressure sore is over the sacrum where the individual is accustomed to sitting in a slumped position with their pelvis posteriorly tilted. It is likely in this situation that as well as direct pressure in the thin tissue over the sacrum, shear forces will also exist as the individual tends to slide anteriorly in the seat. Reclining the back is likely to exacerbate this particular problem by increasing the shear forces (see Ch. 3).

Skin integrity

Damage to the skin tissue can increase the risk of development of pressure sores. For example, the skin may be damaged by sudden forces associated with a clumsy transfer over the wheelchair wheel or by incontinence causing maceration leading to abrasion.

Health and nutritional status

Proteins and vitamins are essential for normal cell metabolism. Poor nutrition reduces tissue viability and therefore results in a decreased pressure tolerance (Mulholland et al 1943). A malnourished individual will also suffer tissue wasting which will result in less tissue bulk to provide padding over bony prominences.

Vascular factors

Any circulatory or peripheral vascular disorders which already reduce supplies of oxygen and nutrients to tissue will obviously compound the problems caused by pressure. The effects of conditions such as cardiovascular disease, arteriosclerosis, diabetes, anaemia and respiratory problems will therefore put the individual at greater risk.

Age-related factors

Some processes associated with ageing put the elderly at greater risk of developing pressure sores. Circulation may be impaired, reducing vital supplies to the tissue. Muscle wastage may occur along with loss of subcutaneous reserves of fat, resulting in less tissue bulk covering bony prominences. Tissue elasticity may be reduced, resulting in tissue being damaged more easily. Activity may be reduced, resulting in less relief to stressed tissues.

MEASURING/ASSESSING RISK
Measurement of extrinsic factors

Pressure measurement

Numerous pressure measurement devices exist although few are suitable for use at the soft tissue/support surface interface associated with wheelchair seating. An ideal pressure monitor would have an infinite number of pressure transducers which would need to be infinitely small, infinitely thin, infinitely flexible and insensitive to changes in temperature, humidity, etc., as well as being practical to use in the clinic environment. In reality such a transducer is not available and it is therefore necessary to accept a degree of compromise.

Several electropneumatic pressure measurement systems are currently available. These are based on a disc-shaped capsule situated at the tissue/support interface being inflated via an external air line until contacts on opposite faces of the capsule separate. It is assumed that the capsule will begin to inflate, and the contacts separate, when the pressure in the capsule exceeds the pressure surrounding it. Hence the pressure measured in the external air line when the contacts separate should be equal to the pressure acting on the capsule. It should be noted that the pressure measured represents an average of the pressure acting over the surface of the capsule and that if there is a steep pressure gradient it is likely that higher pressures than that measured may be acting locally within the area of the capsule. Pressure measurements may

also vary depending on the characteristics of the materials at the interface, although generally such systems provide accurate indication of interface pressure at a particular site.

The most simple devices of this kind include a single sensor capsule of welded plastic connected to a standard sphygmomanometer (or pressure gauge) and hand-held pump. More sophisticated computerized systems include a matrix of small sensors, similar to the one described above, which avoids the need to accurately place the single sensor over the particular site of interest and helps to give an indication of the distribution of pressure over a greater area of the interface. This type of system is generally quick and easy to set up and use in the clinic, and pressure measurements from a large number of sites over the interface can be displayed as a pressure map using histograms or colours to represent pressure bands. Such a static pressure monitor system is shown in Figure 6.7B.

The spacing of the sensors in such systems is critical as pressure concentrations may be missed between sensors if the sensors are spaced too far apart. It is also important to note that if the material in which the matrix of sensors is embedded does not stretch, then the accuracy of pressure measurements made will be limited, especially when the subject is sitting on a soft compliant cushion. Ideally, the sensor matrix should stretch to accommodate the deformation of the cushion as load is applied and if it does not then it will change the characteristics of the cushion which in turn will influence the pressure distribution that was being measured.

Bader & Hawken (1986) developed a system that automatically pumped air into a number of cells in turn and checked the pressure in each by detecting a characteristic change in the pressure–volume relationship which removed the need for electrical contacts on the cell walls. The system could repeatedly cycle around all cells, giving a series of snapshots of the pressure at the interface. Measurements from this type of system (shown in Fig. 6.7A) are generally regarded as relatively accurate although limited in speed and ease of use.

Pressure monitors capable of recording

dynamically changing pressure have also been developed (Bar 1991, Barbenel & Sockalingham 1990, Shaw 1979). Later commercially available versions of this type of device are similar in some ways to the electropneumatic systems above, in that they incorporate a number of plastic capsules positioned at the tissue–support interface and connected via relatively rigid tubes to pressure transducers situated away from the interface. Instead of pumping air into the capsule, however, the capsule and tube are permanently filled with incompressible oil. The pressure acting on the capsule is transmitted directly from the tissue support interface to the pressure transducer and is therefore capable of continuously monitoring the pressure as it changes dynamically. A dynamic pressure monitor system is shown in Figure 6.7C. This type of system lends itself more to the study of pressure variability over a prolonged period of time, which will include the effects of postural adjustment and wheelchair movement. High pressures generated during movement may well compound the insult from static levels of pressure (Bar 1989, 1991).

The accuracy of this sort of system is limited by the fact that the capsule, although thin, still has a significant thickness which may itself influence the pressure being measured. The practicality of such a system in the clinic environment is also slightly reduced by the need to position the individual capsules accurately over anatomical landmarks, and also the limited tube lengths necessary to retain an accurate dynamic response.

There are a number of alternative systems newly available on the market, including some which utilize force sensitive resistor technology. Such systems appear to offer high spatial resolution and sampling rate but concerns exist about the accuracy of early models.

All the pressure measurement systems available have their strengths and weaknesses. When choosing or using a pressure monitor it is important to understand what you want to measure, what you are in fact measuring and what degree of accuracy you can expect with your measurements. Pressure measurements should be inter-

preted carefully and often it is the use of the pressure measurement system for direct comparison (e.g. between different seat configurations, postures or cushions) that is most useful rather than measurement of absolute pressures.

Other measurements

It is more difficult to measure shear stress applied to tissue than it is to measure direct pressure. Transducers have been designed but tend to be rigid devices which are not suited to use at a soft tissue / low density support interface.

Various studies have looked at tissue viability in response to loading by investigating tissue oxygen levels (Newson, Pearcy & Rolfe 1981, Bader 1990, Seiler & Stahelin 1979), tissue vasculature and cutaneous blood flow (Bader, Barnhill & Ryan 1986) and also skin temperature (Davies & Newman 1981). The results of such studies have helped to confirm the potentially damaging effects when external pressure is applied to tissue. However, although the techniques used might help to identify individuals at particular risk, they are not yet sufficiently reliable or practical for routine clinical use.

Measurement of intrinsic factors – risk assessment tools

If pressure sores are to be prevented, it is important to recognize individuals who are at increased risk. These individuals will potentially be sustaining pressures for prolonged periods due to restricted mobility and will also experience one or more of the intrinsic causative factors discussed earlier.

Several risk assessment and scoring scales have been developed which help to identify the nature and severity of the predisposing risk factors, including:

- Norton (Bridel 1993, Norton, McLaren & Exton-Smith 1962)
- Waterlow (Edwards 1995, Waterlow 1985)
- Walsall (Milward 1994)
- Knoll (Hamilton 1992)
- Douglas (Hamilton 1992)
- Gosnell (Hamilton 1992).

Some scales, such as the Norton and Waterlow scales, are based on a scoring system for the most important variables. The lower the score in the case of the Norton scale, and the higher the score in the case of the Waterlow scale, the more the individual is thought to be at risk of developing a pressure sore. Norton, McLaren & Exton-Smith (1962) reported a near linear relationship between the incidence of pressure sores and their clinical score at the time of admission to hospital, although surprisingly little additional evidence is available to conclusively prove the link between risk scores and the potential incidence of pressure sores.

Generally these scales are simple to use and variability between observers is small. There is a danger, however, that too much emphasis may be placed on the total score and not enough emphasis on the individual risks identified, which may be reduced if appropriate action is taken. It is important to note that nearly all the above scales were designed for specific clinical areas with bed-bound patients in mind and not wheelchair users. All risk scales should therefore only be used as a guide and should be interpreted with commonsense.

REDISTRIBUTION OF PRESSURE

As discussed earlier, it is not possible to remove pressure from the equation altogether. It is necessary, therefore, to try to manage pressure by spreading the support over a large area to reduce the pressure at any particular site. An attempt can be made to achieve an even distribution of pressure over the support area. Alternatively, the pressure can be actively redistributed by designing the support so that greater pressure is taken where the tissue is pressure tolerant and less pressure is taken at any sites considered to be at risk.

Before looking at pressure cushions and seating with particular reference to their pressure distributing qualities, some thought should be given to basic considerations like the configuration and size of the wheelchair in relation to the user.

Wheelchair size and configuration

Table 12.2 lists some dangers associated with the use of an inappropriate wheelchair. Pressure sore risk can therefore be reduced with a more appropriate wheelchair prescription.

Pressure-distributing cushions

Wheelchair cushions should ideally perform several functions, including providing a stable postural base and helping to avoid concentrations of pressure. Their potential to achieve the latter depends on their ability to distribute pressure.

Comprehensive guides to specific cushions are available (Tuttiet 1990). The names and compositions of specific cushions tend to change continually and it is therefore important to ensure that information on cushions from the suppliers is kept up to date. The following section lists the generic categories into which most cushions tend to fall and shows photographs of a few examples of each category.

In general, the cushions can be divided into two groups: passive and active.

Table 12.2 Potential effects of inappropriate wheelchair configuration on seat interface pressure

Cause	Potential effect
Wheelchair too narrow	Increased pressure on greater trochanters and lateral aspects of thigh
	Hinders lifting to relieve pressure
	User may be sitting on seat tubes
Wheelchair too wide or seat canvas slack	Increases tendency for canvas to 'hammock' increasing loading taken more laterally and generating shear stresses
Seat depth too short	Reduction in load bearing area leading to increased pressure
Seat depth too long	Likely to encourage pelvis to tilt posteriorly leading to increased pressure in sacral area
Footrests too low or feet unsupported	Increased proportion of load bearing through seat and thighs
Footrests too high	Increased load bearing over ischial tuberosities
Seat/back angle too great	Shearing forces generated as individual has increased tendency to slip anteriorly

Passive cushions

The majority of cushions are passive and again they can be divided into several generic groups depending on their main material content.

Foam

Cushions made from polyurethane and latex foam tend to be simple, lightweight and relatively inexpensive. A wide range of foams are generally available, varying in density, hardness and resilience. Foams with viscoelastic properties (known as plastomer, temper or 'pudgee' foams) are also available, offering improved conformity and improved pressure distribution, particularly over bony prominences (Fig. 12.3).

On the negative side, foam cushions tend to deteriorate and require regular replacement depending on usage and exposure to fluids, sunlight and heat. Another problem is that they act as a thermal insulator and therefore are not efficient at conducting heat away from the body/cushion interface, causing a build up of temperature.

Foam cushions can be cross cut (Figs 12.4, 12.5) to allow them to deform more easily to create a greater support area and reduce surface shear

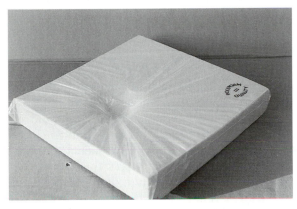

Figure 12.3 A cushion made from foam with viscoelastic properties. The foam has 'memory' characteristics, taking a while to recover following deformation.

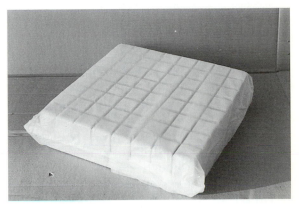

Figure 12.5 A cushion with a cross cut surface. Modular cushion – comprising foam and platilon liner.

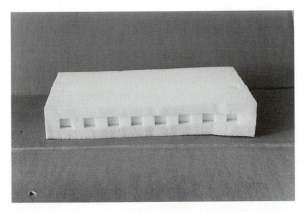

Figure 12.4 A cushion comprising several layers of foam. Section through a Services to Medicine STM 3 cushion – the top layer cross cut and the middle layer cut into a lattice configuration.

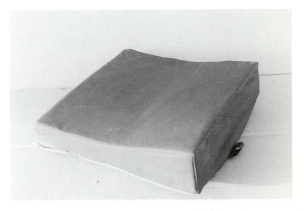

Figure 12.6 A foam cushion with a standard 15 degree ramp. Provides additional support under the anterior part of the thigh which can result in reduction in pressure taken under the ischial tuberosities and also helps posture by encouraging the femurs to be horizontal.

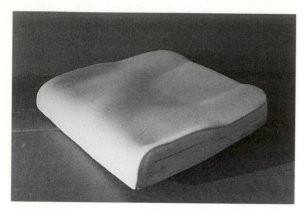

Figure 12.7 A contoured foam cushion. Shaped to the contours of the body and offering increased support area as well as additional support under the anterior part of the thigh and improved pelvic stability.

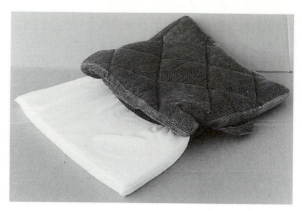

Figure 12.9 High viscosity gel cushion. Spenco Omega 5000 cushion consisting of a block of plastomer polymer.

forces or alternatively they can be actively shaped (Fig. 12.6) or sculptured (Fig. 12.7) to improve posture and pressure distribution (Michael & Walker 1987, Mulcahey & Pountney 1987, Sprigle, Chung & Brubaker 1990, Sprigle, Faisant & Chung 1990). Sections of the cushions are sometimes cut out to relieve pressure under the ischial tuberosities and increase loading under the trochanters, although there is a danger that this may cause shear stresses around the edge of the cut-out section.

Gel

Gels used in cushions can vary in viscosity. The

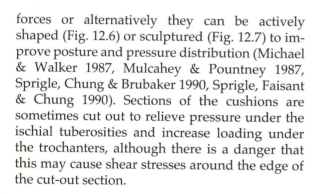

Figure 12.8 A low viscosity gel cushion. Sumed Maxitech cushion – strictly a viscous liquid and aggregate, which behaves like a gel, trapped in a flexible envelope.

lower viscosity gels (Fig. 12.8) behave more like a fluid, while the higher viscosity gels (Fig. 12.9) behave more like a solid. Thixotropic gels theoretically perform like a solid under low pressure and a fluid under high pressure

Gel cushions generally conform well and are efficient at distributing static pressure. The lower viscosity gels have shock absorbency qualities but may leak. The higher viscosity gels are more stable but may result in high dynamic pressures due to their relatively stiff response when subjected to rapid displacements. Thixotropic gels tend to retain the stability of the higher viscosity gels while responding better to the rapid displacements of an active user (Tuttiet 1990).

Gel cushions generally conduct heat well and thus help to avoid a build up of temperature at the body/cushion interface. Their thermal conduction properties also mean that they tend to take on the temperature of the immediate environment and, as a consequence, they can be uncomfortably cold to sit on while slowly warming up after being left in a cold place, such as the back of a car during winter. They tend to be moderately priced, relatively heavy and the gel may deteriorate.

Gel and foam

Some cushions combine gel and foam in layers (Fig. 12.10) or in sponge form (Fig. 12.11) in order

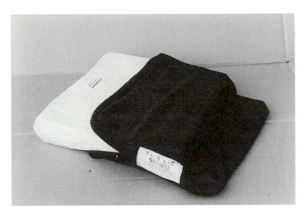

Figure 12.10 A gel and foam cushion. Sumed Ultra 90 cushion – a gel envelope similar to Maxitech trapped between layers of foam.

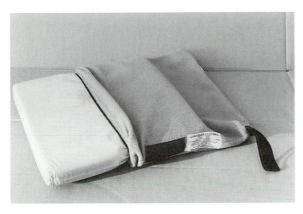

Figure 12.11 A gel and foam cushion. Akros gell-cell cushion – a foam sponge-like matrix impregnated with gel sealed inside a tough vinyl envelope.

to save on weight (in comparison to a gel cushion of the same thickness) and to provide additional support and stability.

Foam and fluid

One well-established range of cushions combines foam and oil-based fluids. The foam base (Fig. 12.12A) is shaped to give firm postural support while the oil-filled pad (Fig. 12.12B) helps to distribute pressure under the ischial tuberosities. These cushions are generally stable and can be customized (Fig. 12.12C) and modified when necessary. When properly prescribed these cushions can be very effective although

relatively expensive and the fluid section can be punctured and leak.

Water

A number of cushions use water instead of gel or oil-based fluids (Fig. 12.13). Although quite good at conducting heat and preventing a build up of temperature, they obviously require waterproof covers, which increases the humidity at the body / cushion interface. If punctured the contents will be lost rapidly. Although liked by some users, these cushions tend to be heavy and are generally less stable than gel cushions.

Air

Some simple air-filled cushions are used widely in nursing care. The air pockets can be either sealed or alternatively fitted with a valve to vary the amount of air and hence pressure inside the cushion. They are generally easy to use and cheap; however, the pressure-distributing qualities are limited by their limited ability to conform.

The more sophisticated air-based cushions have a series of cells, shaped like small balloons, which are interconnected via a series of narrow tubes (Fig. 12.14). The bulbs deform and allow the load to be supported over a relatively large surface area. Some cushions are divided into two or four compartments so that different amounts of air can be trapped in each compartment to improve stability and postural control. These cushions tend to be light in weight, are good at distributing both static and dynamically changing pressures, have a good clinical reputation for pressure sore prevention in high-risk individuals and are reusable if washed properly. However, they are relatively expensive, they can be punctured and they have impermeable covers which can increase the humidity at the seating interface. Care needs to be taken in inflating them appropriately and they require checking regularly. Some users find them unstable although newer designs with four separate compartments and valves provide better stability and allow a limited amount of postural control.

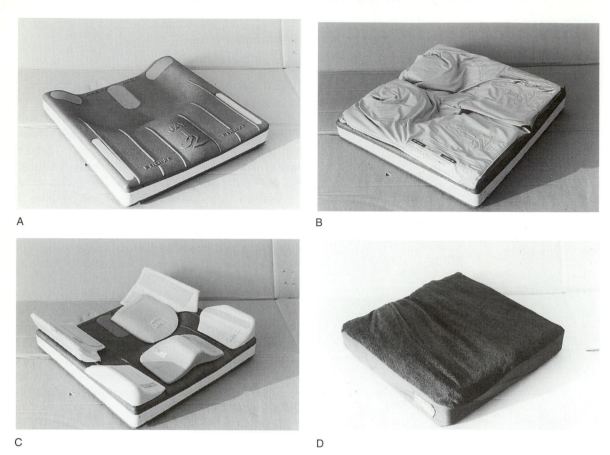

A   B

C   D

Figure 12.12 A foam and fluid cushion Jay 2 cushion. A A foam base shaped to support the thighs and to help to stabilise the pelvis. B Fluid pad which flows and conforms to body shape, increasing support contact area. C Foam base fitted with accessories to improve positioning. D Foam base and fluid pad within stretch cover.

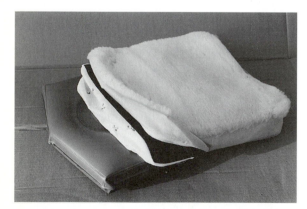

Figure 12.13 A water-based cushion. Dyson Varyflow cushion – consisting of water and a foam base enclosed in PVC envelope. The water is divided into two thigh pads which are interconnected, and a posterior strip. The ischial tuberosities and coccyx rest on the foam base between the water-filled pads.

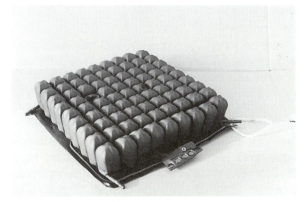

Figure 12.14 A passive air-based cushion. Quadtro Roho cushion – an example from a range of Roho cushions working on a dry flotation principle.

Active cushions

It is interesting to note that, based on calculations of body weight applied to the limited area used in sitting (an example of which was quoted earlier in the chapter), it is unlikely that any cushion could realistically reduce interface pressures below capillary levels despite the claims of some cushion manufacturers.

Where a wheelchair user is unable to adjust position at all, an alternative approach has been the use of cushions that provide intermittent pressure relief by varying the pneumatic inflation pattern of a number of separate cells within the cushion (Fig. 12.15). Any site at the interface is periodically relieved of pressure as the cell supporting it is deflated while the remaining cells support the body. In order to remove the pressure in certain areas it is inevitable that pressure will be increased elsewhere. It is suggested that the intermittent application of pressure to the underlying tissues can improve circulation and hence tissue viability. Many users who have tried this type of cushion are reluctant to give it up. However, the complete system (cushion, pump, battery and battery charger) can be relatively expensive, require regular recharging and be prone to leaks and mechanical breakdown.

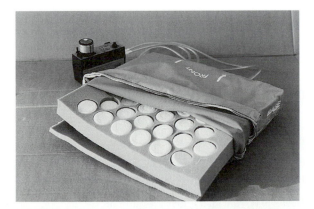

Figure 12.15   An active air-based cushion. Talley base Sequential cushion – deflates each single row of bellows in sequence to relieve pressure over corresponding tissue. Also available with alternating sequence – every alternative row inflates and deflates together.

Other important considerations when choosing a cushion

It is often tempting for a wheelchair user to place their cushion inside a pillow case or under a fleece panel. The pressure-distributing benefits of any of the above cushions will be reduced if the cushion is covered by any material that does not stretch. In order to spread load and hence reduce pressure, the cushion must deform and partially accommodate to the shape of the individual and for this to happen it is necessary for the cover to stretch in two directions. If the cover does not stretch in two directions, tensile stresses will be generated which will increase interface pressure. Terry cloth or dartex are examples of materials that will stretch.

The user will want to know if the cushion cover is waterproof or washable, particularly if incontinence is a factor. Most durable covers which are waterproof are also unfortunately impermeable to gas and often do not stretch. Materials such as platilon which are gas permeable and can stretch but are also waterproof can be used to protect the cushions and allow the use of a normal stretch fabric outer cover. It is important to explain the function of the platilon liner as some users and health care professionals have been known to discard the platilon liner, assuming it to be non-breathable polythene.

The suitability of the height, shape and stability of the cushion for transfers is also worth considering. A difficult transfer can lead to tissue stress and trauma.

Other factors to consider are the life style of the user, the ease of use of the cushion, care and maintenance of the cushion, the range of sizes available and inevitably the cost. For further information please refer to Jane Sutherland's assessment checklist in the 'Wheelchair training resource pack' (Department of Health 1996).

Ideally, once a pressure cushion has been provided it should be reviewed to ensure it is proving successful and any subsequent sores or redness of the tissue should be investigated in order to gain an understanding of the cause. This requires a close working relationship with district nurses and other health care professionals in the community.

Contoured seating

Pressure distribution can also be achieved by contouring a firm support surface to the shape of the individual. This is particularly relevant where individuals have fixed postural deformities.

It may be necessary to partially accommodate certain postural deformities in order to avoid generating high pressures over exaggerated bony prominences. A well contoured surface will help to spread load over a larger area, hence reducing interface pressures. It may be necessary to introduce alternative pressure-distributing materials or rectify the shape to further relieve sites considered to be particularly at risk from pressure.

Alternative pressure management

While the above techniques will help to improve pressure distribution and reduce interface pressure, the duration of any pressure remains of fundamental importance. It has been suggested (Bar 1988), that any postural movement in the wheelchair can act as pressure relief. If the wheelchair user is able to adjust position or even push up to relieve tissues periodically the risk of developing a pressure sore can be dramatically reduced. It is generally recommended that, where possible, adjustments or push ups should be performed every 10–15 minutes.

It might be, therefore, that instead of a different cushion, the wheelchair user needs to be informed of the importance of adjusting position or lifting. A simple timer alarm might be helpful in this respect, as a prompt to remind the user to adjust position or lift.

It may also be helpful to provide information booklets covering self-help advice on preventing pressure sores and reducing the intrinsic risk factors associated with pressure sore development. Such information might include the importance of skin care, diet, cleanliness and wearing appropriate clothing. Examples of such booklets include Department of Health (1994) and Harman (1995).

Finally, although a dependent wheelchair user is likely to spend a significant amount of time in the wheelchair, the provision of a pressure cushion for use in the wheelchair may still be only part of the answer. The user will also inevitably sit or lie on other support surfaces (e.g. an armchair or bed) and there is often a need to liaise with other health care professionals to ensure a 24-hour programme of pressure management.

REFERENCES

Bader D L 1990 The recovery characteristics of soft tissue following repeated loading. Journal of Rehabilitation Research and Development 27(2): 141–150

Bader D L, Barnhill R L, Ryan T J 1986 Effects of externally applied skin surface forces on tissue vasculature. Archives of Physical Medicine and Rehabilitation 67: 807–811

Bader D L, Gant C A 1988 Changes in transcutaneous oxygen tension as a result of prolonged pressures at the sacrum. Clinical Physics and Physiological Measurement 9(1): 33–40

Bader D L, Hawken M B 1986 Pressure distribution under the ischium of normal subjects. Journal of Biomedical Engineering 8: 353–357

Bar C A 1988 The response of tissue to pressure. PhD Thesis, University of Wales

Bar C A 1989 Pressure sores. In: Pathy M S J (ed) Principles and practice of geriatric medicine. John Wiley, Chichester, ch 20.2

Bar C A 1991 Evaluation of cushions using dynamic pressure measurement. Prosthetics and Orthotics International 15: 232–240

Barbanel J C, Sockalingham 1990 Device for measuring soft tissue interface pressure. Journal of Biomedical Engineering 12: 519–522

Bennett L, Kavner D, Lee B Y, Trainer F S, Lewis J M 1979 Shear versus pressure as causative factors in skin blood flow occlusion. Archives of Physical Medicine and Medicine 60: 309–314

Bennett L, Kavner D, Lee B Y, Trainer F S, Lewis J M 1981 Skin blood flow in seated geriatric patients. Archives of Physical Medicine and Rehabilitation 62: 392–398

Bridel J 1993 Assessing risk of pressure sores. Nursing Standard London 7(25): 32–35

Davies N H, Newman P 1981 Pressure sores – thermography as a screening technique. Nursing Times 77(21): 81–84

Department of Health 1993 Pressure sores – a key quality indicator. A guide for NHS purchasers and providers. HMSO, London

Department of Health 1994 Relieving the pressure – your guide to pressure sores. DO14/PS1/1000M

Department of Health 1996 Wheelchair training resource pack (revised DoH 1991 publication). College of Occupational Therapists, London

Dhamic L D, Gopalkrishna A, Thatte R L 1985 An objective study of the dimensions of the ischial pressure point and its correlation to the occurrence of a pressure sore. British Journal of Plastic Surgery 38: 243–251

Edwards M 1995 The levels of reliability and validity of the Waterlow pressure sore risk calculator. Journal of Wound Care 4(8): 373–378

Exton-Smith A N, Sherwin R W 1961 The prevention of pressure sores: significance of spontaneous body movements. Lancet November: 1124–1126

Ferguson-Pell M W, Wilkie I C, Reswick J B, Barbenel J C 1980 Pressure sore development for the wheelchair bound spinal injury patient. Paraplegia 18: 42–51

Fisher S V, Symeke S Y, Apre S Y, Kosiak M 1978 Wheelchair cushion effect on skin temperature. Archives of Physical Medicine and Medicine 59(2): 68–72

Hamilton F 1992 An analysis of the literature pertaining to pressure sores. MSL – assessment scales. Journal of Clinical Nursing Oxford 1(4): 185–193

Harman T 1995 Preventing pressure sores – a patient's guide. Sumed Ltd, Banbury. (Reproduced from Preventing pressure ulcers – a patient's guide. Agency for Healthcare Policy and Research, United States Dept of Health and Human Services)

Hobson D A 1992 Comparative effects of posture on pressure and shear at the body–seat interface. Journal of Rehabilitation Research and Development 29(4): 21–31

Kosiak M 1959 Etiology and pathology of ischaemic ulcers. Archives of Physical Medicine and Rehabilitation 40: 62–69

Kosiak M 1961 Etiology of decubitus ulcers. Archives of Physical Medicine and Rehabilitation 42: 19–29

Krouskop T A 1983 A synthesis of the factors that contribute to pressure sore formation. Medical Hypotheses 11: 255–267

Krouskop T A, Noble P C, Garber S L, Spence W A 1983 The effectiveness of preventive management in reducing the occurrence of pressure sores. Journal of Rehabilitation Research and Development 20(1): 74–83

Michael S J, Walker P S 1990 Clinical trial of body-contoured wheelchair cushioning. Clinical Rehabilitation 4: 229–234

Miller G E, Seale J L 1985 The mechanics of terminal lymph flow. Journal of Bioemechanical Engineering 107: 376–380

Milward P 1994 A community wound care tool. Journal of Community Nursing May: 20–22

Mulcahy C M, Pountney T E 1987 Ramped cushion. British Journal of Occupational Therapy 50(3): 97

Mulholland J H, Tui C O, Wright A M, Vince V, Shafiroff B 1943 Protein metabolism in bedsores. Annals of Surgery 118: 1015

Newson B A, Pearcy M J, Rolfe P 1981 Skin surface pO_2 measurement and the effect of externally applied pressure. Archives of Physical Medicine and Rehabilitation 63: 390–392

Norton D, McLaren R, Exton Smith A N 1962 An investigation of geriatric nursing problems in hospital. National Corporation for Care of Old People. Reissued 1975. Churchill Livingstone, Edinburgh

Reswick J B, Rogers J 1976 Experiences at Rancho Los Amigos Hospital with devices and techniques to prevent pressure sores. In: Kennedi R M, Cowden J M, Scales J T (eds) Bedsore biomechanics. MacMillan, London, pp 301–310

Romanus E M 1976 Microcirculatory reactions to controlled tissue ischaemia and temperature. In: Kennedi R M, Cowden J M, Scales J T (eds) Bedsore biomechanics. MacMillan, London, pp 79–82

Seiler W O, Stahelin H B 1979 Skin oxygen tension as a function of imposed skin pressure: implication for decubitus ulcer formation. Journal of American Geriatricians Society 27: 298–301

Shaw B H 1979 A simple laboratory instrument for giving continuous readout of interface pressure. Engineering in Medicine 8: 105–106

Sprigle S, Chung K C, Brubaker C E 1990 Reduction of sitting pressures with custom contoured cushions. Journal of Rehabilitation Research and Development 27(2): 135–140

Sprigle S, Faisant T E, Chung K C 1990 Clinical evaluation of custom-contoured cushions for the spinal cord injured. Archives of Physical Medicine and Rehabilitation 71: 655–658

Touche Ross 1993 The cost of pressure sores. Touche Ross, London

Tuttiet S 1990 Wheelchair cushions: Summary report, 2nd edn. DoH Disability Equipment Assessment Programme. HMSO, London

Waterlow J A 1985 Risk assessment card. Nursing Times November: 27

13

Powered wheelchairs and outdoor mobility

INTRODUCTION

The development of the powered wheelchair began with the application of a car starter motor to the tubular cross frame of the wheelchair, with the power derived from a car battery. With the development that subsequently followed, the cross frame of the wheelchair was removed and the space beneath the seat became available to hold equipment or the battery (Warren 1990). An electrically driven chair was described in the USA in 1915, which could reach 4.5–5 miles/h (7.25–8 km/h), with acceleration being achieved by the depression of a foot pedal (Anon 1915). Also, Carter in London produced motorized wheelchairs in 1916, to meet the demands of the large number of surviving paraplegics and amputees from the First World War (Kamenetz 1969) and subsequently, those who went further than 3 miles (4.8 km) to work at this time were provided with motorized chairs by the Red Cross (Guttmann 1964, Jolly 1964).

With the further increase in the survival of people with physical disabilities in the 1960s and 1970s, the demand for powered wheelchairs increased (Bennett-Wilson 1986). Manual wheelchairs have improved dramatically over the last 20 years but for some people the powered chair is more functional for their needs. Improvements in powered wheelchairs have led to models being less cumbersome or heavy, to more varieties and improvements in the batteries which has meant recharging is needed less frequently and they have a longer life (Letts 1991). The use of a powered wheelchair in the community setting allows both the user and their carers to be more independent and to be more functional in their environment, improving their quality of life. As the built environment becomes more accessible to wheelchair users, the independence allowed to those using powered chairs also increases. This includes schools, workplaces, shops, recreational areas and public places.

It has been said that perhaps no single piece of equipment makes a greater contribution to implementing the five basic rights for disabled people. These basic rights, as outlined by the USA's Department of Health and Human Services, are the freedom: to life, to learn, of movement, to work and for independent living (Breed & Ibler 1982). Powered wheelchairs also increase the individual's self-image and activity with their peers and reduce negative behaviours present in some individuals.

ISSUE OF SUPPLY

In the UK in 1986, there were on average 72 powered wheelchair users per 10 000 population (Royal College of Physicians 1987). In 1992/93 the total figure was 8434, in 1993/94, 8449 and in 1994/95, 9441. However, this figure is only for those users who have received indoor powered models from the NHS, as these were the only models available from the NHS until April 1996. (Since April 1996, powered indoor/outdoor models have been available from the NHS for those who meet the local service's criteria; see Ch. 1.) These figures do not include private purchases and indoor/outdoor or outdoor users. A typical NHS wheelchair service serving a population of 220 000 had between 50 and 60 indoor powered users at any one time (Ham 1995).

Increasingly, marginally dependent users are purchasing powered chairs in the form of scooters or three wheelers. Such people are generally able to walk indoors, perhaps using a mobility aid, but require assistance outdoors. Such vehicles do not hold the same stigma as a wheelchair for the elderly.

Powered wheelchair equipment must be part of the rehabilitation programme integrated into the total care plan (Warren 1990). It is issued to individuals who are generally completely dependent or with limited independence who are unable to propel a manual wheelchair. If the user is able to effectively operate a manual wheelchair then such supply may be appropriate. However, the user may be unable to use a manual chair successfully due to: physical factors, fatigue, breathlessness or motor incapacity. Powered models should be issued to enhance the individual's quality of life, independence, functional capabilities and independent mobility, and should not leave the individual so exhausted that it is difficult for them to perform other tasks. Independent mobility should be a right not a privilege (Letts 1991) and it should be as efficient as possible, not leaving the individual exhausted (Trefler et al 1993). Ideally, children should be able to keep up with their peers both at school, and in the community, and adults should be able to keep up with their schedules, both at work and socially. The importance of the user being independently mobile in their own environment cannot be overstated (Trefler et al 1993). Powered models should not be denied to users for the reason that they do not encourage exercise. Mobility and the development of muscle strength and exercise tolerance should not be confused with each other (Trefler et al 1993).

Age should not be a factor in the issue of a powered wheelchair. Young children and the elderly alike will benefit from a powered wheelchair which will make them more independent; the children in their schools with their peers and the elderly possibly by simply augmenting their mobility with a simple scooter. The introduction of powered mobility at the time in the child's development pattern that coincides as closely as possible to when they would have begun independent mobility as an able-bodied child is recommended (Warren 1990). It is important that the child understands the dangers involved, is able to recognize dangers and understands safety precautions and the limitations of the model provided. It is also important that all the carers involved with the child, both at home and at school, are involved in the discussions and contribute to any decisions that are made. Environmental controls or computer interfaces should be considered at this time also.

It is usual for the individual to have both a powered and a manual wheelchair which are used for different purposes. For some, the manual wheelchair allows greater manoeuvrability within the home or workplace and the powered wheelchair allows greater distances to be travelled outdoors. For others the powered wheelchair allows independence indoors whereas a manual model allows safe travel outdoors with an attendant or greater transportability than a powered chair would allow. It should be noted that an individual's horizons increase with age and outside activities, for example college and work, and decrease again when they became elderly (Trefler et al 1993).

CRITERIA FOR ISSUE

Some users, as in the UK, will have to meet the criteria laid down for the issue of a powered wheelchair from, for example, the government or NHS or from a charity. (Such criteria for issue in one wheelchair service is given in Box 13.1.) In other countries the criteria may be set by other bodies, for example insurance companies. For others the purchase will be privately (4% of all users in the UK) or through a charitable organization. However the equipment is obtained, full assessment of the individual's needs and requirements in all the aspects of their daily life will ensure that the correct prescription requirements, and therefore model and accessories, are recommended and purchased.

ACCESS TO WORK SCHEME (formerly the Manpower Service Commission)

Assistance is available for the equipment needed for an individual to carry out their work if they are unemployed, employed or self employed. (The period necessary to qualify varies with each group.) If a wheelchair is required that cannot be provided by the local wheelchair service and it is essential to enable the individual to carry out their work, then an application can be made through the Disability Employment Adviser (DEA) at the local Jobcentre (Wells 1996). The DEA will assist with an Access to Work application. If a wheelchair is required, a PACT (the

---

Box 13.1   Newham Wheelchair Service: eligibility criteria

1. Be severely and permanently restricted in mobility.
2. Be unable to walk/self-propel a wheelchair effectively within the home.
3. Have potential to benefit from, and have permanent need for, an indoor/outdoor powered wheelchair (EPICIC) which will increase mobility leading to improved quality of life. This includes clients with progressively disabling diseases.
4. Be medically fit to independently control a powered wheelchair indoor and outdoors. For example: free from conditions causing loss of consciousness (epileptic seizures in waking hours within the last 3 years); free from any combination of medical conditions and/or treatments likely to make independent powered wheelchair control unsafe.
5. Be safety aware of the environment. For example, can read a car number plate at 120 m (40 feet). No major neglect or inattention; no perceptual or spatial awareness problems; have demonstrated in a driving test and by other means that they have the insight and dexterity to independently operate an EPICIC safely and responsibly.
6. Have a local outside environment which is accessible by an EPICIC and compatible with its use.
7. Have a suitable home environment which includes: adequate storage space for the EPICIC; adequate space for movement of the wheelchair within the home; storage area with a power supply for a battery charger or is suitable for adaptation as agreed by the user, property owner and relevant authorities.
8. Be able to ensure that the EPICIC will be maintained adequately personally or by a carer.
9. Agree to comply with the Wheelchair Service conditions of loan and will take out: insurance to cover third party liability, and theft and damage; take out membership of a breakdown/recovery service.
10. If subsequently the user fails to meet any one of these criteria, the wheelchair may be withdrawn. This may be determined by regular reviews.
11. The assessors may seek further medical advice about individual patients from their GP or consultant if deemed necessary.

placement, assessment, counselling team) assessor will carry out an assessment in the workplace and recommend a wheelchair, the funding arranged depending upon need. For example, if the individual is employed, they currently find the first £300 and then 80% of the remaining amount between £300 and £10 000 is paid and the full amount over £10 000 up to £21 000. If self employed, the individual pays the first £100 and then PACT pays 90% of the amount between £100 and £10 000 and the full amount to £21 000. The remainder must be found through the employer, charity or by the individual. The chair belongs to either the individual, the employer or PACT by agreement. Once the guarantee runs out the individual is responsible for the repairs and, if and when a replacement is required, another application is made. There are no restrictions on where the chair is used but it must essentially be for work and unavailable from the NHS. (Full details are available from the local Jobcentre and in the College of Occupational Therapists' wheelchair training resource Pack 1996).

ASSESSMENT

In general terms, the user has to have a desire and motivation to move in the environment either greater distances or faster than they could before. The seating position of the wheelchair is important for safety, function and postural support. The ability of the user to move the device through space and to be responsive to what they meet is also important, as is the need for the user to be spatially aware of the surroundings and to be able to operate the device safely. The position and shape of the joystick could make a great deal of difference for the user and, if incorrect, could even lead to rejection. Control of powered wheelchairs is generally through the hand and a joystick but if this is not suitable for the individual, head, foot, chin, suck-blow and more sophisticated designs such as head switches are also available. It is important that powered wheelchairs (preferably three models) are tried in the environment that they are to be used in before they are purchased or issued. Such home demonstrations of this type of equipment

should be standard practice. Training in the various environments in which the wheelchair is to be used, or transported, is essential following issue (Trefler et al 1993).

For powered assessments and advice to be given to users, it is essential that a wheelchair team is available that is familiar with the current market and the features available on power models, and ideally in an environment where models for trial are available at the time of the assessment. The individual using the mobility device should outline the requirements for use.

The assessment should include the user's disability requirements, their social, transportation and environmental needs and awareness of the finances available. Manual equipment is usually also required by the user and often some type of seating system is required for postural support or as a pressure-relieving cushion in order to use the controls. The cost of providing and maintaining a powered system is three times that of a manual one (Warren 1990).

The initial assessment of the user will include:

- disability
- age
- height
- weight
- physical limitations to include
  — joint range
  — muscle weakness and tone
  — balance
  — coordination
  — transfers
  — pain
  — fatigue
  — vision
  — visual perception
  — hearing
  — concentration
  — reaction time
  — epilepsy and seizure control
- cognition
- intellectual function
- hand dominance
- sensory impairment
- skin breakdown
- any psychological factors.

Transfers, position of the brakes, and type of tyres that can be altered by the manufacturer should also be considered. The home environment should also be assessed, noting doorway widths, direction of opening, steps or slopes to be negotiated and turning space, as this will be greater than that required for a manual chair and floor coverings, alerting the potential user to the extra general wear and tear and dirt on the carpet of an in/outdoor model. Assessment of the following should also be included: bathroom/toilet access, kitchen access, ceiling lifts capacity and size, communal lifts, recharging of the batteries, storage and access (Medical Devices Directorate 1993, Research Institute for Consumer Affairs 1996, Wells 1996). (Examples of assessment forms from Newham Wheelchair Service are given in Appendix 2.)

Information on the design, necessary and possible alterations, the space required for turning and dimensions for access to the home are given in other texts (International Organization for Standards 1982) and from the Centre for Accessible Environment. Also, Care and Repair, a charity which receives some government funding, may be able to assist if modifications to the home are required.

The transportation needs of the user and carer also need to be considered. This may be a car with a boot, a hatchback car, an estate car, a van, a coach or ambulance or a taxi. If the model is required to fold, how many parts are there? What is their size, shape, weight and lifting points? Which is the heaviest part? Is the re-assembly foolproof or at least within the ability of the carer? Has the carer the sufficient mental and physical ability to handle the chair through dismantling and re-assembly? Where is the model to be used? Is this indoors only, indoors and outdoors or only outdoors? The user should always make the final decision regarding the model and needs to take this responsibility (Trefler et al 1993).

TRIALLING AND TRAINING

Once the user's needs and requirements have been assessed, models should be selected to try with the user. Before contacting individual suppliers and dealers, it is useful to look to reference sources that are available where models are described and can be compared with each other (College of Occupational Therapists 1996, Kelsall, Houghton & Cochrane 1993, Wells 1996).

Once a model or models are selected, trialling of the chair in use is essential and this should take place in a safe and spacious environment initially. If trialling is not in the user's own environment, once a model has been selected it should then be tried at home and other places of use before the item is purchased. A checklist of all the possible places the item will be used for each user should be drawn up to ensure suitable models are purchased. Too commonly training, review and a lack of instruction and information are missing when powered wheelchairs are issued (Beaumont-White & Ham 1996).

A stable base or seating system and position should first be obtained before the position of the joystick is assessed. This ensures the user can concentrate on the controls with the minimum of effort. Training and supervision will be needed over a number of sessions, as there is a learning curve and the process takes time. The process includes:

- driving skills
- avoidance of obstacles and hazards
- moving in space
- perceptual skills, especially spatial
- knowing where they are
- noting how controllable and not excitable the user is
- reaction in crisis
- using the chair in the dark
- travelling down a sloped-edged pavement
- climbing kerbs
- descending curves
- crossing the street
- turning about
- how to ask for help
- maintenance requirements.

Supervision, once the model is issued, is vital also for both the user and the carer. Safety is paramount and it is therefore essential to increase the individual's awareness to this, especially if it is to be their first experience in the wider environment. The user's confidence will increase once they feel safe in the environment in which they are to use the chair.

Both the therapist and the rehabilitation engineer (RE) have a role to play in the provision and handover of the powered chair. This includes:

- assessement
- trial
- seating systems and modifications if applicable
- training in use
- instruction regarding maintenance and repair
- annual checks of the battery (which is a statutory requirement in the UK)
- regular checks to ensure the equipment is meeting the user's needs
- equipment updates.

Control boxes leave the factory preset to an average setting. The settings can, however, be altered for the individual by turning up or down the setting to make the chair more or less responsive in the required direction. If the control box is altered, a sticker should be placed on it by the RE to ensure that it is corrected before issuing to someone else. The settings can be recorded in the user's notes on the manufacturer's setting card and altered at review as the user improves or if they deteriorate.

Regardless of technical development, assessment and training, the use of a powered wheelchair will continue to carry safety risks. Specific guidance to the users should be used to modify those risks whenever possible (Hays, Jaffe & Ingman 1985). (A checklist is given in Box 13.2.)

MODELS

Three types of powered wheelchair are available. These are: indoor, indoor/outdoor and outdoor models. The models vary in the design of both the chassis and seating, specific features and complexity, weight, size, power, turning circle, speed and the different terrains on which they can travel. There are both three- and and four-wheeled powered wheelchairs available and they may either be attendant or user controlled, or both.

Box 13.2 Powered wheelchair process check list

- Physical condition and full assessment
- Seating position
- Cushion
- Control system
- Transfer method
- Trial of chair
- Indoors – check size, obstacles, doorways, turning circle
- Outdoors – kerbs, jolts, soft grass, rough ground
- Distance required to travel
- Manoeuvrability in shops
- Is protection available?
- Lights
- Carer
- Charging method
- Dismantle
- Transport, vehicles, taxis, cars
- Storage
- Battery life
- Maintenance/servicing
- Handover (rehabilitation engineer)
- Training/supervision

Indoor models

Indoor models are the smallest, compact and least complex (Fig. 13.1). The wheelbase tends to be short so that the turning circle is small for domestic use, increasing their manoeuvrability.

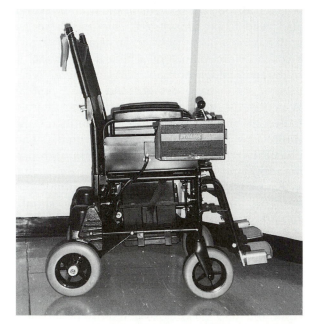

Figure 13.1 Indoor powered model: note the small wheels.

Such chairs are very manoeuvrable on smooth surfaces but a slight gradient can cause problems. The wheels are small and may be without tread to provide a better interface with flooring, carpets, etc. Tyres with tread are available for these chairs, especially if they are travelling on some pavement between buildings for example, and these are often called snow tyres. These models are designed based on manual models and therefore tend to be easily transportable and collapsible for storage purposes. There are a number of design variations available. In general the range is approximately 6 miles (9.5 km).

Indoor/outdoor models

Indoor/outdoor models are also compact but they are larger than the indoor models (Fig. 13.2). They generally have small wheels at the front and larger wheels at the back of the chair and the tyres have a tread to ensure the terrain travelled is gripped. Some models are foldable and are relatively easy to dismantle for travel and to load into a vehicle. The carer should be assessed for this task as some of the models break down into a

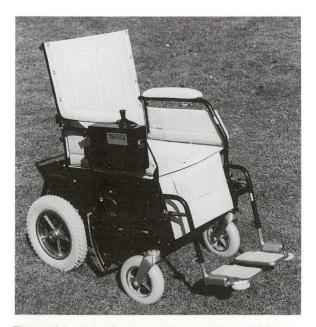

Figure 13.2 Indoor/outdoor model: note the size of the tyres.

number of smaller parts and some parts, especially the drive wheels, can be fairly heavy to lift. When transporting a powered chair in a car, at least four lifting sequences are entailed to put the whole model into a vehicle and the carer should be aware that the batteries will weigh approximately 22 lb (10 kg) each (Disabled Living Foundation 1993).

The range is generally between 4 and 30 miles (6.5 and 48 km). Such wheelchairs have more supportive seating than a scooter and require less physical effort to control the vehicle compared to a scooter. The turning circle is larger than the indoor models but they remain manoeuvrable in confined spaces, but this must be assessed carefully in the individual's home. Most indoor/outdoor wheelchairs feature a kerb climber to ascend a kerb. When descending a kerb, this should be done backwards. When such chairs are used indoors and outdoors, users have to be reminded to provide an area where the chair can be cleaned before it moves into the house to avoid dirt on carpets and floors.

Further information is also available from the 'Wheelchair training resource pack' (College of Occupational Therapists 1996) available from the College of Occupational Therapy, with training materials and reports on powered pilot schemes. Also 'Which one should they buy?' (Medical Devices Directorate 1993) is available from the Medical Devices Directorate.

Outdoor models

Outdoor models are the largest, most robust and the heaviest but they are able to travel across rough terrain, climb kerbs and descend kerbs forward and they have the power to travel long distances (between 30 and 62 miles (48 and 100 km) before recharging is necessary (Fig. 13.3). There is limited dismantling of these models and the turning circle is large and large amounts of space are required for storage. The seating system is generally more comfortable than the simpler models, often with built-in suspension, and accessories such as hoods are often available. Many of these models can be driven on the road, in which case they should have bicycle type red

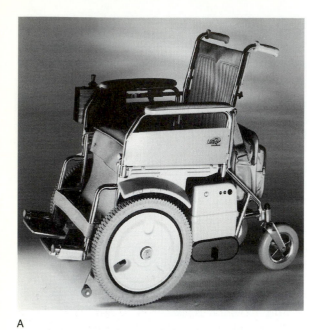

A

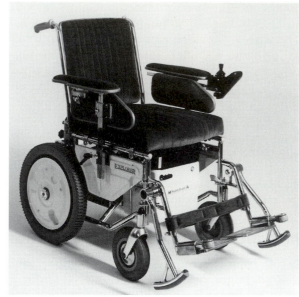

B

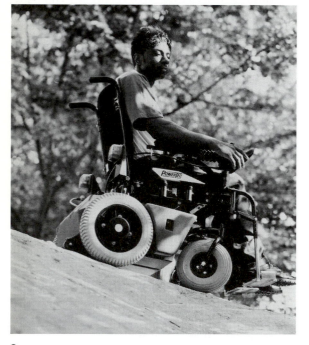

C

Figure 13.3(A–C) Outdoor models: note the size of the tyres (A,B with permission from Huntleigh Mobility; C with permission from Sunrise Mobility).

reflectors on the rear aspect and lights in the front. Many also have a horn or similar to attract attention and they can travel at 6–8 miles/h (10–13 km/h) on roads and 4 miles/h (6.5 km/h) on the pavements (Research Institute for Consumer Affairs 1996).

Spinal cord injured users

In a recent survey it was found that the spinal cord injured users below the level T1 favoured the outdoor models. The key areas of preference included: a firm seat base onto which the cushion can be placed, pneumatic tyres for a more comfortable ride outdoors or microcellular tyres for greater manoeuvrability with less maintenance, kerb climbers and tilt in space if appropriate. Although folding frames were commonly purchased, they were rarely folded, as it was not found to be necessary with the transportation vehicles they chiefly used. The batteries were also found to be too heavy for their carers to handle in general. Reclining backrests and elevating legrests were issued but again not used regularly (Curtin 1993).

Scooters

Scooters have been available since the 1960s with front-wheeled drive for indoor use and, from the 1980s, more powerful models for outdoor use were introduced.

Many three-wheeled scooters are available for both indoor and outdoor use (Fig. 13.4). They are basically a chair on a platform with a power supply. The outdoor models are larger and, although sturdier, may not be suitable indoors. The scooters are steered like a tricycle with handlebars or a tiller on which the controls are situated. No complex types of controls are available generally. The seat rotates to enable the user to transfer. The seating system is very simple and so not suitable for those users who require postural support or for prolonged use. Although such models are popular with the elderly to increase their mobility outdoors, the users must have good function of the upper limbs, balance and trunk control as the armrests do not touch the user's body. They are less supportive than a wheelchair and good spatial perception is important as they are less stable than a traditional wheelchair. Most scooters turn with the back wheels at the centre of the turning circle, therefore the radius is the length of the chassis. Scooters are able to climb 3 inch (8 cm) kerbs and

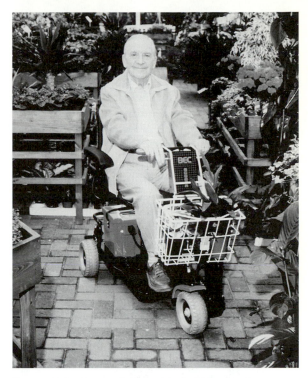

Figure 13.4   Scooter (with permission from Sunrise Mobility).

some outdoor models are able to descend kerbs forwards, although the stability of the user may be a problem and care should be taken when turning corners or travelling down slopes (Weyers & Massie 1986).

Front wheel drive scooters have small wheels which limit kerb climbing, but they are lighter, smaller, less powerful and have less ground clearance. Rear wheel drive scooters have greater traction, as the weight and centre of gravity is close to the drive wheel. Three-wheeled versions tend to be less stable than four-wheeled models but they are more manoeuvrable. Care is always needed with kerbs and uneven ground when using a scooter.

To use a powered wheelchair, scooter or buggy on the road the user must be aged 14 years or over (Kelsall 1996).

Add-on power packs

Although manufacturers of wheelchairs take no responsibility when modifications or additional items are placed on a wheelchair, the power pack is a useful addition to the power range to supplement manual power (Fig. 13.5). It provides a means of adding electric propulsion to an existing general purpose folding wheelchair. The weight of such devices is approximately 4 lb (1.8 kg). The system requires the user to have the ability to propel the wheelchair manually, as this provides the means of stopping, steering or reversing the wheelchair. The added power eases the difficulty with hill climbing and negotiating obstacles, for example. Control of the wheelchair is dependent upon both the manual dexterity and unimpaired mental function of the user and so careful assessment of the user's ability is necessary. It is especially useful when the wheelchair is to be used for different purposes and where there is limited space in the home. For example, a user may have a manual model which

they use satisfactorily in the home; however for outings, the user is unable to self-propel long distances due to their physical condition, or the user's weight and the carer's health or physique does not allow them to push the chair for long distances. The add-on power pack is therefore added to assist the carer. Another example of need may be for an attendant chair when storage, supply or finances are not available for an attendant-powered model. The conversion of the manual chair does have some problems. The device does put additional stress on the frame and the tyres wear out quickly as the chair is not really designed to be converted.

More elaborate power chairs that climb stairs, elevate the seat, stand up and tilt are available, but these are chairs designed to meet a specific and not general need (Kelsall 1996). Further information about such models is available

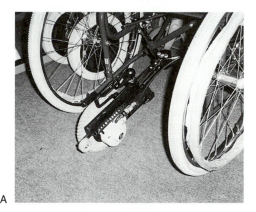

A

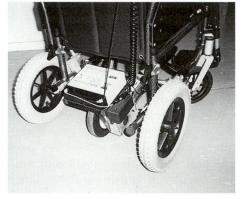

B

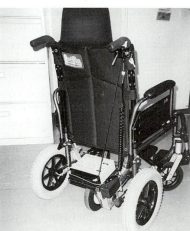

C

Figure 13.5(A–C)   Power pack add-on unit with permission from TGA Electric Leisure.

from the nearest Disability Living Centre or the Disabled Living Foundation.

General features

General features such as the frame type, wheels, tyres, footrests and plates, armrests, backrests, seat unit, manual brakes and accessories, should be assessed, as with a manual wheelchair. Other features are specific to powered chairs.

Power brakes/drive brakes

These brakes come into operation when the control box/joystick are released. They can be disengaged to manually push the powered chair.

Kerb climbers

An arc or wheel of metal set between the front wheels or at either side of the front wheels can enable a wheelchair user to climb kerbs and allow the user greater access in the environment. The need and position of the kerb climbers should be assessed at the time of the initial assessment, as the position may interfere with transfers. This is often the case with kerb climbers that are centrally located, whereas those positioned at the side may interfere with access and may be difficult to reposition if they are knocked backwards in order to get close up to something. However, for some users they are not suitable and the action is daunting (Research Institute for Consumer Affairs 1996). Some users find kerb climbers difficult to use and uncomfortable, as a jolt often occurs as the devices hit the kerb to be climbed. For example, such individuals may have poor balance, painful joints, sensory loss or slow reactions. Kerb climbers are available to allow the user to climb kerbs from 2 inches (5 cm) to 4–5 inches (10–13 cm). Kerbs are always climbed frontways but not all models allow the user to come down a kerb forwards. Often coming down the kerb has to be accomplished backwards and if this is the case the user must be able to turn the upper body around to ensure the pathway for travel is clear. Such models tend to be cheaper but are not suitable for every user.

Although the advice given to users with different models varies, generally to climb a kerb, the front castors have to be facing the kerb squarely with the forks trailing behind (Weyers & Massie 1986). Some models have to have full power to climb the kerb and with other models it can be done more slowly, and the procedure is smoother with some models than with others. The kerb climbers are generally detachable to allow the chair to be folded for transportation or storage. Trial of the chair with this equipment is essential.

Type of drive

Front wheel drive wheelchairs are more manoeuvrable and tend to be used where longer distances are travelled, or outdoors on rugged ground. They are in the minority in the UK. If there are large wheels at the front they are good kerb climbers, but transfers may be difficult. Steering is by the rear castors which increases the turning circle and therefore this is a characteristic the user needs to learn.

Rear wheel drive wheelchairs are easier to control and therefore recommended for users with poor control and poor balance. If kerb climbers are added with these models, the descent is backwards. Such chairs are more common in the UK with a greater number of models available.

Wheels and castors

Generally for indoor use, models are found with four small wheels with solid tyres and smooth treads in order to give a smooth ride but with little grip. Models with small front wheels and larger rear wheels are used indoors and outdoors and generally include kerb climbers. Models which have castors or wheels that swivel are difficult to use on slopes but the castors may be more satisfactory indoors. Models that have large front wheels and small rear wheels tend to have outdoor rough tread on the tyres and models that have four large wheels with thick outdoor tread have a turning circle that is too large for use indoors but is suitable for outdoor use. Inflatable tyres are generally found to be best on rough ground.

The indoor lighter models can produce difficulties if the user's posture is asymmetrical and the weight is over to one side, which can affect the steering and turning corners.

Controls

Powered wheelchairs may be controlled or driven in a number of ways. Users must try a variety of controls to see which ones suit them. These include the following:

Joystick. The standard method used is where the device controls the direction not the speed of the chair. It is recommended that the joystick is held between the 'V' of the thumb and the index finger for ease and comfort (Disabled Living Foundation 1993).

Proportional controls. Here the joystick controls the direction and the speed. It may also have an acceleration limiter fitted, for users with involuntary movements or tremors. Such controls are not suitable for people with poor control, especially where there are obstacles to negotiate.

Swash plates. This is a box which the user presses at different edges to go in different directions. Pushing the front edge of the box starts the chair.

Chin switches. Very little pressure is required for this device to control the chair. A special mounting bracket is required to attach the device to the chair and it can be contolled by the chin, tongue or hand. Also chin-operated eight-way joysticks are available. These are small and light.

Suck/puff. These switches are controlled with different combinations of sucks and puffs (Research Institute for Consumer Affairs 1996).

Head switches. These are shaped around the head as headrests. The most common type has the forward switch behind the head, left and right at the appropriate side and the reverse position is located at the front end of the side supports. There are, however, other designs, for example the Peach Tree which is a flat pad which is clicked a number of times to set. The head is then moved away and the further forward the user moves the faster they go. The user does not touch the pad to steer, but as the head is turned, the chair turns. In another design a small single switch is operated with any part of the body, for example the tongue, finger tip, elbow, and there is also a direction panel which is clicked to change direction. Foot controls are also available and with the advance in electronics today very sophisticated switches are available for people who have very little or virtually no movement. There are specialist centres around the UK available for such assessments. For example the Mary Marlborough Centre in Oxford, the Wolfson Centre in London and the Chailey Heritage in Sussex.

Attendant. Here the control box is usually mounted in the traditional position on the armrest but the joystick or control lever is located near the push handles for the attendant to operate. A model does not need to be either attendant or user controlled but may have both on the same chair, for different needs and circumstances; for example, when the user becomes tired or uses the model outside in unfamiliar environments.

Special devices are also developed by specialist engineering centres to meet the individuals' needs, for example necklace switches. Control levers can be located both at the side of the chair or centrally or at any variation of the two depending on the user's needs.

Batteries and chargers

A battery is a heavy and expensive part of a powered wheelchair and needs replacing approximately every 2 years. Such wheelchairs operate on the energy stored in batteries, typically 12-volt batteries which are similar to those used in cars. Car batteries require a heavy current to the starter motor for a few seconds, and use up only a fraction of the energy stored with a low depth of discharge during normal use. However, wheelchair batteries use up nearly all of their stored energy in use and then require long periods of recharge, a so-called deep discharge. Car batteries give poor performance in these conditions. 'Trickle' chargers were used but it was important that this type of charger was switched off once the charging was complete which was inconvenient to users. Subsequently, 'motive' power or traction batteries have been developed for use with wheelchairs, which enables them to tolerate repeated deep cycles of discharge and charge. Developments in these chargers ensured that overcharging did not occur if they were left switched on for longer than the recommended period.

Until recently the majority of powered wheelchairs were powered by liquid electrolyte, deep cycle, 'wet' lead acid batteries. They are economical to use but require regular attention, are unpleasant to handle and not considered safe for transportation (Fisher, Garrett & Seeger 1988). They do however have a large mileage range (Curtin 1993). In these batteries, the water decomposes to hydrogen and oxygen and therefore distilled water needs to be added regularly. If this topping up does not occur, the lead plates become exposed to air and are ruined, reducing the battery's capacity. Reading the battery's specific gravity is a reliable method to determine the amount of energy left in the battery.

Today sealed, gel-electrolyte or valve-regulated batteries are more commonly used. They are more expensive, but are compact, neat and safer in handling, as the risk of acid burns through spillage is removed. Therefore the gel will not spill in transport situations, making their use more accessible for users in public vehicles. These gel batteries prevent the unacceptable build up of gas pressure. The units do not need routine maintenance but do require extra care with charging and they should be used with chargers that have controlled maximum voltage. The chargers should be clearly labelled to ensure the correct equipment is used together. The capacity of a new gel-type battery is not reached until the battery has been cycled a few times. The wheelchair should always be made inoperable while charging is taking place. This is done automatically by the chair's electronic system (Department of Health/Medical Devices Directorate 1992). Gel batteries have a reduced mileage range compared to the wet type (Curtin 1993) and have been found to have a shorter life which

is not as long as some manufacturers state (Fisher, Garrett & Seeger 1988). The correct type of charger should always be used and the battery charger should charge the battery completely within 8 hours otherwise the battery will degrade faster.

Most powered wheelchairs will climb a 1 : 6 slope without losing speed. However, the battery power will be reduced in such situations and the range will therefore also be reduced (Disabled Living Foundation 1993). This is obviously a problem in hilly areas.

Maintenance and repairs

It is essential that powered wheelchairs are serviced at least annually. This is for statutory reasons regarding the batteries in the UK (National Prosthetic and Wheelchair Services Report 1993–1996) and also as a preventive practice to insure against breakdowns and accidents. In some areas, the rehabilitation engineer or therapist will check the powered user annually to ensure the equipment is still appropriate, that it meets the needs of the user and that the repairs and maintenance have been satisfactorily carried out (Ham 1995). For NHS users this is currently a 'free at the source of delivery' service but for both private purchasers and charities, this additional cost must be taken into account when calculating the cost of issuing such equipment or when receiving a chair from a charity. The maintenance costs will not be obvious in the first year or two, but can be very heavy after that, especially if the chair is being used for long distances. In the UK the service and maintenance may be carried out by the approved repairer service or by the supplier or distributor of the equipment.

Road use

Through the Road Traffic Statutory Instrument No. 2268 (1988), the definitions below are used for pavement vehicles.

Class 1

Not mechanically propelled, i.e. self-propelled or attendant-controlled models.

Class 2

Not mechanically propelled and incapable of a speed greater than 4 miles/h (6.4 km/h) on the level under its own power. Such models are allowed to be used in public places by those with a physical defect or disability. The brakes should hold the vehicle on a 1 : 5 gradient and no lights are required. But if there is no pavement, and the vehicle should go on the road, a single white light at the front and a red reflector at the rear is required (Research Institute for Consumer Affairs 1996, Wells 1996). The vehicles should weigh less than 250 lb (113 kg) when empty. No driving licence or statutory visual acuity test are required in the UK but it is suggested that a distance vision equivalent to Snellens Chart 6/60 should be the minimum for safely moving models outdoors in public places.

Class 3

Mechanically propelled and capable of more than 4 miles/h (6.4 km/h) but less than 8 miles/h (12.8 km/h). The user should be over 14 years of age and also have a physical disability. Again no driving licence is required to use one of these models but it is recommended that the user is able to read a number plate at a distance of 40 feet (12 m). Again insurance is not compulsory but it is recommended. The speed allowed on the pavement for these models is 4 miles/h (6.4 km/h) and 8 miles/h (12.8 km/h) on the road. A light, a horn, indicators and a rear view mirror are also required on these models. The brakes are as in Class 2 and the maximum empty weight allowed is 350 lbs (150 kg) (Medical Devices Directorate 1993, Wells 1996).

OTHER ASPECTS OF POWERED AND OUTDOOR WHEELCHAIR USE

Insurance

Although insurance is not compulsory for class 2 or 3 models, it is recommended that users insure for at least third party cover, i.e. accidental damage the user may cause other people and their property as a result of using the wheelchair.

Such models are also subject to theft, and insurance against this, as well as loss, fire and damage, is also advised (Wells 1996). If the chair is purchased through the Motability scheme then it has to be fully insured before it is delivered to the user. A number of companies are available for such insurance and their numbers are increasing. They cover both the equipment and costs arising because of the involvement of carers and assistants. Such companies are listed in other publications (Wells 1996).

Safety and training

The user should be taught how to handle the equipment in all situations, how to cope with obstacles, pedestrians and other traffic, and how to deal with regular battery charging. To check that a user has reached a minimum standard of safety, the Royal Society for the Prevention of Accidents (RoSPA) silver or gold tests may be used. For example these include:

- Reading a number plate at 44 feet (13.5 m)
- switching the vehicle on and off
- travelling in straight lines forwards and backwards
- turning left and right
- turning around
- carrying out an emergency stop
- demonstrate awareness of other road and pavement users
- using the chair in a confined space
- going up and down kerbs
- crossing the road via a pedestrian crossing
- demonstrating knowledge of the Highway and Green Cross code
- demonstrating knowledge of battery care and maintenance.

Some of the national voluntary groups run training sessions or they may be able to assist the local service by giving a contact for a local trainer.

Disability living allowance (DLA)

The DLA is a tax free benefit for people who need help with personal care, with getting around or with both. It is made up of two components, the care component and the mobility component, which is for people aged 5 or over. Both components are for people disabled before the age of 65. There are two rates of the mobility component depending upon the impairment. The higher rate applies if the person is unable or virtually unable to walk, has had both legs amputated at or above the ankle, was born without legs or feet, is both deaf and blind and needs care and attention whilst outdoors or is severely mentally impaired and displays severe behavioural problems (Department of Transport 1996). The lower rate applies when the person can walk but needs supervision out of doors. The conditions have to have lasted 3 months and will continue for at least 6 months. If the individual receives the higher rate or receives the war pensioner's mobility supplement, then they can apply to Motability, a voluntary organization, for help in hiring a new car, buying on hire purchase new or used cars or wheelchairs on preferential terms (Department of Health 1996). Motability has its own lease scheme which runs over a 3-year period and its own hire purchase scheme also.

Orange Badge scheme

This scheme provides a national arrangement of parking concessions for people with severe walking disabilities who travel either as drivers or passengers, registered blind people, and people with very severe upper limb disabilities who regularly drive a vehicle but cannot turn a steering wheel by hand. It allows badge holders to park closer to their destination but the national concessions only apply to on-street parking. To qualify for an Orange Badge the user will: receive the higher rate of the DLA (mobility component), be registered blind, use a vehicle supplied by a government department, get a grant towards the vehicle, receive a war pensioner's mobility supplement, have a severe disability in both upper limbs or have a permanent or substantial disability which means they are unable to walk or have considerable difficulty walking (Department of Transport 1996).

Travel in general

Although the provision for wheelchair users on all types of transport is improving, there are still limitations as far as access and space are concerned. Users should be advised to contact the service they intend to use for more details. Such addresses are given in detail in other publications (Department of Health 1996, Department of Transport 1996, Wells 1996).

Private assessments

Private assessments are available in some areas from the local wheelchair service. In other areas this is not the case. At some Disability Living Centres, assessments are available with therapists in post at the centres. At a few centres test tracks are also available. The mobility centres that are located across the country also carry out such assessments, often with a charge. These include Banstead Mobility Centre (a charity and part of the mobility forum) in Surrey, Treloar Disability Assessment Unit in Alton in Hampshire (a charity), the Mary Marlborough Centre in Oxford, and MAVIS, the mobility advice and vehicle information service in Berkshire. Details of such centres are given in other publications (Department of Health 1996, Department of Transport 1996, Research Institute for Consumer Affairs 1996, Wells 1996).

Private purchases

Many users unable to fund the powered chair themselves and who do not qualify for one under the NHS, may gain help with the purchase from charities and trusts (Wells 1996). These charities and trusts may be connected to the area they have worked or served in, may be national charities or trusts connected to their disability or may be local charities. The *Directory of Grant Making Trusts Handbook* (Charitable Aids Foundation 1997) which is available from the local library, may be of assistance in locating such sources.

Many manufacturers belong to the British Surgical Trades Association (BSTA) and many retailers belong to the British Association of

Wheelchair Distributors (BAWD). Both of these organizations operate codes of practice and standard warranty conditions which aim to promote members' responsibility to the public at large and the ultimate users of their products in particular. Such standards serve to ensure that services provided by members conform to service standards and include such items as: not calling at users' homes without an appointment, no pressure to buy, a range of models should be shown and advice given, demonstration of the use of the model and a full instruction manual and full service and repair facilities. A list of companies in the association are available in other publications (Wells 1996). Suppliers also often run wheelchair loan schemes for which a deposit and a charge are made.

Second-hand purchases

If a wheelchair is no longer required or a second-hand model is required, it may be sold or purchased through a number of channels. For example, the *RADAR Monthly Bulletin*, the *Disability Equipment Register* (Research Institute for Consumer Affairs 1996), *Disability Now* magazine, the *Disabled Driver* magazine, *Exchange and Mart* newspaper, the Disabled Living Foundation noticeboards, through the local wheelchair service noticeboards, local newspapers and noticeboards and through some local distributors and manufacturers.

Dial-a-Ride

Most large urban areas and many small towns in the UK have a Dial-a-Ride scheme. It may be known by other terms such as Ring-a-Ride or Dial-a-Journey also. This is a door-to-door public transportation service in the form of a small bus, for disabled people who are unable or find it difficult to use conventional buses and trains because of their disabilities. It was founded by users and continues to offer a user-controlled service, though funded by a government grant.

Escorts and companions may travel with the passenger and usually pay the same fare, which is comparable to that of a bus journey of the same length. Dogs and other animals may also be transported if the other passengers do not object and they are well secured or boxed. The service runs daily (except Christmas Day in some areas) from the early morning, usually 6 a.m., to the late evening and often as late as 2 a.m. Trips are booked normally 48 hours in advance but other bookings are available depending upon availability. Bookings are made by phone and the procedure is clearly described in the information given to all users of the service. The service is available to all locations and for all journeys that would not be covered by other transportation systems, for example the local authority or hospital transportation, for specific purposes. For some battery-powered wheelchairs and scooters that cannot be adequately secured, or if there is insufficient space, they may be refused (Dial-a-Ride 1995).

Shopmobility

Many towns have large pedestrianized shopping areas and a growing number of shopmobility schemes have been set up to give disabled people the maximum mobility when they shop there. The National Federation of Shopmobility is a charity with a membership of about 120 schemes and has information on schemes throughout the country and produces a directory of the towns where there are schemes operating. Each scheme is run independently so the availability varies (Wells 1996). Powered and manual wheelchairs as well as electric scooters are available on loan, with proof of identity, a nominal returnable deposit, leaving the car parking ticket or car keys, for example. If enough warning is given, an escort can often be provided to help with shopping. The scheme also often links up with the Dial-a-Ride scheme for those without their own cars (Department of Transport 1996).

Community transport

Local community transport organizations usually have a pool of vehicles which they will hire out to local member groups or associations, with or without a driver, depending upon

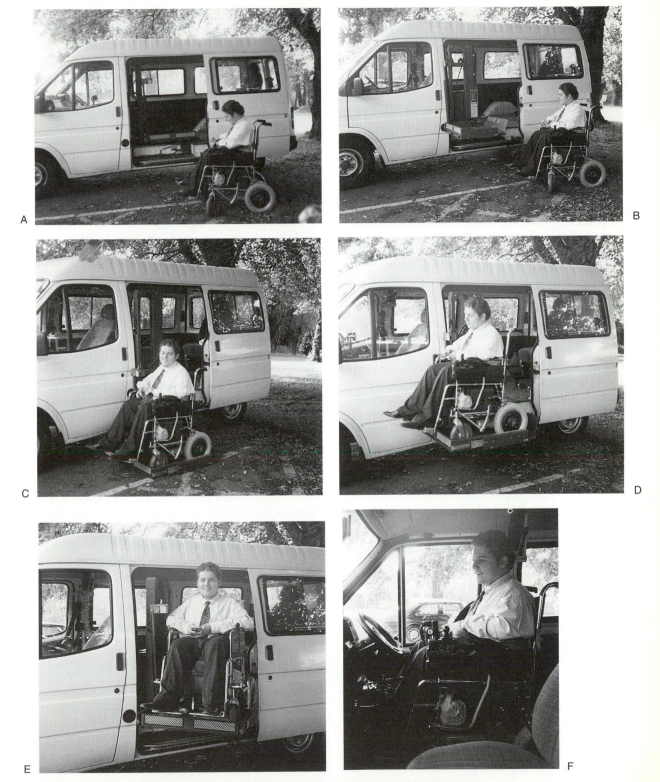

Figure 13.6(A–F)   Transportation: one method illustrated to increase the user's independence.

the particular community transport group. The vehicles are generally wheelchair accessible (Department of Transport 1996).

Department of Transport

The Department of Transport in the UK has a Mobility Unit which produces information that is useful and informative for professionals and users alike. Such publications include: *Door to Door*, *Its not my problem*, the Disability Discrimination Act, Transport Bulletins, Mobility Policy, information on the Low-floor bus, train and taxi schemes and videos and training materials are also available. The 2-yearly Mobility Roadshow which is held at Crowthorne, Berkshire is organized through this department.

Transportation

Some users will use their allowances for the purchase of a suitable vehicle to accommodate their disability and chosen method of transportation to increase their independence. Space for access when the vehicle is parked, the method of access into the vehicle from the side or the back, for example, and the driving method have to be carefully selected (see Fig. 13.6 A–F).

Within vehicles it is essential to stress the importance of safe transportation of wheelchairs. Users with developmental disabilities sitting in wheelchairs often lack the balance skills or protective responses necessary to avoid injury during routine swerving, let alone collisions (DiGaudio & Msall 1991). Some wheelchairs have been crash tested and the manufacturer's literature clearly indicates this with fixing points or attachments. The majority are not and manufacturers are now also stating that their models are not covered for clamping either. All wheelchairs should be securely restrained to the structure of the vehicle with the correct straps (Department of Transport 1993), so that in the event of a collision there is reduced risk of the seat being ripped out of the floor of the vehicle. The individual should be independently secured (McMillan 1992), wearing a safety belt that is also attached to the vehicle and not the adjacent seat. It should be remembered that body-restraining straps are issued for use at walking speed, i.e. 4 miles/h (6.44 km/h), not for vehicle restraint. All items that are attached to the wheelchair in the static or walking mode should be clearly reviewed before they are transported on a vehicle. This may include the removal of trays and supports, for example. The correct use of tail lifts when transporting wheelchairs and the occupant is important and staff involved with this should be correctly trained and made aware of the dangers that may occur. When boarding an individual using a non-standard wheelchair (Department of Transport 1993), a powered or lightweight model for example, it may be advisable to remove the user first as the weight and shape of the chair may create difficulties.

A wheelchair can constitute a mass two to three times that of a person in a crash and is therefore a formidable missile inside a vehicle. Even an emergency stop at 7.5 miles/h (12 km/h) will create chaos amongst passengers who cannot brace themselves (Wevers 1983). The orientation of the individual in transportation is also important. They should be front or rearward facing and never side facing as this position can cause injury in the event of harsh braking or collision. It is essential that persons dealing with wheelchair occupants work closely with the transportation departments involved in their locality.

REFERENCES

Anon 1915 Evolution of the wheelchair. Scientific American 112: 497–502

Beaumont-White S, Ham R O 1997 Powered wheelchairs: are we enabling or disabling? Prosthetics and Orthotics International 21: 62–73

Bennett-Wilson A Jr 1986 Wheelchairs: a prescription guide. Rehabilitation Press, USA

Breed A L, Ibler I 1982 The motorised wheelchair: new freedom, new responsibility, new problems. Developmental Medicine and Child Neurology 24: 366–371

Charitable Aids Foundation 1997 Directory of grant making trusts. Charities Aid Foundation, Tunbridge Wells, Kent

College of Occupational Therapists 1996 Wheelchair training resource pack. (Revised DSA 1991 Publication.) College of Occupational Therapists, London.

Curtin M 1993 Powered wheelchairs and tetraplegic patients: improving the service. British Journal of Occupational Therapy 56(6): 204–226

Department of Health/Medical Devices Directorate 1992 Wheelchair battery charging and maintenance. Wheelchair evaluation centre MDD/DTS/IB (doc E4 10/92). Department of Health, London

Department of Health 1996 A practical guide for disabled people. HMSO, London

Department of Transport 1993 'It's not my problem'. The transportation of children with special needs. Department of Transport, London

Department of Transport 1996 Door to door, 5th edn. HMSO, London

Dial-a-Ride 1995 Going places, a guide to your service. St Margarets, London

DiGaudio K M, Msall M E 1991 Guidelines for safer transportation of children in wheelchairs. American Journal of Diseases of Children 145: 653–655

Disabled Living Foundation 1993 Wheelchair information. DLF, London

Fisher W E, Garrett R E, Seeger R R 1988 Testing of gel-electrolyte batteries for wheelchairs. Journal of Rehabilitation Research and Development 25(2): 27–32

Guttmann L 1964 Symposium on the wheelchair, London 1993. Paraplegia 2(1)

Ham R O 1995 Newham Wheelchair Service, Annual Report. St Andrew's Hospital, London

Hays R M, Jaffe K M, Ingman E 1985 Accidental death associated with motorised wheelchair use: a case report. Archives of Physical Medicine and Rehabilitation 66: 709–710

International Organisation for Standards 1982 Needs of people in buildings. Design guidelines. ISO, Geneva

Jolly D W 1964 Symposium on the wheelchair, Ministry practice, London 1963. Paraplegia 2: 20

Kamenetz H L 1969 The wheelchair book. Charles C Thomas, Springfield, Illinois

Kelsall A 1996 What to look for in an outdoor powered wheelchair, scooter or buggy. British Journal of Therapy and Rehabilitation 3(9): 507–513

Kelsall A D, Houghton R H, Cochrane G M 1993 Wheelchairs, 7th edn. Equipment for disabled people series. Disability Information Trust, Nuffield Orthopaedic Centre, Oxford

Letts R M 1991 Powered wheelchairs and other mobility aids. In: Letts R M (ed) Principles of seating the disabled. CRC Press, Florida, pp 265–286

McMillan P H 1992 A survey of transportation for children in wheelchairs. British Journal of Occupational Therapy 55: 179–182

Medical Devices Directorate 1993 Which one should they buy? Medical Devices Directorate, MDD/M93/01. Department of Health, London

National Prosthetic and Wheelchair Services Report 1993–1996 DoH funded project. College of Occupational Therapists, London

Research Institute for Consumer Affairs 1996 Powered wheelchairs, scooters and buggies. A guide to help you choose. RICA, London

Royal College of Physicians 1987 Physical disabilities in 1986 and beyond. Royal College of Physicians, London

Trefler E, Hobson D A, Taylor S J, Monahan L C, Shaw C G 1993 Seating and mobility for persons with physical disabilities. Therapy Skill Builders, University of Tennessee, Memphis

Warren C G 1990 Powered mobility and its implications. Journal of Rehabilitation Research and Development (Clinical Supplement 2) March: 74–85

Wells J 1996 Choosing a wheelchair. The Royal Association for Disability and Rehabilitation (RADAR), London

Wevers H W 1983 Wheelchair and occupant restraints systems for transportation of handicapped passengers. Archives of Physical Medicine and Rehabilitation 64: 374–377

Wayers J, Massie B 1986 Wheelchairs and their use. RADAR, London

14

Training issues for therapists and wheelchair users

INTRODUCTION

Training is defined in the English dictionary as 'practical education; a course of exercise for developing physical strength, endurance or dexterity'. This definition describes well the needs of the professional involved in the process of wheelchair prescription and provision as well as the wheelchair user. Each group has significant differing and additional needs, but even so, both professional and user require an appropriate level of training if there is to be a satisfactory outcome from the assessment, prescription and provision process. This chapter looks specifically at both the needs and the availability of appropriate education and training for both therapists and wheelchair users. Additional details can be found in the Further reading at the end of the chapter, as well as Appendix 3.

EDUCATION AND TRAINING FOR THERAPISTS

'The first step is to improve the training for all those who may become involved in wheelchair assessment and prescription at some time in their career.' This statement is taken from the McColl report, paragraph 94 (McColl 1986). In the summary of the final recommendations, the McColl committee specifically identified the need for improved training for therapists and GPs, whilst training for medical students is referred to elsewhere in the review.

At the time this was written, therapists played

a very minor role in the prescription process for wheelchairs. In most cases therapists were responsible for identifying the wheelchair requirements for their 'patients', though it was the consultant or GP who in theory agreed the prescription and signed the form. If a client required further assessment, this would be carried out at the nearest Artificial Limb and Appliance Centre (ALAC) by the medical officer and technical officer. Prescription was based on size and weight of user, with little or no account being taken of need, environment, ability or user preference. The Department of Health and Social Services (DHSS) saw its responsibility as ending with the provision of mobility. Any other activities carried out in the wheelchair were seen as being the responsibility of other departments (Mitchell 1984).

Requests from therapists for modifications to improve individual function were often inappropriate on a technical basis and because of their limited knowledge of wheelchair equipment, therapists often failed to see the difficulties that could be created by even a minor modification; for example, raising an armrest would prevent the user sitting close to a table and could reduce efficiency for self-propelling. Technical officers on the other hand would sometimes initiate a change of prescription without realizing the clinical implications of the change; for example, providing a reclining backrest for improved comfort could increase spasm, cause shear and reduce function. Many of these problems arose due to poor communication between ALAC staff (technical officers) and clinicians (therapists). Apart from signing the referral form, involvement by doctors was minimal and GPs are, even now, often unaware of the wheelchair users registered with their practice. This is not surprising as wheelchair users, whilst having limited walking ability, are not ill and do not necessarily require the services of a doctor any more frequently than their able-bodied counterparts. By recommending that wheelchair assessment should be carried out closer to the user's home environment, the McColl committee recognized the need for greater involvement of therapists and better home assessments. There was, however,

an assumption that most therapists had adequate knowledge to cope with this responsibility and that additional information on equipment would be sufficient to improve prescription standards, as at this time (1987) the range of wheelchair models available through the DHSS was extremely limited and, certainly, many therapists considered they had sufficient knowledge to assess and prescribe accurately and appropriately.

National resources for wheelchair training

Few resources specific to wheelchair training were available at the time of the reorganization of the service in England. This fact was readily acknowledged by the Disablement Services Authority (see Ch. 1), who addressed the matter by funding a multidisciplinary group with a part-time coordinator, to compile a 'Wheelchair training resource pack'. The original pack was completed and distributed to the 14 health regions in England at the end of 1989. This material was not intended as a complete training course, but contained a range of information in the form of written materials, slides with tapes and scripts, videos, booklets and an informative bibliography that could be used as a basis for setting up training sessions tailored to local need (Wells 1991). Each region was given the opportunity of an 'introductory offer' for identified staff to attend a 1- or 2-day awareness training session and explanation of the pack contents and purpose. It was envisaged that by starting with small teams of trainers which included experienced occupational therapists and physiotherapists, whose backgrounds were in either health or community work, the information would be 'cascaded' down through the different levels of service to embrace all who worked with wheelchair users and were involved either as assessors or carers. This indeed happened and continues to happen in a number of areas, though inevitably standards are not uniform and the opportunity for training and level of expertise available to therapists is variable and dependent on the level of resources in any one place.

At the demise of the DSA in 1991, a further 500

resource packs were funded and distributed by the Department of Health to the newly established 169 district wheelchair services, all social service departments, as well as some voluntary organizations and training centres for therapists (Department of Health 1991). This was partly in recognition of the difficulties being experienced in many of the services following the introduction of the NHS and Community Care Act (1990) with the subsequent total reorganization of the National Health Service, and partly to ensure that training was continued and supported as demands on the service increased. The original training resource packs are still available at main wheelchair service centres, though additional and revised information was produced supported by a Section 64 grant in 1996 and is available from the College of Occupational Therapists (Department of Health 1996).

Present education and training opportunities for therapists

Many wheelchair services in England organize training courses for local postgraduate therapists and other professionals. Some services provide additional training for carers and voluntary groups, though the content and standard of all training is very variable and depends heavily on the knowledge, experience, interest and availability of individual trainers as well as the funding levels at each centre. There is wide variation in the level of expertise seen in assessors around the country and, as stated in the McColl report, ongoing training is essential to maintain high standards of prescription. This view has been widely supported, with additional emphasis being placed on the fact that appropriate training will also ensure good use of scarce budgets and supplies (Ham 1993).

National standards for wheelchair therapists

The absence of nationally recognized training standards for wheelchair therapists is a matter for concern that is shared by professionals and users alike. Many of the complaints received are related to cases when users have expressed dissatisfaction with the level of assessment received (Lecouturier & Jacoby 1995, Smith & Goddard 1994). Although the professional bodies representing therapists have recognized validation procedures to approve the standard of undergraduate training for occupational therapists and physiotherapists, lack of a national curriculum results in wide variation in both content and time allocated to specific topics. This was clearly demonstrated in a survey of all training centres by Silcox (1995).

As part of a Department of Health funded project based at the College of Occupational Therapists from 1993 to 1996, lecturers from higher education centres attended a meeting to discuss with members of a training committee guidelines for the education of students of occupational therapy and physiotherapy. The proposed guidelines were divided into four sections, allowing easy integration of basic material into existing higher education modules. Each section was divided into: aims; learning outcomes; recommendations, and references. The final document was published as part of the project report (College of Occupational Therapists 1995) and signalled the way towards ensuring all newly qualified therapists obtained a basic level of awareness and understanding in wheelchair matters (Box 14.1).

Future training trends for therapists

The introduction of two new government schemes, one for the provision of indoor/outdoor powered wheelchairs (HSG(96)34) and the other for vouchers (HSG(96)53), raised expectations for users and professionals and rapidly increased the demands placed on the wheelchair therapists, highlighting the need for improved and continuing training. Although both sets of guidelines made reference to the need to review staffing levels and training, the decision to implement these recommendations was left to the discretion of the individual health commissioners in consultation with wheelchair services. In practice, it has been found that few therapists have had the opportunity to undergo additional

---

Box 14.1   Summary of aims in the four sections from 'Guidelines for the education of students of occupational therapy and physiotherapy' (College of Occupational Therapists 1995)

Experiential
- Practical and safe handling of a wheelchair in all environments
- Understanding safety factors and legislation influencing prescription
- Identifying issues experienced daily by wheelchair users and their carers
- Attitudes of others to user and carer

Assessment
- Principles of assessment. Recording and interpreting relevant facts and figures
- Awareness of posture; causes and prevention of deformity and tissue trauma
- Involvement of others in assessment
- Identifying problems of inadequate assessment and inappropriate prescription

Equipment
- Knowledge of standard equipment; identify components; influence on user and performance
- Ability to set up and adjust a wheelchair; care and handling
- Understanding the properties of pressure-relieving cushions
- Awareness of guidelines affecting provision, manufacture and transportation of wheelchairs

Organizational
- Awareness of current structure, function and remit of NHS wheelchair service
- Importance of liaising with other agencies – voluntary and statutory
- How to access the contract repairer
- Awareness of professional responsibilities; documentation. Other sources of provision

---

training. This is not entirely due to funding problems. The majority of services are dependent on a single-handed therapist and absence for training can quickly have an adverse affect on all service users. There is also a noticeable absence of suitable courses readily available. Consequently, some services liaised and organized their own training assisted by staff from local mobility centres and suppliers (Fig. 14.1A–D), whilst others are learning by trial and error.

The pace of change has quickened in recent years and advances in technology have resulted in a rapidly growing and changing range of wheelchair equipment appearing on the market. This is coupled with greater opportunities for wider travel being available to disabled people and, indeed, an increase in the numbers of severely handicapped and elderly people living in the community. In addition to the growing range of clinical demands being placed on therapists, many of those directly responsible for a wheelchair service are expected to negotiate service and equipment contracts, set up audit procedures and monitor the service to ensure that it is cost effective and meeting the needs of the users. As with all aspects of rehabilitation, much of the expertise required is gained on the job, though basic clinical, technical and equip-

ment knowledge, and information is essential before the additional skills can be developed. The independent status of universities who provide higher education, coupled with the independent nature of the NHS trusts, makes it difficult to obtain national agreement on the standards of training and competence required by a wheelchair therapist. However, there are now signs that due to continuing pressure from both those working in the field and service users, action may be taken to establish a recognized qualification as part of continuing professional development for wheelchair therapists in the near future.

Other sources for information and training of therapists (see Useful addresses)

Appropriate courses in this field are few and far between though some have been developed in response to demand in certain areas. A 3-day wheelchair and seating course, supported by the Scottish Seating and Wheelchair Group, has been available as part of the National Prosthetic and Orthotic training programme at Strathclyde University for several years. The National Posture and Mobility Group, a society in England which is open to all professionals, holds an

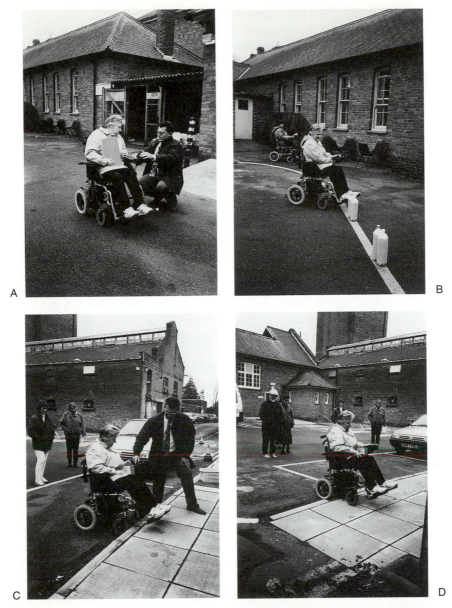

Figure 14.1 A group of wheelchair therapists receive practical training and experience the problems that can be encountered when handling an electrically powered indoor/outdoor chair (EPIOC). (A) Receiving instruction in setting the control box. (B) Negotiating a series of obstacles. (C) Learning how to approach the kerb. (D) Mounting a 4 inch (10 cm) kerb using kerb climbers.

annual 2-day scientific meeting which offers an opportunity to learn of new developments, participate in discussions and workshops on posture, mobility and associated matters and to meet others with a similar interest. On a smaller scale,

CIGOPW, a clinical interest group in orthotics, prosthetics and wheelchairs for occupational therapists, issues a quarterly newssheet for members and arranges study days relating to wheelchair and seating issues. Independently run courses are available throughout the country. Some concentrate on clinical issues and assessment of posture and mobility, others are equipment focused and provide up to date information on the rapidly increasing range of models and accessories now being marketed. At present none of these are accredited with higher education.

Opportunities do indeed exist. When time and funding allow, many wheelchair services will organize ongoing training sessions and regular updates for therapists assessing in their area. International conferences on rehabilitation increasingly include sessions relating to wheelchairs and seating for those who can find the resources and time to attend, but acquiring these resources can create a hurdle, particularly when there is little support from higher managers and no official recognition from the professional bodies concerned. Until this support and recognition is achieved, there will continue to be concern and lack of confidence from users in the level of advice being provided by professionals.

TRAINING OPPORTUNITIES FOR WHEELCHAIR USERS

Whilst recognizing the need for improved education for therapists, practical training is also required by wheelchair users if optimum benefit and enjoyment is to be gained from their wheelchair. The majority of less active and able users receive adequate information and training from their wheelchair service in different formats, including face to face instruction as well as provision of a users' handbook (see Further reading). However, active full-time users, whether with a powered wheelchair or high performance model, as well as many of their carers, frequently fail to receive the necessary practical training in handling skills and caring for their wheelchair. Many wheelchair therapists do not have adequate

skills, experience or time to support this level of instruction for new users. Suitable courses or individual tuition are not readily available locally though there are some specialist centres and an increasing number of independent centres now providing some form of training for users and carers. For anyone purchasing or being issued with an active user or powered outdoor wheelchair, training should be sought to ensure confidence and safety in its use, and to enable each individual to obtain maximum benefit from the equipment provided. School children attending special schools are generally given instruction and practice in the use of their wheelchair as part of the curriculum and many schools arrange for the children to take part in the Royal Society for the Prevention of Accidents (RoSPA) training and awards schemes. This encourages the children to improve their handling skills and understand that by regular care of the equipment, improved performance and safety will be achieved. These tests can be compared to the cycling proficiency tests run by RoSPA for able-bodied children. Taking part in the schemes provide the children with a challenge and an additional incentive to make the best use of their wheelchair. Local road safety officers may also be willing to assist in this way or provide further information.

Not everyone has the strength, ability or incentive to become an Olympic or marathon competitor, but failure to provide training appropriate to the needs of each user quickly reduces the value of the equipment as well as the opportunity for each individual to reach their full potential and level of ability. Neither is it cost effective from the health service point of view if expensive equipment is assessed to be needed, issued and then inappropriately used. Improvements in availability and standards of wheelchair training for users is a question for professionals and users alike to address.

REFERENCES

College of Occupational Therapists 1995 Guidelines for the education of students of occupational therapy and physiotherapy. College of Occupational Therapists, London

Department of Health 1991 Wheelchair training resource pack. Department of Health, London (Available on loan from local wheelchair services)

Department of Health 1996 Wheelchair training resource pack revision. Revised 1991 DoH publication. College of Occupational Therapists, London

Ham R 1993 Monitoring wheelchair and seating provision. Clinical Rehabilitation 7: 139–145

Lecouturier J, Jacoby A 1995 Study of user satisfaction with wheelchair provision in Newcastle. Centre for Health Services Research, University of Newcastle upon Tyne

McColl 1986 Review of artificial limb and appliance centre service, vol 1. HMSO, London

Mitchell J 1984 Wheelchairs and the discharge of personal responsibility. Physiotherapy 7(12): 467–472

Silcox L 1995 Assessment for the prescription of wheelchairs: what training is available to therapists. British Journal of Occupational Therapy 58(3): 115–118

Smith S, Goddard T 1994 Wheelpower? Case studies from users and providers of the NHS wheelchair services. The Spastics Society, London

Wells J 1991 How to set up a training course. In: Department of Health 1991 Wheelchair training resource pack. Department of Health, London (Available on loan from local wheelchair services)

FURTHER READING

Handbooks for users and carers

British Red Cross 1990 People in wheelchairs. Hints for helpers. British Red Cross, London

Getting about with your wheelchair 1992 DHA, Oaktree Lane Centre, Birmingham

RADAR 1994 Getting the best from your wheelchair. RADAR, London

Scriptograph 1990 What everyone should know about assisting a wheelchair user. Scriptographic Publications, Alton, Hants

Appendices and glossary

Appendix 1
Levels of lying and sitting ability: adults and children

Reproduced from McCarthy G T (ed) 1992 Physical disability in childhood. Churchill Livingstone, Edinburgh, pp 404–408, with permission from Chailey Heritage and Churchill Livingstone.

Levels of lying ability in supine and prone positions: children

Supine

Level 1
Placeable but unable to maintain

Unable to maintain supine when placed except momentarily and then very asymmetrically. Body follows head turning in a total body movement and therefore rolls into and maintains side-lying. Weightbearing through lateral aspect of head, trunk and thigh. Neck extended with chin poke.

Level 2
Able to maintain position when placed

Settles on back when placed. 'Top heavy'. Weightbearing through upper trunk, head. Pelvis tilted posteriorly. Shoulder girdle retracted. Asymmetrical posture – head to one side, difficulty in turning it side to side – bottom moves laterally as the head is turned giving 'corkscrew' appearance.

Level 3
Able to maintain position. Beginning longitudinal weight shift

Maintains supine position with neutral pelvic tilt, hip abduction, shoulder girdle neutral. Symmetrical posture but top heavy. Chin tucked, not retracted – head in midline and able to move freely side to side without lateral movement of bottom. Able to track visually and make eye contact. Weightbearing through pelvis and shoulder girdle giving general curvature to trunk – with 'pot belly' lateral profile. Beginning of unilateral grasp to side of body and takes fist and objects to mouth. Longitudinal weight shift begins. May roll into prone due to lack of lateral weight shift.

Level 4
Able to maintain position. Beginning lateral weight shift

Symmetry of posture and midline play is seen at this level. Pelvis anteriorly tilted, shoulder girdle protracted. Chin retracted. Shoulders flexing and adducting allowing midline play above chest with hands together; feet also together. Symmetrical posture. Weightbearing through upper trunk and pelvis. Definite lordotic curve. 'Free' pelvic movement beginning, allowing child to touch knees with hips flexed (but not toes). Alternatively can extend hips and knees; rests in crook lying. Beginning unilateral leg raise – independence of limbs from trunk. Adept finger movements towards end of this stage.

Level 5
Consistently moving out from lying position. Beginning to attain lying postures

'Free' movement of shoulder girdle and pelvis on trunk. Pelvis has full range of movement allowing child to play with toes with legs extended and rolls into side-lying. Side-lying functional. Can return to supine. Weightbearing either on shoulder girdle and pelvis or on central trunk only and playing between these postures. Efficient limb movement – hand play and prehensile feet – crossing midline.

Level 6
Consistently moving between lying postures and into sitting

Pelvic and shoulder girdle moving freely. Consistent ability to roll into prone by achieving side-lying as in Level 5 and then anteriorly tilting pelvis on trunk and extending hips.

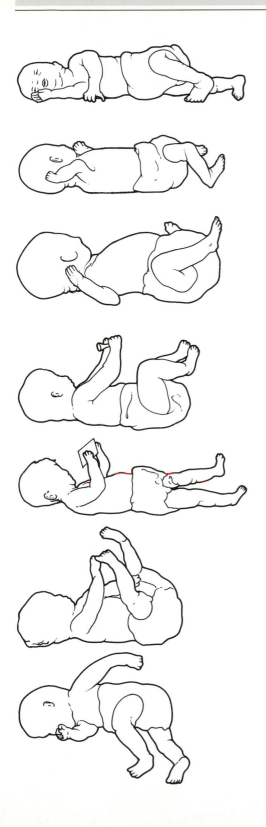

Level 1
Placeable but unable to maintain

Level 2
Able to maintain position when placed

Level 3
Able to maintain position. Beginning longitudinal weight shift

Level 4
Able to maintain position. Beginning lateral weight shift

Level 5
Consistently moving out from lying position. Beginning to attain lying postures

Level 6
Consistently moving between lying postures and into sitting

Prone

Level 1
Placeable, but unable to maintain

Top heavy. Unstable with tendency to topple. Weightbearing through face, shoulders and chest. Pelvis posteriorly tilted. Hips and knees flexed. Shoulder girdle retracted, shoulders flexed and adducted. Asymmetrical posture and head to one side.

Level 2
Able to maintain position when placed

Settles when placed. More generalised weightbearing than Level 1. Weight-bearing through chest, upper abdomen. Pelvis posteriorly tilted. Shoulder girdle retracted, shoulders flexed and adducted. Head to one side but beginning to lift it from floor with 'flat back' profile but not sustaining. Asymmetrical posture, bottom moving laterally as head turns side to side.

Level 3
Able to maintain position. Beginning longitudinal weight shift

Maintains prone position with neutral pelvis, shoulder girdle beginning to protract. Symmetrical weightbearing through abdomen, lower chest and knees and thighs. Maintains head lift from floor with total trunk curvature – head in line with spine. Rocking longitudinally. No lateral weight shift and therefore often topples into supine when lifts head and chest up.

Level 4
Able to maintain position. Beginning lateral weight shift

Pelvis anteriorly tilted but not 'anchoring'. Shoulder girdle protracted, weight-bearing through abdomen and thighs, varying between forearm and hand prop-ping with shoulders elevated. Head and upper trunk movement dissociated from lower trunk allowing lateral trunk flexion with lateral weight shift = begin-ning of pivoting. Angular lateral profile of upper chest and bottom. Unilateral leg kicking. Hand and foot play is midline.

Level 5
Consistently moving out from lying position. Beginning to attain lying postures

Pelvis anteriorly tilted. Shoulder girdle protracted – hand propping with extended elbows and lumbar spine extension. Weightbearing through iliac crests and thighs and lower abdomen. Pelvic anchoring and upper body movement (extension and rotation) upon it. Deft pivoting with lateral trunk flexion and moving backwards on floor. Purposeful roll prone into supine.

Level 6
Consistently moving between lying postures and into sitting

'Free' movement of pelvis and shoulder girdle. Beginning to weightbear on all fours – anteroposterior rocking on all fours.

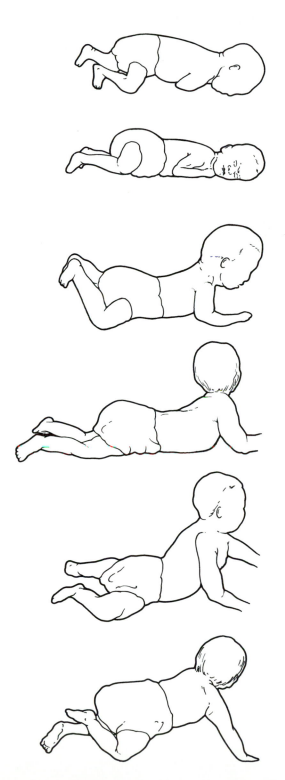

Level 1
Placeable, but unable to maintain

Level 2
Able to maintain position when placed

Level 3
Able to maintain position. Beginning longitudinal weight shift

Level 4
Able to maintain position. Beginning lateral weight shift

Level 5
Consistently moving out from lying position. Beginning to attain lying postures

Level 6
Consistently moving between lying postures and into sitting

Levels of sitting ability with an individual placed on a flat box of the correct height, feet on floor: adults

Level 1
Unplaceable

Wriggles and slides and cannot be placed in a sitting position

Level 2
Placeable, not able to maintain position

Can be placed in a sitting position but needs holding to stay in position – at best can balance momentarily

Level 3
Able to maintain position but not move

When placed in a sitting position can just keep balance as long as there is no movement

Level 4
Able to maintain position and move within base

Once placed in a sitting position can sit independently and can move trunk forward over sitting base but cannot recover balance after reaching to one side

Level 5
Able to maintain position and move outside base

Can sit independently, can use either hand freely to the side of the body and can recover balance after leaning or falling to either side

Level 6
Able to move out of position

Can sit independently and can transfer weight across the surface of a seat but cannot regain a correct sitting position

Level 7
Able to attain position

Can regain sitting position after moving out of it

Appendix 2
Examples of assessment and referral forms

G.P. REFERRAL FOR SUPPLY OF AN N.H.S. WHEELCHAIR

This form should be used when a client needs a wheelchair because of **permanent illness or disability**. ALL sections to be completed.

Clients Surname (Mr/Mrs/Miss/Ms) ....

Forename ....   N.H.S. No. ....

Address..   Tel No. (home)...................

..............................Post code...............   Tel No. (work)....................

Day centre attended if any..

D.O.B. ....   Height.............   Weight ....

Diagnosis and relevant clinical features ....
....

Why is chair required? ....

Does the client already have an N.H.S. Wheelchair   Y( )   N( )
The client requires a wheelchair for use: INDOORS ( )   OUTDOORS ( )

ASSESSMENT IS REQUIRED FOR:
Manual Self Propelling Wheelchair (folding)   ( )
Is person medically fit to propel? ....

Manual Wheeled Pushchair (folding)   ( )
Who will push, are they fit enough?........................

Powered Indoor Chair   ( )
Any fits or blackouts?...
Any cognitive or visual impairments?.....................
Pacemaker fitted? If so when ....

Other (please specify)...

Additional information ....

Referring G.P. Name .... Tel No..............

Address..
....

Signature ....   date............
For return address please see overleaf   Ref: GPREF

A simple level 1 wheelchair referral form for use by a GP. (Reproduced with permission of Merton & Sutton Wheelchair Service.)

WHEELCHAIR - REFERRAL / PRESCRIPTION FORM
Oxfordshire Wheelchair Service
at the Mary Marlborough Centre
Nuffield Orthopaedic Centre NHS Trust
Windmill Road, Headington, Oxford OX3 7LD
(01865 227273)

Date Received

OWS Ref: ....
For OWS Office Use

Please Print Clearly

Background Details

Surname: ....
Forename *(In Full)*: ....
Title: ....

Date of Birth: .... / .... / ....

Home Address: ....
....
....
Post Code: ....
Telephone No: ....

Has the client's address changed since last in contact with OWS?   *Yes*: ☐   *No*: ☐

G.P.: ....
Address: ....
....
Telephone No: ....

Delivery Address (if different to above): ....
....
Telephone No: ....

Special delivery instructions:...
....

Medical Background (including disability):

Physical Information

General

Height: ....

Weight: ....

Basic Sitting Measurements

Hip Width (a): ....

Thigh Length (b): ....

Calf Length (c): ....

Walking Ability (e.g. range):

Method of Transfer

    From the front: ☐   *From the Side (removable armrests req'd)*: ☐

    Other (please specify): ☐ ....

a

b

c

A level 2 wheelchair assessment/referral form. (Reproduced with permission of the Oxfordshire Wheelchair Service at the Mary Marlborough Centre, Nuffield Orthopaedic Centre (NHS) Trust.)

WHEELCHAIR USE

How often will the wheelchair be used?

Every day: ☐   *More than once a week:* ☐   *Once a week or less:* ☐

For how long will the wheelchair normally be used at any one time?

More than 6 hours: ☐   *From 3 to 6 hours:* ☐   *Less than 3 hours:* ☐

Where will the wheelchair be used most?

Indoors at home: ☐   *Outdoors only:* ☐   *Indoors & Outdoors:* ☐

Are there any specific factors about the client's home (or other places where the wheelchair will be used) which should be taken into consideration?

Are there any specific factors associated with the transportation of the wheelchair which should be taken into consideration?

How will the wheelchair be propelled?

Additional Information (e.g. fitness of attendant):

By the User: ☐

By an Attendant: ☐

Category of Need (please tick one box only)

- Totally dependent upon a wheelchair for mobility due to permanent disability: ☐

- Totally dependent upon a wheelchair for a limited period occurring within a log term disability: ☐

- Non dependent, but requires a wheelchair for daily use: ☐

- Non dependent, but requires a wheelchair for 1-3 days per week throughout the year: ☐

- Non dependent, but requires access to a seasonal loan scheme (May to October): ☐

A level 2 wheelchair assessment/referral form (cont'd).

RECOMMENDATIONS

Provision of Equipment

If you are an OWS registered assessor and you wish to recommend a suitable wheelchair and/or accessories please give as much relevant informations as possible (e.g w'chair model, size, etc.).

Please note that in order to recommend a pressure distributing cushion it will now be necessary to complete a separate form specifically for pressure distributing cushions.

Wheelchair:

Accessories:

Further Assessment

Further assessment required? *Yes*: ☐   *No*: ☐

If Yes, please tick one or more boxes:

- *Non powered Wheelchair*: ☐
- *Powered Wheelchair*: ☐
- *Special Seating*: ☐
- *Pressure Relieving Cushion*: ☐
- *Other (please specify)*: ☐ ....

Additional information about client that might be relevant:

A level 2 wheelchair assessment/referral form (cont'd).

ARRANGING AN APPOINTMENT (if required)

Who should be present at the assessment?   Please state contact number / availability:

Is the client able to travel to the OWS?   *Yes*: ☐   *No*: ☐

If necessary it may be possible to arrange a visit to the client's home or an alternative location although the waiting time for such an appointment is likely to be slightly longer.
Which type of appointment is preferred (please tick one box):

        OWS Clinic: ☐

        Home visit: ☐

        Other Location: ☐ ....

Please indicate appropriate means of transport to OWS clinic, if necessary:

    Please tick one box: *Own Transport*: ☐   *Hospital Car*: ☐

                               Ambulance -2 man: ☐   *Ambulance -tail lift*: ☐

If transport requested, will client be accompanied?   *Yes*: ☐   *No*: ☐

Will the client need assistance to transfer?   *Yes*: ☐   *No*: ☐
If yes, please give details of method: ....
                               ....

Other information about client to be taken into account when arranging the appointment:

DETAILS OF ASSESSOR

Name: ....

Profession: ....

No. on OWS Register of Assessors: ....

Contact Location: ....
....

Contact Telephone No: ....

Availability: ....

Signature: ....   Date: ....

- *Please complete the form and return it to the OWS address above.*
- *Please print clearly. Incomplete or illegible information will need to be checked and is likely to lead to a delay in provision of equipment to the client.*
- *Please refer to OWS policy guidelines when recommending equipment for a client.*

A level 2 wheelchair assessment/referral form (cont'd).

TAYSIDE REHABILITATION ENGINEERING SERVICES
SEATING ASSESSMENT FORM

DLFC Seating No: ....

Name: ....

D.O.B: ....   Sex: ....   Marital Status: ....

Address: ....   Change of Address: ....
....
....
....
Tel. No: ....   Tel. No: ....

Occupation: ....

Therapist: ....   Therapist: ....
Address: ....   Address: ....
....
....
Tel. No: ....   Tel. No: ....

G.P: ....
Address: ....
....
....
Tel. No: ....

Other Carers (e.g. relative, nurse, teacher): ....
....
....
....

Diagnosis and Related Conditions:

Communication Ability (and Comprehension):

Referring Authority: ....

A level 3 seating assessment form. (Reproduced with permission of the Tayside Rehabilitation Engineering Services.)

page 2

SUMMARY OF PREVIOUS SEATING ASSESSMENTS

1:   Date .... /......... /..........   Present: ....

Problem:

Objectives:

Proposed Seating:

2:   Date .... /......... /..........   Present: ....

Problem:

Objectives:

Proposed Seating:

A level 3 seating assessment form (cont'd).

page 3

3:   Date: .... /......... /..........   Present: ....

Problem:

Objectives:

Proposed Seating:

4:   Date: .... /......... /..........   Present: ....

Problem:

Objectives:

Proposed Seating:

5:   Date: .... /......... /..........   Present: ....

Problem:

Objectives:

Proposed Seating:

A level 3 seating assessment form (cont'd).

page 4

SEATING ASSESSMENT - Medical Factors

Date : ...... / ...... / ......

Previous Surgery: ....
....
....

Neurological Summary:
    Spinal Lesion: ....
....

    Motor Deficit: ....
....

    Sensory Deficit (location): ....
....

    Excess Sweating (location): ....
....

    Epilepsy: ....
    Other: ....
....

Pressure Sores:
    Previous Sores: ....
    (location, cause, scarring) ....
....

    Current Sores: ....
    (location, cause, scale) ....
....

    Susceptibility: ....

Incontinence:
    Urinary/Faecal? ....
    Management: ....

Respiratory Problems:
(cause, posture)

Pain/Discomfort:
(location, cause, posture)

Behavioural Problems:

Devices Prescribed:

Other information:
(e.g. oedema or significant trends)

A level 3 seating assessment form (cont'd).

Subsequent Assessments: page 5

2:   ...... / ...... / ......   3:   ...... / ...... / ......   4:   ...... / ...... / ......   5:   ...... / ...... / ......

A level 3 seating assessment form (cont'd).

page 6

SEATING ASSESSMENT - Physical Data 1 of 3   Date: ...... / ...... / ......

SUPINE (pelvis as reference):   Left   /   Right

Hips: Dislocation / Subluxation
         (apparent shortening):   ....
                                    ....

         Maximum   Flexion: ....
                   Extension: ....

         Maximum   Abduction: ....
                   Adduction: ....

         Rotation Internal: ....
                   External: ....

Femurs: Bowing / Shortening: ....

Knees: Maximum   Flexion: ....
                   Extension: ....

Ankle: Maximum   Plantarflexion: ....
                   Dorsiflexion: ....

Trunk: Rib Deformity: ....
                              ....

PRONE (pelvis as reference):

         Scoliosis   Lordosis / Kyphosis
comments: ....
          ....
          ....

A level 3 seating assessment form (cont'd).

page 7

Subsequent Assessments:

2: ...... / ...... / ......   3: ...... / ...... / ......   4: ...... / ...... / ......   5: ...... / ...... / ......

A level 3 seating assessment form (cont'd).

page 8

SEATING ASSESSMENT - Physical Data 2 of 3   Date: ...... / ...... / ......

SITTING UPRIGHT   (in optimum posture with the pelvis as near vertical
                         as possible -   reference now vertical/horizontal)

Pelvic orientation:

Obliquity (coronal plane)   ASIS Down   L / R   ....degrees

Rotation (transverse plane):   ASIS Anterior   L / R   ....degrees

Tilt (sagittal plane):   ASIS wrt ITs   Ant / Post ....degrees

		Left / Right
		Left	Right

Hips: Maximum   Flexion:
                         Abduction:
                         Adduction:

Knee: Maximum   Flexion:

Ankle: Maximum   Dorsiflexion:
                         Plantarflexion:

Upper Limbs:
              Positioning of Shoulders:
                              Elbows:
                              Wrist:

Spine (drawing if different from prone):
              Scoliosis: Lordosis / Kyphosis

Is the spinal deformity flexible or structural? ....
....
....
Other comments: ....
....
....

A level 3 seating assessment form (cont'd).

page 9

Subsequent Assessments:

2: ...... / ...... / ......   3: ...... / ...... / ......   4: ...... / ...... / ......   5: ...... / ...... / ......

A level 3 seating assessment form (cont'd).

page10

SEATING ASSESSMENT - Physical Data 3 of 3   Date: ...... / ...... / ......

SITTING ABILITY and STABILITY

Trunk Stability:
    Degree of stability: ....
    Direction of instability: ....
    Cause of instability: ....

Head Stability:
    Degree of stability: ....
    Direction of instability: ....
    Cause of instability: ....

Overall Sitting Ability:
    Chailey Score: ....
    Ability to make voluntary movements (eg pushups): ....
    ....
    ....

Transfer Ability:
    Method (assisted?) : ....
    Influences: ....
    ....

Walking Ability
    Comment: ....
    ....

Other Information: ....
    ....
    ....
    ....

PATTERNS, REFLEXES and MUSCLE TONE

Patterns   (Specify eg extensor, flexor): ....
    ....
    ....
    ....

Reflex   (Specify Presence and Severity):
    The Moro Response: ....
    Positive Supporting Reaction:...
    The Galant Response: ....
    A.T.N.R: ....
    S.T.N.R: ....
    Tonic Labyrinthine Reflex: ....
    Other: ....
    ....
    ....

Muscle Tone (Specify eg hyper / hypotonic, dystonic and postural influence):
    ....
    ....
    ....
    ....

A level 3 seating assessment form (cont'd).

page 11

Subsequent Assessments:

2:   ...... / ...... / ....   3:   ...... / ...... / ....   4:   ...... / ...... / ....   5:   ...... / ...... / ....

A level 3 seating assessment form (cont'd).

page 12

SEATING ASSESSMENT - Activities   Date: ...... / ..... / ......

Specify environments: Primary: Secondary:

Environmental Considerations: ....
(eg space, door widths, lifts, ...
  indoors/outdoors, flooring) ....
                             ....
                             ....

Activities of Daily Living:
Dressing: ....
                             ....

Eating: ....
                             ....

Toileting: ....
                             ....

Bathing: ....
                             ....

Functional Activities:
Specify: ....
(include laterality)   ....
                             ....
                             ....
                             ....

Furniture Considerations: ....
(eg table height)   ....
                             ....
                             ....

Communication:
Method(s):   ....
                             ....

Equipment: ....
                             ....

Mobility:
Method of Propulsion: ....
                             ....

Transfer: ....
                             ....

Transport: ....
                             ....

Other Proposed Activities:
Specify: ....
                             ....
                             ....

Other Information:
Specify: ....
                             ....
                             ....

A level 3 seating assessment form (cont'd).

page 13

Update changes to environment:

Tertiary:	Change:	Change:

....
....
....
....
....

....
....

....
....

....
....

....
....

....
....
....
....

....
....
....

....
....
....

....
....
....
....
....

....
....
....

A level 3 seating assessment form (cont'd).

NEWHAM WHEELCHAIR SERVICE

ELECTRIC (EPIC) WHEELCHAIR ASSESSMENT FORM

Name:_____Referrence Number:_____

Referred By:_____

Date & Place of Assessment:_____

Assessor: _____

Current Chair (s) , Cushion On Issue:
Reason for Referral:
Users Expectations or Goals:
Does the User live alone?
Who will be in charge of looking after / maintaining an electric chair? (give name contact number and relation to user):
Is that person present now?
How long would the user be likely to spend in the chair a day?
Centres / School / College attending:
Transport methods used:
Manual Wheelchair (use, problems and propulsion method):
State of continence:

ref:RH/AH/elec.ass/May 96

An electric (EPIC) wheelchair assessment form (with permission from Newham Community Health Services NHS Trust).

PHYSICAL ASSESSMENT:

HEIGHT:	Feet:	Metres:	WEIGHT:	Stone:	Kg:

EYE SIGHT:	PERCEPTION:

DOMINANT FUNCTIONAL HAND:	PINCH GRIP:

OTHER CONTROL METHOD POSSIBLE:

HEAD CONTROL:

TREMOR:

PATTERNS OF TONE: (State any effect on posture or function)

	RANGE OF MOVEMENT	TONE	STRENGTH
HEAD & NECK			
RIGHT UL			
LEFT UL			
TRUNK			
DEFORMITIES			

IS THE CONDITION STATIC:

SPECIAL POSTURAL NEEDS:

ADL:

DRESSING:
GETTING INTO / OUT OF BED:
COOKING:
FEEDING:
WASHING:
TOILETTING:
TRANSFERS:

An EPIC electric wheelchair assessment form (cont'd).

EQUIPMENT CONSIDERATIONS:
(STATE MODIFICATIONS)

CHAIR MODEL:
SEAT SIZE:
CUSHION:
BACK REST:
ARM REST:
LEG REST:
FOOT REST:
WHEELS / CASTORS:
TYRES:
BRAKES:
ACCESSORIES:
SPECIAL SEATING EQUIPMENT:
TYPE OF CONTROL:
LOCATION OF CONTOL:

An EPIC electric wheelchair assessment form (cont'd).

ENVIRONMENTAL ASSESSMENT:

1. Where is the chair intended to be used (state rooms. centre's school, college):

2. How will the batteries be charged (socket location, voltage, room, length of time etc.):

3. If wet acid batteries are being considered, is that room well ventilated?

4. Is the wall socket easily accessible (note any obstrictions):

5. Floor coverings (type, thickness, additional rugs, location):

6. Door widths (state minimum width, location, check hall ways):

7. If the chair will not pass through all door /hall ways, what alterations are made to improve the situation?

8. If the chair is to be used on more than one level, what alterations have been / are going to be carried out to allow safe passage (give rough dates, location and gradient of ramps):

9. If there are steps, how canthey be safeguarded from accidentally driving down / into them?

10. Heating (state type and location):

11. Fireguards (give location):

12. Where is the chair to be stored?

ADDITIONAL INFORMATION:

COMMUNICATION AIDS ON ISSUE / ORDER:
WHO ELSE IS INVOLVED WITH THIS?
ENVIRONMENTAL CONTROLS CONSIDERED / ON ISSUE / ORDER:
WHO ELSE IS INVOLVED?
OTHER ONGOING PLANS:
CAN WE IMPROVE / MEET THE USERS EXPECTATIONS / GOALS BY PROVIDING AN ELECTRIC CHAIR?
OTHER COMMENTS:

An EPIC electric wheelchair assessment form (cont'd).

PLAN OF ACTION:

EQUIPMENT TRIAL DATE:
EQUIPMENT REQUEST DATES:
IS IT LIKLY THAT THE CONTROL BOX WILL NEED PROGRAMMING TO SUIT THE USER?
NUMBER OF THERAPY SESSIONS PLANNED:
WHO NEEDS TO BE PRESENT AT THESE SESSIONS?
DATE OF REVIEW:
DATE OF ANNUAL CONTRACT REPAIRER CHECK:

SIGNATURE:
DATE FORM COMPLETED:

An EPIC electric wheelchair assessment form (cont'd).

NEWHAM WHEELCHAIR SERVICE

ELECTRIC (EPIOC) WHEELCHAIR ASSESSMENT FORM

Name:	Reference Number:

Diagnoses / Disability:

User Requirements:

Vision: (6/60)

Visual Perception:

Hearing:

Concentration:

Cognition /Learning New Tasks / Memory:

General Tiredness / Specific Fatigue:

Pain: (if any)

Carer Details: (ability, age, fitness, health, availability)

Previous Vehicle Experience:

Social / Environmental Consideration:

Storage:

An electric (EPIOC) wheelchair assessment form (cont'd).

Physical Assessment:

1. **Joint Restrictions / Range of Movement:**

Neck:

Trunk:

Shoulders:

Elbows:

Wrist:

Hands: (dominate side)

Hips:

Knees:

Ankles:

2. **Muscle Tone:**

Left Upper Limbs: **Right Upper Limbs:**

Left Lower limbs: **Right Lower Limbs:**

Neck:

Trunk:

3. **Sitting Balance :**

4. **Co-Ordination:**

5. **Spatial Awareness:**

6. **Sensory Impairment / Pressure Areas:**

An EPIOC electric wheelchair assessment form (cont'd).

7.   **Standing Balance: (if appropriate)**

8.   **Walking Ability:**

9.   **Exercise Tolerance / SOB:**

10.   **Transfer Method (aided / unaided)**

11.   **Height:**

Thigh Length: **Lower Leg Length:**

Back: **Arm Rest:**

12.   **Weight:**

Seat Width:

13.   **Seating Needs:**

An EPIOC electric wheelchair assessment form (cont'd).

Social / Environmental Requirements:

1. **Type of Home:**
2. **Access:**
3. **Storage Area:**
4. **Charge Area:**
5. **Area of Use: How Often and Distance Travelled**
6. **Types of Terrain:**
7. **Shopping:**
8. **Kerb Climbing:**
9. **Transportation Method: (if any)**

An EPIOC electric wheelchair assessment form (cont'd).

Method of Selection:

1. **Sift:**

    Vehicle Type:

    User Requirements:

    Size Required:

    Performance:

2. **Static Demonstration:**

    Access:

    Seating:

    Controls / Operation:

3. **Home Demonstration:**

    Storage Area to Pavement:

    Variety of Surfaces (grass, gravel, cobbles, unmade road, pavement)

    Crossing Road:

    Into room / doorway:

    Obstacles:

    Kerbs:

    Return to storage area:

    Charging:

    Carer:

    Dismantle:

    Load / Unload: (if appropriate)

    Charging:

    Everyday Maintenance:

4. **Insurance:**

    ref:power.ass

An EPIOC electric wheelchair assessment form (cont'd).

HOW TO CHOOSE A POWERED VEHICLE

Date: June 1997

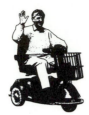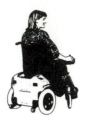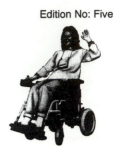

Edition No: Five

STAGE ONE Ask yourself the following questions:

1. Do I want to use it all day, everyday? (If yes, the vehicle must be comfortable, durable and easy to maintain.

2. Do I want to use it only indoors, mainly outdoors or only outdoors? (Remember, you may need to take it into a shop or inside a friend's house).

3. Do I need to go over the grass, or gravel, or up and down hills, or up and down kerbs? (Kerb climbing is never as comfortable as it looks!)

4. Do I need a vehicle with a hood or can I manage with extra clothing in bad weather? Do I need a waterproof seat cover if I leave the vehicle outside the shop?

5. Do I need to take the vehicle inside a car and, if so, how often, which car and who is going to put it in? Does it fold? (A hatchback with a low sill is best). Should it be powered up ramps or hoisted in? (An estate with level access is easiest).

6. Where am I going to keep and charge the vehicle when not in use? (These vehicles need to be stored under cover). Will I need help to charge and maintain the vehicle?

7. How far will I go in a single journey or during each day? (Remember age of battery, weight of user, type of road/floor surface, hills, kerbs and cold weather may all adversely effect the maximum range of a single battery charge).

8. Would it be an advantage if I could travel at up to 8mph (13kph) on the road as well as up to 4mph (6kph) on a pavement?

9. How much can I afford to pay? (Remember you must put by money for replacement batteries and other maintenance and you should take out insurance cover).

STAGE TWO

Having asked yourself these questions, now look at the chart overleaf to find out which vehicles best meet you requirements.

Edited By:

Damson Way
Fountain Drive
Carshalton
Surrey
SM5 4NR

Published by:

 SUNRISE MEDICAL

Sunrise Medical Ltd
High Street
Wollaston
West Midlands
DY8 4PS
England

Questionnaire for the user to consider prior to assessment. (Reproduced with permission of Banstead Mobility Centre and Sunrise Medical Ltd.)

Appendix 3
Training information

For contact addresses for organizations, societies, etc. listed here, refer to Useful addresses.

Training information for therapists

- Details of local courses available from nearest wheelchair service.
- National Centre for Training and Education in Prosthetics and Orthotics, University of Strathclyde – source of training outside NHS.

Training information for users

- Disabled Living Centres – information and full address list for UK from the Disabled Living Centres Council, London.
- Banstead Mobility Centre, Surrey.
- Treloar Disability Assessment Centre, Hants.
- RoSPA, Safety Education Department, Birmingham.
- Additional information available from National Voluntary Groups, e.g. Association for Spina Bifida and Hydrocephalus, Spinal Injuries Association, Scope.

University courses

- MSc courses in rehabilitation may include modules relevant to wheelchairs and seating. Some modules can be attended as a single training session without further commitment to the degree. Contact individual universities or see relevant journals.

Commercial firms

- May provide relevant courses based on equipment. Advertised through wheelchair centres, therapy departments and relevant journals.

Appendix 4
Useful addresses

Age Concern England
Astral House
1268 London Road
London SW16 4ER
Tel: 0181 679 8000

AIC, Adverse Incident Centre
Hannibal House
Elephant and Castle
London SE1 6QT
Tel: 0171 972 8080

Alzheimer's Disease Society
Gordon House
10 Greencoat Place
London SW1P 1PH
Tel: 0171 306 0606

Arthritis Care
18 Stephenson Way
London NW1 2HZ
Tel: 0171 916 1500

Ankylosing Spondylitis International Federation (ASIF)
5 Grosvenor Crescent
London SW1
Tel: 0171 235 9585

ASBAH, Association for Spina Bifida and Hydrocephalus
ASBAH House
42 Park Road
Peterborough PE1 2UQ
Tel: 01733 555988

Banstead Mobility Centre
Damson Way
Orchard Hill
Carshalton
Surrey SM5 4NR
Tel: 0181 770 1151

British Diabetic Association
19 Queen Ann Street
London W1M 0BD
Tel: 0171 323 1531

British Polio Fellowship
Ground Floor, Unit A
Eagle Office Centre
Runway
South Ruislip
Middlesex HA4 6SE
Tel: 0181 842 1898

British Standards Institution
389 Chiswick High Street
London W4 4AL
Tel: 0181 996 9000

Brittle Bone Society
Ward 8, Strathmartine Hospital
Strathmartine
Dundee DD3 0PG
Tel: 01382 817771

British Surgical Trade Association (BSTA) (including British
Association of Wheelchair Distributors [BAWD])
Director
1 Webb Court, Buckhurst Avenue
Sevenoaks
Kent TN13 1LZ
Tel: 01732 458868

Care and Repair
Castle House
Kirtley Drive
Nottingham NG7 1LD
Tel: 0115 979 9091

Carers National Association
20/25 Glasshouse Yard
London EC1A 4JS
Tel: 0171 490 8898

Centre for Accessible Environment
Nutmeg House
60 Gainsford Street
London SE1 2NY
Tel: 0171 357 8182

Chartered Society of Physiotherapists
14 Bedford Row
London WC1 4ED
Tel: 0171 346 5282

College of Occupational Therapists
6–8 Marshalsea Road
Southwark
London SE1 1HL
Tel. 0171 306 6666

CORE, Centre of Rehabilitation Engineering
Kings' Healthcare Rehabilitation Centre
Bowley Close
London SE19 1SZ
Tel: 0171 346 3700

DIAL UK
Park Lodge
St Catherine's Hospital
Tocklink Road
Doncaster DN4 8QN
Tel: 01302 310123

DoT (Department of Transport) Mobility Unit
1st Floor
1–11 Great Minster House
76 Marsham Street
London SW1P 4DR
Tel: 0171 271 5256

Directory of Grant Making Trusts
Charities Aid Foundation
25 King's Hill Avenue
West Malling
Kent ME19 4TA
Tel: 01732 520000

Directory of Social Change
24 Stephenson Way
London NW1 2DP
Tel: 0171 209 5151

DLCC, Disabled Living Centre Council
First Floor
Winchester House
11 Cranmer Road
London SW9 6EJ
Tel: 0171 820 0567

DLF, Disabled Living Foundation
380 Harrow Road
London W9 2HU
Tel: 0171 289 6111

Friedreich's Ataxia Group
Copse Edge
Thursley Road, Elstead
Godalming
Surrey GU8 6DJ
Tel: 01483 417111

Headway, National Head Injuries Association
King Edwards Court
7 King Edward Street
Nottingham NG1 4EW
Tel: 0115 912 1000

Help the Aged
St James's Walk
London EC1R 0BE
Tel: 0171 253 0253

Huntington's Disease Association
108 Battersea High St
London SW11 3HP
Tel: 0171 223 7000

Imperial Cancer Research Fund
PO Box 123
44 Lincoln's Inn Fields
London WC24 3PX
Tel: 0171 242 0200

ISPO (International Society for Prosthetics and Orthotics)
Membership Secretary, UK Branch
Dr C. Stewart
Dundee Limb Fitting Centre
Broughty Ferry
Dundee DD5 1AG
Tel: 01382 730104

MAVIS (Mobility Advice and Vehicle Information Service)
Department of Transport
Transport and Road Research Laboratory
Crowthorne
Berkshire RG11 6AV
Tel: 01344 661000

MDA, Medical Devices Agency
Hannibal House
Elephant and Castle
London SE1 6QT
Tel: 0171 972 8000

MDA Wheelchair Evaluation Centre
241 Bristol Avenue
Bispham
Blackpool FY2 0BR
Tel: 01253 596000

MERU, Medical Engineering Resource Unit
Manager
8 Damson Way
Fountain Drive
Carshalton
Surrey SM5 4NR
Tel: 0181 770 8284

Mobility Roadshow Unit
1/11 Great Minster House
76 Marsham Street
London SW1P 4DR
Tel: 0171 271 5232

Motability
Goodman House
Station Approach
Harlow
Essex CM20 2ET
Tel: 01279 635666

Motor Neurone Disease Association
38 Hazlewood Road
Northampton NN1 1LN
Tel: 01604 250505

Multiple Sclerosis Society
25 Effie Road
Fulham
London SW6 1EE
Tel: 0171 610 7171

Muscular Dystrophy Group
7–11 Prescott Place
London SW4 6BS
Tel: 0171 720 8055

NACVS (National Association of Councils for Voluntary
Services)
3rd Floor
Arundel Court
177 Arundel Street
Sheffield S1 2NU
Tel: 0114 278 6636

National Centre for Training and Education in Prosthetics
and Orthotics
University of Strathclyde
Curran Building
131 St James Road
Glasgow G4 0LS
Tel: 0141 552 4400
RECAL and Library Services, Tel: 0141 548 3814

National Council for Voluntary Organisations
Regents Wharfe
8 All Saints Street
London N1 9RL
Tel: 0171 713 6161

National Society for Epilepsy
Ansley House
Hanover Square
Leeds
Tel: 01345 089599

NHS Supplies Authority
Wheelchair Purchasing Centre
80 Lightfoot Street
Chester CH2 3AD
Tel: 01244 505000

NPMG, National Posture and Mobility Group
Dr A. Turner-Smith (Secretary)
King's Healthcare Rehabilitation Centre
Bowley Close
London SE19 1SS
Tel: 0171 346 3736

Osteoporosis

National Osteoporosis Society
PO Box 10
Radstock
Bath
Avon BA3 3YB
Tel: 01761 471104

ParentAbility
6 Forest Road
Crowthorne
Berkshire RG11 7EH
Tel: 01344 773366

Parkinson's Disease Society of the UK
22 Upper Woburn Place
London WC1H 0RA
Tel: 0171 383 3513

RADAR, Royal Association for Disability and Rehabilitation
12 City Forum Road
250 City Road
London EC1V 8AF
Tel: 0171 250 3222

REMAP
National Organizer
Eur. Ing. J.J. Wright
Hazeldene
Ightham
Sevenoaks
Kent TN15 9AD
Tel: 01732 883818

RESMaG, Rehabilitation Engineering Service Managers'
Group
P. Richardson (Chair)
Kings' Healthcare Rehabilitation Centre
Bowley Close
London SE19 1SZ
Tel: 0171 346 3700

Rett Syndrome Association, UK
29 Carlton Road
London N11 3EX
Tel: 0181 361 5161

RoSPA, Royal Society for the Prevention of Accidents
Edgbaston Park
353 Bristol Road
Birmingham B5 7ST
Tel: 0121 248 2000

SCOPE
12 Park Crescent
London W1N 4EQ
Tel: 0171 636 5020

Scoliosis Association (UK)
2 Ivebury Court
325 Latimer Road
London W18 6RA
Tel: 0181 964 5343

Spinal Injuries Association
Newpoint House
76 St James Lane
London N10 3DF
Tel: 0181 444 2121

SSWG, Scottish Seating and Wheelchair Group
Dr G. Bardsley
Tayside Rehabilitation Engineering Services
Broughty Ferry
Dundee DD5 1AG
Tel: 01382 73104

STEPS
15 Statham Close
Lymm
Cheshire WA13 9NN

Stroke Association
CHSA House
Whitecross Street
London EC1Y 8JJ
Tel: 0171 490 7999

Tissue Viability Society
Secretary
Wessex Rehabilitation Association
Salisbury District Hospital
Salisbury
Wiltshire SP2 8BJ
Tel: 01722 336262

Treloar Disability Assessment Centre
Lord Mayor Treloar National Specialist Centre
Holybourne
Alton
Hants GU34 4EN
Tel: 01420 547400

Tuberous Sclerosis Association
Little Barnsley Farm
Catshill
Bromsgrove
Worcestershire B61 0NQ
Tel: 01527 871898

UK Forum of Mobility Centres
Mrs M Cornwell
Banstead Mobility Centre
Damson Way
Orchard Hill
Carshalton
Surrey SM5 4NR
Tel: 0181 770 1151

Whizz-Kidz
215 Vauxhall Bridge Road
London SW1V 1EN
Tel: 0171 233 6600

Glossary of wheelchair-related terms

Organizations and societies

The contact points referred to in these glossary entries can be found in Appendix 4.

AIC	Adverse Incident Centre. Previously known as NATRIC. Responsible for investigating adverse incidents (accidents/defects, etc.) that could affect the health and safety of patients and equipment users. All adverse incidents relating to wheelchair equipment should be reported. This is generally the responsibility of the rehabilitation engineer. (*Contact: MDA, AIC*)
BAWD	British Association of Wheelchair Distributors. A section of BSTA – an association of suppliers for special physical needs. Members are from some of the leading wheelchair distributors in the UK and conform to a strict code of practice. They are encouraged to liaise with people and organizations working in the field of wheelchair provision and use. (*Contact: Director, BSTA*)
ALAC	Artificial Limb and Appliance Centre. Responsible for providing the wheelchair and other associated services in England until 1987.
CIGOPW	A clinical interest group for occupational therapists with a special interest in orthotics, prosthetics, wheelchairs and seating. Quarterly newssheet and study days during the year. (*Contact: College of Occupational Therapists*)
DLCC	Disabled Living Centre Council. A council for the many Disabled Living Centres found across Britain. Advisers on a range of equipment for disabled people. Many employ therapists and provide training sessions for professionals and users. (*Contact: DLCC*)
DoT Mobility Unit	Department of Transport Mobility Unit. Responsible for transport policy as it affects the mobility of elderly and disabled people. Provides a range of information and guidance on public transport, access and the environment. Videos and training information available. (*Contact: DoT Mobility Unit*)

DSA — Disablement Services Authority. A special health authority set up by the government in 1987 for a 3-year period. Purpose: to plan and implement the transfer of the wheelchair service (and other ALAC services) from a centrally controlled organization to local services focused on users, their mobility and wider rehabilitation needs

ISO — A world federation of national standard bodies (ISO member bodies) who prepare international standards. (*Contact: British Standards Institution*)

ISPO — International Society for Prosthetics and Orthotics with additional interest in wheelchairs and seating. Quarterly magazine; scientific meetings; conferences. (*Contact: ISPO Membership Secretary, UK Branch*)

MDA — Medical Devices Agency. An agency of the Department of Health, responsible for ensuring safety and quality of all medical devices used in the UK. Wheelchair Evaluation Section based in Blackpool. (*Contact: MDA*)

MERU — Medical Engineering Resource Unit. Provides a design and manufacturing service for disabled children living in the Merton and Sutton Health Authority. Willing to provide information and advice to others. (*Contact: MERU*)

Mobility Centres — Ten accredited centres in the UK that offer a free information service on any aspect of outdoor mobility for disabled drivers, passengers and wheelchair users. Also undertake assessments for people wishing to choose a manual or powered wheelchair. Some offer driving lessons and others provide training to wheelchair users. (*Contact: Chairman of UK Forum*)

NAIDEX — A national exhibition of equipment for disabled people and rehabilitation, including wheelchairs and mobility aids, car conversions, etc.

NATRIC — National Reporting and Investigation Centre. (*Contact: MDA, AIC*)

NPMG — National Posture and Mobility Group (England). A society for all professionals working in the field of wheelchair posture and mobility. Annual 2-day conference; newssheet. (*Contact: NPMG*)

NWSSCG — The National Wheelchair and Special Seating consultative group. A committee made up of representatives from wheelchair services. Originally set up to look at purchase of equipment in relation to clinical need. Members advise the NHS Supplies (wheelchairs) on appropriate equipment for national contracts. (*Contact: NHS Supplies*)

PACT — Placing, Assessment and Counselling Team based at the Local Employment Office, the DEA (Disability Employment Adviser) provides information and support for disabled people returning to or seeking work. (*Contact: Local Employment Office*)

RADAR — Royal Association for Disability and Rehabilitation. Provides free information on all matters concerning disabled people; campaigns on political issues; acts as an adviser to government; produces a range of booklets; guidelines; factsheets and regular news bulletin. (*Contact: RADAR*)

RECAL — Information service for professionals working in prosthetics, orthotics, wheelchairs and seating. Members receive fortnightly listing of newly published articles from the scientific, medical and relevant technical literature. Undertakes comprehensive search for additional fee. (*Contact: National Centre for Training and Education in Prosthetics and Orthotics*)

REMAP — A charity which designs, manufactures and supplies technical aids to disabled persons where there is no suitable commercial item available. (*Contact: REMAP*)

RESMaG — Rehabilitation Engineering Service Managers' Group. Members represent every region in the country. Regular meetings; provide advice to REs (Rehabilitation Engineers); set standards for training; collect and disseminate information. (*Contact: RESMaG*)

REview — Newsletter produced by Centre of Rehabilitation Engineering (CORE). Provides link between fragmented services and disseminates service and technical developments. (*Contact: CORE*)

RoSPA — Royal Society for Prevention of Accidents. Organizes proficiency tests for wheelchair users and advises on safety issues. (*Contact: RoSPA*)

SSWG — Scottish Seating and Wheelchair Group. A society for professionals working in the field of wheelchairs and special seating. Regular meetings and training for members, networking and advice. (*Contact: SSWG*)

Equipment

Accessories — Items added to a wheelchair. See under separate names, e.g. tray, headrest, etc.

Anti-tip bars/levers — Short bars generally with small wheel on end. Fitted into lower tubes at the back of the seat. Used as stabilizers to prevent backward tipping. Removable for more experienced users

Armrests —
1. Adjustable: Offered as an option on many models. Height adjustable.
2. Desk arms: Shortened pad length to allow closer access to table or work surface
3. Mobile arm support: Designed to be fitted to wheelchair or static stand. Three hinged sections: proximal, distal and arm trough. Used to provide support and function for people with upper limb weakness, e.g. MND, poliomyelitis, rheumatoid arthritis

Basic wheelchair — Centrally folding frame. Most commonly used with self-propelling and attendant-pushed wheelchairs. With or without folding backrest; removable armrests; removable footrests. Modular versions available with choice of wheel size; armrests, castors, etc.

Bexhill armrest	An 'L' shaped arm support. Designed for use with hemiplegics to support paralysed arm
Calf strap	Alternative to heel loop to keep the feet from slipping backwards off the footplate and catching on the castor wheels
Chailey Skates	Foot-shaped supports fitted to footplates to hold feet in correct position. Made by several manufacturers
Custom made seat	Supportive seat made to individual shape or size, e.g. matrix, lynx, moulded seat insert. Used for persons with complex postural problems and fixed deformities
Elevating legrests (ELR)	Replace standard footrests. Can be raised and lowered. Fitting an elevating legrest will lengthen the chair even when in the lowered position. Difficult for the user to operate independently. Increases turning space required
EPIC	Electrically powered indoor (wheel)chair. Available through NHS to people unable to walk or self-propel indoors. Operates with battery
EPIOC	Electrically powered indoor/outdoor (wheel)chair. Provided to wheelchair users in Scotland since 1992, available in England since 1996
Folding frame	Centrally folding wheelchair frame. Commonly with folding backrest and removable footrests and armrests, e.g. basic model
Footstraps	Ankle strap and/or toe strap. Fitted to footplate to secure feet. Essential for people using a kneeblock to maintain leg in correct alignment
Head control	1. Headrest. Fitted to back of chair to provide support for relaxing or protection when travelling in a wheelchair in a car, minibus, etc. Can be a flat pad or shaped support with side wings. May also be angle adjustable
	2. Head support. Used to hold head upright for persons with low tone and flopping heads. Support from front; generally with chin rest and strap around neck to hold in position or type of collar, e.g. Headmaster collar; Hensinger; Lecky dynamic head control and others
High-performance wheelchair	Describes wheelchair with adjustable position of rear wheel to reduce stability for competent user. Enables user to balance on the back wheels for kerb climbing or negotiating rough ground. Seat angle; height; position of front castor may also be adjustable to improve performance of wheelchair. Sometimes called an active user wheelchair
Interface	The mechanism that joins a seating system to a wheelchair, e.g. a board, clips or frame
Kneeblock	Shaped to the knees and adjustable in height

	and preferably in depth and angle. Used as a counterforce for someone using a seating system with sacral support. Purpose is to hold the head of femur in correct alignment to the acetabulum, prevent pelvic rotation and reduce possibility of hip dislocation
Lightweight wheelchair	Made from lightweight materials, e.g. carbon fibre; titanium. Generally used by very active users, e.g. spinal injuries. Adjustable stability as with 'high-performance' wheelchairs. These are not necessarily sports chairs which are generally custom made to the particular sport and expensive
Pelvic pads	Pads fitted to each side of a wheelchair or seating system that support the pelvis and help to maintain the user in midline
Pelvic strap	Attached at seat level to back corners; preferably at a 45 degree angle to the seat. Adjusted to correct length to hold pelvis back in wheelchair and maintain correct pelvic position. Sometimes called lap strap, or waist strap, when fitted higher on the chair frame
Quick release wheels (QRW)	Wheels – generally self propelling – that can be removed quickly from the chair by pressing a button or clip. Commonly found on rigid frame chairs, sports chairs, high-performance chairs
Reclined backrest	Angle of backrest in relation to seat is greater than 90 degrees from upright. May be fixed or adjustable. Increases overall length of wheelchair. Depending on angle of recline, rear wheels may be set back to provide stability. Also anti-tipping levers to prevent backward tipping
Rigid frame	Fixed frame as often seen on modern style, high-performance wheelchairs. Does not centrally fold. Commonly has quick release wheels and backrest folds forward on to seat
Stumpboard	Fitted in place of a footrest for an amputee without his or her prosthesis. Supports the stump after an amputation
Tray	Standard tray generally used for carrying goods or meals. Shaped tray. Supports forearms. Used for postural support to prevent slumping, assist head control, enable change of position with forward support as seen in the Putney Alternating Position chair. Correct height is important
Thoracic pad	Pads fitted to the wheelchair or seating system to support the trunk; assist maintenance of an upright symmetrical posture and prevent falling sideways
Tilt in space	Angle between seat and backrest remains fixed but position of seat is tilted backwards. Described as tilt in space
Wheelie	Balancing on rear propelling wheels. This enables the skilled user to move more easily over rough ground and up kerbs

Index

Page numbers in bold type refer to illustrations, tables and boxes.